Neonatal Nutrition: Evidence-Based Recommendations for Common Conundrums

Editors

BRENDA B. POINDEXTER
AMY B. HAIR

CLINICS IN PERINATOLOGY

www.perinatology.theclinics.com

Consulting Editor
LUCKY JAIN

September 2023 • Volume 50 • Number 3

ELSEVIER

1600 John F. Kennedy Boulevard ● Suite 1800 ● Philadelphia, Pennsylvania, 19103-2899

http://www.theclinics.com

CLINICS IN PERINATOLOGY Volume 50, Number 3
September 2023 ISSN 0095-5108, ISBN-13: 978-0-323-94021-4

Editor: Kerry Holland
Developmental Editor: Karen Justine S. Dino

Clinics in Perinatology (ISSN 0095-5108) is published quarterly by Elsevier Inc., 360 Park Avenue South, New York, NY 10010-1710. Months of issue are March, June, September, and December. Business and Editorial Offices: 1600 John F. Kennedy Blvd., Ste. 1800, Philadelphia, PA 19103-2899. Customer Service Office: 3251 Riverport Lane, Maryland Heights, MO 63043. Periodicals postage paid at New York, NY and additional mailing offices. Subscription prices are $341.00 per year (US individuals), $713.00 per year (US institutions), $387.00 per year (Canadian individuals), $872.00 per year (Canadian institutions), $461.00 per year (international individuals), $872.00 per year (international institutions), $100.00 per year (US and Canadian students), and $195.00 per year (International students). International air speed delivery is included in all Clinics subscription prices. All prices are subject to change without notice. **POSTMASTER:** Send address changes to *Clinics in Perinatology*, Elsevier Health Sciences Division, Subscription Customer Service, 3251 Riverport Lane, Maryland Heights, MO 63043. **Customer Service: Telephone: 1-800-654-2452** (U.S. and Canada); **1-314-447-8871** (outside U.S. and Canada). **Fax: 1-314-447-8029. E-mail: journalscustomerservice-usa@elsevier.com** (for print support); **journalsonlinesupport-usa@elsevier.com** (for online support).

Reprints. For copies of 100 or more, of articles in this publication, please contact the Commercial Reprints Department, Elsevier Inc., 360 Park Avenue South, New York, NY 10010-1710. Tel. 212-633-3874; Fax: 212-633-3820; E-mail: reprints@elsevier.com.

Clinics in Perinatology is also published in Spanish by McGraw-Hill Interamericana Editores S.A., P.O. Box 5-237, 06500 Mexico D.F., Mexico.

Clinics in Perinatology is covered in *MEDLINE/PubMed (Index Medicus) Current Contents, Excepta Medica, BIOSIS and ISI/BIOMED.*

Contributors

CONSULTING EDITOR

LUCKY JAIN, MD, MBA
George W. Brumley Jr Professor and Chairman, Department of Pediatrics, Emory University School of Medicine, Pediatrician-in-Chief, Children's Healthcare of Atlanta, Atlanta, Georgia, USA

EDITORS

BRENDA B. POINDEXTER, MD, MS
Marcus Professor of Pediatrics, Division of Neonatology, Department of Pediatrics, Children's Healthcare of Atlanta, Emory University School of Medicine, Atlanta, Georgia, USA

AMY B. HAIR, MD
Associate Professor of Pediatrics, Division of Neonatology, Baylor College of Medicine, Texas Children's Hospital, Houston, Texas, USA

AUTHORS

MANDY BROWN BELFORT, MD, MPH
Department of Pediatric Newborn Medicine, Brigham and Women's Hospital, Harvard Medical School, Boston, Massachusetts, USA

CYNTHIA BLANCO, MD
The University of Texas Health Science Center at San Antonio, San Antonio, Texas, USA

KRISTA BONAGURIO, RDN
The University of Texas Health Science Center at San Antonio, San Antonio, Texas, USA

KARA L. CALKINS, MD, MS
Division of Neonatology and Developmental Biology, Department of Pediatrics, Neonatal Research Center of the UCLA Children's Discovery and Innovation Institute, David Geffen School of Medicine, UCLA, Los Angeles, California, USA

ALVIN CHAN, MD, MPH
Division of Gastroenterology, Department of Pediatrics, David Geffen School of Medicine UCLA, Los Angeles, California, USA

TANIS R. FENTON, PhD, RD
Cumming School of Medicine, University of Calgary, Calgary, Alberta, Canada

TING TING FU, MD
Assistant Professor of Pediatrics, Division of Neonatology, Perinatal Institute, Cincinnati Children's Hospital Medical Center, Department of Pediatrics, University of Cincinnati College of Medicine, Cincinnati, Ohio, USA

PARVESH M. GARG, MD
Wake Forest School of Medicine, Brenner Children's Hospital, Atrium Health Wake Forest Baptist, Winston-Salem, North Carolina, USA

LAURA GOLLINS, MBA, RDN, CNSC, FAND
Department of Pediatrics, Division of Neonatology, Baylor College of Medicine, Texas Children's Hospital, Houston, Texas, USA

SHARON GROH-WARGO, PhD, RDN
MetroHealth Medical Center, Case Western Reserve University School of Medicine, Cleveland, Ohio, USA

SHRUTI GUPTA, MD
Associate Professor, Department of Pediatrics, Yale School of Medicine, New Haven, Connecticut, USA

AMY B. HAIR, MD
Associate Professor of Pediatrics, Division of Neonatology, Baylor College of Medicine, Texas Children's Hospital, Houston, Texas, USA

ROSA K. HAND, PhD, RDN, LD, FAND
Department of Nutrition, Case Western Reserve University, Cleveland, Ohio, USA

IMRAN M. ILAHI, DO
Department of Pediatrics, Northwestern University Feinberg School of Medicine, Ann & Robert H. Lurie Children's Hospital of Chicago, Chicago, Illinois, USA

ELENA ITRIAGO, MD
Department of Pediatrics, Section of Neonatology, Baylor College of Medicine, Texas Children's Hospital, Houston, Texas, USA

HEIDI KARPEN, MD
Associate Professor of Pediatrics, Associate Program Director, Neonatal-Perinatal Medicine Fellowship Training Program, Emory University/Children's Healthcare of Atlanta, Atlanta, Georgia, USA

JASMEET KATARIA-HALE, MD
Department of Pediatrics, Division of Neonatology, Mission Hospital, Asheville, North Carolina, USA

KATERINA KELLAR, MD
Pediatric Resident, The University of Texas Health Science Center at San Antonio, San Antonio, Texas, USA

CAMILIA R. MARTIN, MD, MS
Division of Neonatology, Department of Pediatrics, Weill Cornell Medicine, New York, New York, USA

LEONOR ADRIANA MASSIEU, RD, LD, CNSC
Department of Pediatrics, Section of Neonatology, Baylor College of Medicine, Texas Children's Hospital, Houston, Texas, USA

JENNIFER MCALLISTER, MD, IBCLC
Associate Professor of Clinical Pediatrics, Department of Pediatrics, University of Cincinnati College of Medicine, Cincinnati Children's Hospital Medical Center Perinatal Institute, Cincinnati, Ohio, USA

STEPHANIE MERLINO BARR, MS, RDN, LD
MetroHealth Medical Center, Case Western Reserve University School of Medicine, Cleveland, Ohio, USA

ALVARO G. MOREIRA, MD, MSc
Associate Professor, Pediatrics, The University of Texas Health Science Center at San Antonio, San Antonio, Texas, USA

NISHA REDDY PANDILLAPALLI, MBBS
Pediatrics, The University of Texas Health Science Center at San Antonio, San Antonio, Texas, USA

RAVI M. PATEL, MD, MSc
Department of Pediatrics, Associate Professor of Pediatrics, Emory University, Children's Healthcare of Atlanta, Atlanta, Georgia, USA

KRYSTLE PEREZ, MD MPH
Assistant Professor of Pediatrics, Division of Neonatology, Department of Pediatrics, University of Washington, Seattle, Washington, USA

BRENDA B. POINDEXTER, MD, MS
Marcus Professor of Pediatrics, Division of Neonatology, Department of Pediatrics, Children's Healthcare of Atlanta, Emory University School of Medicine, Atlanta, Georgia, USA

MURALIDHAR H. PREMKUMAR, MD
Department of Pediatrics, Section of Neonatology, Baylor College of Medicine, Texas Children's Hospital, Houston, Texas, USA

JANICE RAUCCI, PharmD, BCPPS
Ann & Robert H. Lurie Children's Hospital of Chicago, Chicago, Illinois, USA

STEFANIE RIDDLE, MD
Associate Professor of Clinical Pediatrics, Division of Neonatology, Department of Pediatrics, University of Cincinnati College of Medicine, Cincinnati Children's Hospital Medical Center, Cincinnati, Ohio, USA

DANIEL T. ROBINSON, MD, MSc
Department of Pediatrics, Northwestern University Feinberg School of Medicine, Ann & Robert H. Lurie Children's Hospital of Chicago, Chicago, Illinois, USA

SAMANTHA ROGERS, RD, CDN, CNSC
NewYork-Presbyterian Food & Nutrition Services, NewYork-Presbyterian Hospital/Weill Cornell Medical Center, New York, New York, USA

SARA ROSTAS, PharmD, BCPPS
NewYork-Presbyterian Department of Pharmacy, NewYork-Presbyterian Hospital/ Komansky Children's Hospital, New York, New York, USA

ARIEL A. SALAS, MD, MSPH
Division of Neonatology, Department of Pediatrics, Heersink School of Medicine, Associate Professor of Pediatrics, The University of Alabama at Birmingham, Birmingham, Alabama, USA

ANAND SALEM, DO
Department of Pediatrics, Emory University, Children's Healthcare of Atlanta, Atlanta, Georgia, USA

ANNE L. SMAZAL, MD, MS
Department of Pediatrics, Northwestern University Feinberg School of Medicine, Ann & Robert H. Lurie Children's Hospital of Chicago, Chicago, Illinois, USA

SAHARNAZ TALEBIYAN, MD
Department of Pediatric Newborn Medicine, Brigham and Women's Hospital, Boston, Massachusetts, USA

SARAH N. TAYLOR, MD
Professor, Department of Pediatrics, Yale School of Medicine, New Haven, Connecticut, USA

KIMBERLY FERNANDEZ TRAHAN, MD
Department of Pediatrics, Section of Neonatology, Baylor College of Medicine, Texas Children's Hospital, Houston, Texas, USA

COLM P. TRAVERS, MD
Assistant Professor of Pediatrics, Division of Neonatology, Department of Pediatrics, Heersink School of Medicine, The University of Alabama at Birmingham, Birmingham, Alabama, USA

GREGORY C. VALENTINE, MD, MED, FAAP
Assistant Professor of Pediatrics, Division of Neonatology, Department of Pediatrics, University of Washington, Seattle, Washington, USA

LAURA WARD, MD, IBCLC
Associate Professor of Clinical Pediatrics, Department of Pediatrics, University of Cincinnati College of Medicine, Cincinnati Children's Hospital Medical Center Perinatal Institute, Cincinnati, Ohio, USA

SCOTT WEXELBLATT, MD
Associate Professor of Clinical Pediatrics, Department of Pediatrics, University of Cincinnati College of Medicine, Cincinnati Children's Hospital Medical Center Perinatal Institute, Cincinnati, Ohio, USA

Contents

During the fetal-to-neonatal transitional period, extremely preterm newborns undergo significant intrabody fluid shifts and resulting weight loss due to increased insensible fluid losses due to immature skin, kidneys, among other factors. These ongoing physiologic changes make fluid and nutritional management complex in the neonatal-to-fetal transitional time period for extremely premature newborns. However, limited literature exists to guide optimal practices for providers caring for this population. Here, we review the evidence on optimal fluid and nutritional management during the fetal-to-neonatal transition of extremely preterm newborns.

Use of parenteral nutrition (PN) in the neonatal intensive care unit (NICU) requires evaluating the need for central venous catheters, potential drug incompatibilities, unintentional exposures, and suboptimal energy and nutrient intake during the transition to full enteral nutrition. Risks of photooxidation reactions in PN components, refeeding syndrome, and excess early amino acid intake should prompt the reevaluation of routine practices. The goal of this paper is to review the practicalities, challenges, and conundrums of administering PN in the NICU.

Intravenous lipid emulsions (ILEs) are a source of nonprotein calories and fatty acids and help promote growth in preterm infants and infants with intestinal failure. An ILE dose and oil source determines its fatty acid, phytosterol, and vitamin E delivery. These factors play a role in the infant's risk for essential fatty acid deficiency and cholestasis, and help modulate inflammation, immunity, and organ development. This article reviews different ILEs and their constituents and their relationship with neonatal health.

Inadequate intake of calcium and phosphorus during the perinatal period can result in metabolic bone disease (MBD), characterized by decreased bone mass, altered bone mineralization, and increased risk for fractures. Preterm neonates have higher risk of developing MBD. Treating MBD involves ensuring adequate calcium and phosphorus intake, early fortification, and vitamin D supplementation. Health care providers should closely monitor nutrient intake, postnatal growth, and screening of preterm neonates at risk for MBD. This review summarizes the critical roles of calcium and phosphorus in regulating bone physiology, how they regulate bone formation and resorption, and their influence on overall bone health.

Establishing full enteral nutrition in critically ill preterm infants with immature gastrointestinal function is challenging. In this article, we will summarize emerging clinical evidence from randomized clinical trials suggesting the feasibility and efficacy of feeding interventions targeting the early establishment of full enteral nutrition. We will also examine trial outcomes of higher volume feedings after the establishment of full enteral nutrition. Only data from randomized clinical trials will be discussed extensively. Future opportunities for clinical research will also be presented.

Human milk is the preferred diet for very preterm infants due to short-term and long-term benefits for health and neurodevelopment. Fortification of human milk is required to deliver sufficient nutrients to attain recommended growth targets during the neonatal hospitalization. Intrinsic variability in human milk composition poses a challenge in clinical practice because some infants fail to meet recommended nutrient intakes even with existing approaches of standard (fixed-dose) and adjustable fortification. Individually targeted fortification is an emerging strategy to minimize nutrition delivery gaps through application of point-of-care human milk analysis and has potential to improve growth and related outcomes.

Multicomponent fortification is the standard of care to support short-term growth in preterm infants receiving human milk. There is no consensus regarding the optimal timing, method, or products used to fortify human milk. Both bovine milk-based and human milk-based human milk fortifiers are safe options, though increased fortification and enrichment may be needed to achieve adequate growth. Additional studies are needed to evaluate newer fortifier products and fortification strategies.

> Nutrition management of the high-risk infant after hospital discharge is complicated by the infant's dysfunctional or immature oral feeding skills, nutritional deficits, and the family's feeding plan. Although evidence is limited, available studies point to developing an individualized nutritional plan, which accounts for these factors; protects and prioritizes the family's plan for breastfeeding; and promotes an acceptable growth pattern. Further research is needed to identify the type and duration of posthospital discharge nutrition to optimize high-risk infant neurodevelopment and body composition. Attention to infant growth, lactation support, and safe feed preparation practices are critical in the transition to home.

> Necrotizing enterocolitis (NEC) is a leading cause of morbidity and mortality in preterm infants. Severe anemia and red blood cell (RBC) transfusion are associated with gut inflammation and injury in preclinical models and observational studies. However, there is uncertainty about the causal role of these factors in the pathogenesis of NEC. Observational studies have shown that withholding feeding during RBC transfusion may reduce the risk of NEC, although confirmatory data from randomized trials are lacking. In this review, we summarize data on feeding during RBC transfusion and its role in NEC and highlight ongoing randomized trials.

> Necrotizing enterocolitis (NEC) is a neonatal disease with high mortality and morbidity. There is a lack of evidence-based recommendations on nutritional rehabilitation following NEC, and much of the current practice is guided by institutional policies and expert opinions. After a diagnosis of NEC, infants are exposed to an extended period of bowel rest and a prolonged course of antibiotics. Recognizing the patient characteristics that predict nutritional tolerance, early initiation of enteral nutrition, minimizing periods of bowel rest and antibiotic exposure, and standardization of dietary practices are the mainstay of post-NEC nutrition.

> Perioperative malnutrition in infants with congenital heart disease can lead to significant postnatal growth failure and poor short- and long-term outcomes. A standardized approach to nutrition is needed for the neonatal congenital heart disease population, taking into consideration the type of cardiac lesion, the preoperative and postoperative period, and prematurity. Early enteral feeding is beneficial and should be paired with parenteral nutrition to meet the fluid and nutrient needs of the infant.

PROGRAM OBJECTIVE

The goal of *Clinics in Perinatology* is to keep practicing perinatologists, neonatologists, obstetricians, practicing physicians and residents up to date with current clinical practice in perinatology by providing timely articles reviewing the state of the art in patient care.

TARGET AUDIENCE

Perinatologists, neonatologists, obstetricians, practicing physicians, residents and healthcare professionals who provide patient care utilizing findings from *Clinics in Perinatology*.

LEARNING OBJECTIVES

Upon completion of this activity, participants will be able to:

1. Recognize the importance of optimal nutrient delivery during the neonatal period and how it impacts long-term outcomes.
2. Discuss factors that make nutritional management complex for extremely premature newborns and their families.
3. Review the practicalities, challenges, and conundrums of administering parental nutrition in the NICU and data that supports the early commencement of enteral feeds.

ACCREDITATION

The Elsevier Office of Continuing Medical Education (EOCME) is accredited by the Accreditation Council for Continuing Medical Education (ACCME) to provide continuing medical education for physicians.

The EOCME designates this journal-based CME activity for a maximum of 14 *AMA PRA Category 1 Credit*(s)™. Physicians should claim only the credit commensurate with the extent of their participation in the activity.

All other health care professionals requesting continuing education credit for this enduring material will be issued a certificate of participation.

DISCLOSURE OF CONFLICTS OF INTEREST

The EOCME assesses conflict of interest with its instructors, faculty, planners, and other individuals who are in a position to control the content of CME activities. All relevant conflicts of interest that are identified are thoroughly vetted by EOCME for fair balance, scientific objectivity, and patient care recommendations. EOCME is committed to providing its learners with CME activities that promote improvements or quality in healthcare and not a specific proprietary business or a commercial interest.

The planning committee, staff, authors, and editors listed below have identified no financial relationships or relationships to products or devices they or their spouse/life partner have with commercial interest related to the content of this CME activity:

Mandy Brown Belfort, MD, MPH; Krista Bonagurio, RDN; Alvin Chan, MD, MPH; Tanis R. Fenton, PhD, RD; Kimberly Fernandez Trahan, MD; Ting Ting Fu, MD; Parvesh M. Garg, MD; Laura Gollins, MBA, RDN, CNSC, FAND; Sharon Groh-Wargo, PhD, RDN; Shruti Gupta, MD; Rosa K. Hand, PhD, RDN, LD, FAND; Imran M. Ilahi, DO; Elena Itriago, MD; Lucky Jain, MD, MBA; Jasmeet Kataria-Hale, MD; Katerina Kellar, MD; Michelle Littlejohn; L. Adriana Massieu, RD, LD, CNSC; Jennifer McAllister, MD, IBCLC; Stephanie Merlino Barr, MS, RDN, LD; Alvaro G. Moreira, MD, MSc; Nisha Reddy Pandillapalli, MBBS; Krystle Perez, MD, MPH; Brenda B. Poindexter, MD, MS; Muralidhar H. Premkumar, MD; Janice Raucci, PharmD, BCPPS; Stefanie Riddle, MD; Samantha Rogers, RD, CDN, CNSC; Sara Rostas, PharmD, BCPPS; Ariel A. Salas, MD, MSPH; Anand Salem, DO; Anne L. Smazal, MD, MS; Jeyanthi Surendrakumar; Saharnaz Talebiyan, MD; Colm P. Travers, MD; Gregory Valentine, MD, MPH; Laura Ward, MD, IBCLC; Scott Wexelblatt, MD

The planning committee, staff, authors, and editors listed below have identified financial relationships or relationships to products or devices they or their spouse/life partner have with commercial interest related to the content of this CME activity:

Cynthia Blanco, MD: Research: Prolacta

Kara L. Calkins, MD, MS: Instituitional Principal Investigator: Mead Johnson Nutrition; Advisor: Fresenius Kabi, Mead Johnson Nutrition

Amy B. Hair, MD: Research: Prolacta

Heidi Karpen, MD: Research: Prolacta

Camilia R. Martin, MD, MS: Instituitional Principal Investigator: Mead Johnson Nutrition; Advisor: Lactalogics, Inc., Plakous Therapeutics, Vitara Biomedical, Inc

Ravi M. Patel, MD, MSc: Consultant: Noveome

Daniel T. Robinson, MD, MSc: Institutional Principal Investigator: Mead Johnson Nutrition; Advisor: Fresenius Kabi

Sarah N. Taylor, MD: Institutional Principal Investigator: Ferring Pharmaceuticals, Pfizer, Prolacta; Research: Mead Johnson Nutrition

UNAPPROVED/OFF-LABEL USE DISCLOSURE
The EOCME requires CME faculty to disclose to the participants:
1. When products or procedures being discussed are off-label, unlabelled, experimental, and/or investigational (not US Food and Drug Administration [FDA] approved); and
2. Any limitations on the information presented, such as data that are preliminary or that represent ongoing research, interim analyses, and/or unsupported opinions. Faculty may discuss information about pharmaceutical agents that is outside of FDA-approved labelling. This information is intended solely for CME and is not intended to promote off-label use of these medications. If you have any questions, contact the medical affairs department of the manufacturer for the most recent prescribing information.

TO ENROLL
To enroll in the *Clinics in Perinatology* Continuing Medical Education program, call customer service at 1-800-654-2452 or sign up online at http://www.theclinics.com/home/cme. The CME program is available to subscribers for an additional annual fee of USD 254.00.

METHOD OF PARTICIPATION
In order to claim credit, participants must complete the following:
1. Complete enrolment as indicated above.
2. Read the activity.
3. Complete the CME Test and Evaluation. Participants must achieve a score of 70% on the test. All CME Tests and Evaluations must be completed online.

CME INQUIRIES/SPECIAL NEEDS
For all CME inquiries or special needs, please contact elsevierCME@elsevier.com.

CLINICS IN PERINATOLOGY

SERIES OF RELATED INTEREST

Obstetrics and Gynecology Clinics of North America
https://www.obgyn.theclinics.com

THE CLINICS ARE AVAILABLE ONLINE!
Access your subscription at:
www.theclinics.com

Foreword

Feeding a Newborn Shouldn't be That Complicated

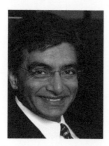

Lucky Jain, MD, MBA
Consulting Editor

Years ago, when we were expecting our first child, my wife and I asked my mom for advice about feeding issues and how she had managed to raise four children with relative ease. "What advice?" "You were exclusively breast-fed until you were one. You turned out okay, didn't you?" To this day, I have never forgotten that conversation. "And don't forget the importance of mom's diet. What she eats during pregnancy and nursing has long-lasting impact on the baby!"

Much of that advice holds true even today. But then, I wasn't born premature, and not very many early preterm babies survived in the 50s! Few good alternatives to breast milk were available in much of the world, and malnutrition was rampant. Newborn care has become much more complex since then, with a vast majority of preterm babies and those with birth defects surviving. Their nutritional needs have become complex as have the techniques used to deliver needed nutrition enterally and parenterally.

There is renewed interest in maternal nutrition and its impact on fetal development, particularly development of the brain. **Fig. 1** shows highly represented terms in a recent nutrition article about impact of nutrition on fetal neurodevelopment.[1] They speak to the importance of maternal environment in the development of the offspring. Postnatal nutrition represents a continuum, and there is a clear movement toward standardizing nutritional management of the baby through evidence-based pathways. In his bestselling book, *The Checklist Manifesto*, Dr Atul Gawande reminds us that we should not accept mediocre care and the high rate of errors in medicine.[2] Even in the face of complexity, or even more to deal with them, he emphasizes the need for uniform care through guidelines, checklists, and care paths that are readily available to practitioners. Rightly so, this forms the backbone of quality improvement efforts in holistic management of NICU babies.

Clin Perinatol 50 (2023) xv–xvi
https://doi.org/10.1016/j.clp.2023.05.002
0095-5108/23/© 2023 Published by Elsevier Inc.

perinatology.theclinics.com

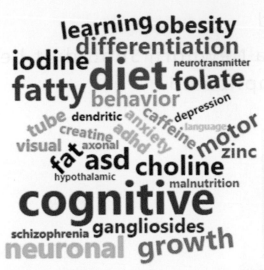

Fig. 1. The nutrients and neurodevelopmental outcomes most frequently encountered during review of related articles. (*From* Cortes-Albornoz MC, Garcia-Guaqueta DP, Velez-van-Meerbeke A, Talero-Gutierrez CT. Maternal Nutrition and Neurodevelopment: A Scoping Review. Nutrients 2021, 13, 3530.)

This current issue of the *Clinics in Perinatology* focuses on common controversies and conundrums in neonatal nutrition and emphasizes evidence-based pathways to resolve them. Drs Poindexter and Hair are to be congratulated for engaging top experts in the field to assemble a top state-of-the-art offering. As always, I am grateful to the authors for their valuable contributions and to my publishing partners at Elsevier (Kerry Holland and Karen Justine S. Dino) for their help in bringing this valuable resource to you.

Lucky Jain, MD, MBA
Department of Pediatrics
Emory University School of Medicine
Children's Healthcare of Atlanta
2015 Uppergate Drive Northeast
Atlanta, GA 30322, USA

E-mail address:
ljain@emory.edu

REFERENCES

1. Cortes-Albornoz MC, Garcia-Guaqueta DP, Velez-van-Meerbeke A, et al. Maternal nutrition and neurodevelopment: a scoping review. Nutrients 2021;13:3530. https://doi.org/10.3390/nu13103530.
2. Gawande A. The checklist manifesto. Chicago: Profile Books; 2011.

Preface

Using Evidence to Address Differences in Opinions and Practice in Neonatal Nutrition

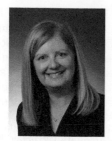
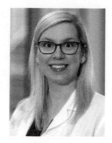

Brenda B. Poindexter, MD, MS   Amy B. Hair, MD
Editors

The field of Neonatology continues to change over time, as there are advances in maternal care and technology used in the Neonatal Intensive Care Unit (NICU) with infants of younger gestational age surviving. When the first NICUs were established, there were limited options in how to provide nutrition to these infants. There was not parenteral nutrition, which is a vital component of care today when infants are unable to tolerate enteral nutrition. Mothers were encouraged to provide breast milk in the past, but there were not high-functioning human milk pumps available until more recently. Formulas, used if breast milk was unavailable, were very limited 30 years ago. Nutritional care of NICU infants has evolved over time with the invention of parenteral nutrition, human milk fortifiers, and specialized formulas.

While nutrition is a vital component of the care of the neonate, there is a lag in research and evidence on how to provide the most appropriate nutrition for high-risk infants in the NICU. In addition, due to lack of evidenced-based practice in the past, there are myths and fallacies that have developed in the nutritional care of the neonate. In the absence of evidence, NICUs created their own practices and protocols. Fortunately, there has been a significant increase in neonatal nutrition research over the past 10 years, which is changing and guiding nutrition practice.

The goal of this issue of *Clinics in Perinatology* titled "Neonatal Nutrition: Evidence-Based Recommendations for Common Conundrums" was designed to address common myths, fallacies, and conundrums in neonatal nutrition from experts in the field. The focus is preterm infants and special populations of high-risk infants, such as infants with congenital heart defects or intestinal disease.

Topics were chosen based on differences in opinions and practice in the NICU. These topics are addressed using evidence-based recommendations and based on

Clin Perinatol 50 (2023) xvii–xviii
https://doi.org/10.1016/j.clp.2023.05.001
0095-5108/23/© 2023 Published by Elsevier Inc.

a review of the literature. When evidence is limited, guidance in practice is provided. The articles offer key recommendations from experts in the field. These articles are meant to help with clinical practice at the bedside. In addition, future research questions are identified specifically in areas that require more research to provide evidence-based recommendations.

We would like to thank the authors that contributed to this issue, many of whom who are mentors, collaborators, and friends of the coeditors. The authors are thought leaders in the field, and we hope that this body of work will inspire the promotion of evidence-based neonatal nutrition.

Brenda B. Poindexter, MD, MS
Marcus Professor of Pediatrics
Division of Neonatology
Department of Pediatrics
Children's Healthcare of Atlanta and
Emory University School of Medicine
2015 Uppergate Drive Northeast
Atlanta, GA 30322, USA

Amy B. Hair, MD
Associate Professor of Pediatrics
Division of Neonatology
Baylor College of Medicine
Texas Children's Hospital
6621 Fannin Street
MC: A5590
Houston, TX 77030, USA

E-mail addresses:
brenda.poindexter@emory.edu (B.B. Poindexter)
abhair@texaschildrens.org (A.B. Hair)

Early Fluid and Nutritional Management of Extremely Preterm Newborns During the Fetal-To-Neonatal Transition

Gregory C. Valentine, MD, MED[a],*, Krystle Perez, MD, MPH[a],
Amy B. Hair, MD[b]

KEYWORDS

- Neonate • Nutrition • Prematurity • Weight loss

KEY POINTS

- There is a relative paucity of data on optimal nutritional and fluid management of extremely preterm newborns during the fetal-to-neonatal transitional period.
- The optimal range of physiologic maximal weight loss (MWL) may be an important marker to guide fluid management, with an MWL between 5% and 15% from birthweight associated with reduced adverse in-hospital health outcomes.
- The association between time to regain birthweight and short- and/or long-term health outcomes of extremely preterm newborns remains ill-defined, requiring further research.
- Evidence for use of serum sodium as a proxy for weight loss and overall hydration status during the fetal-to-neonatal transitional period is lacking; serum sodium values may not be ideal markers of overall hydration status during the fetal-to-neonatal transition period of extremely preterm newborns due to physiologic intrabody fluid shifts, immature kidneys unable to retain sodium, higher insensible water losses, and parenteral fluid administration of varying sodium quantities.

INTRODUCTION

Immature organ systems impair preterm newborns' ability to breathe adequately, thermoregulate, engage in oral feeding, and concentrate urine resulting in early challenges in fluid and electrolyte management (**Fig. 1**).[1–8] The extra- and intracellular fluid shifts between and within body compartments during the fetal-to-neonatal transition lead to alterations in weight and electrolytes.[9,10] Maintaining homeostasis during this

[a] Division of Neonatology, Department of Pediatrics, University of Washington, Box 356320, RR542 HSB, Seattle, WA, USA; [b] Department of Pediatrics, Division of Neonatology, Baylor College of Medicine, Texas Children's Hospital, 6621 Fannin Street, Suite W6104, Houston, TX 77030, USA
* Corresponding author. University of Washington, Box 356320, RR542 HSB, Seattle, WA 98195-6320.
E-mail address: gcvalent@uw.edu

Clin Perinatol 50 (2023) 545–556
https://doi.org/10.1016/j.clp.2023.04.002
0095-5108/23/© 2023 Elsevier Inc. All rights reserved.
perinatology.theclinics.com

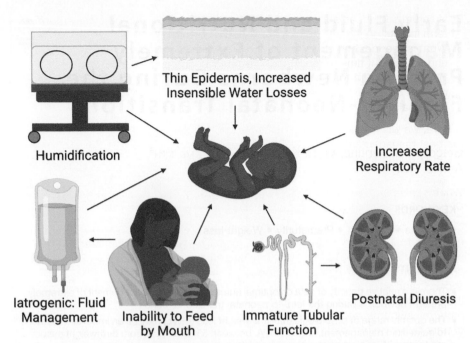

Fig. 1. Reasons for impaired homeostasis of the extremely preterm newborn. There are numerous reasons for impaired homeostasis of the extremely preterm newborn during the fetal-to-neonatal transitional period and include increased insensible water losses through a thin epidermis, changes in humidification practices (radiant warmer vs humidified incubator), differences in clinical prescription of total fluids, inability to feed by mouth with limited suck-swallow reflex development, immature renal tubular function with inadequate sodium retention and increased postnatal diuresis, and underlying tachypnea increasing insensible fluid losses. Created with Biorender.com.

transitional period is further complicated by high insensible water losses that occur as a consequence of the inherent immature skin integrity, respiratory distress, and high urine output that become more substantial with increasing degree of prematurity (see **Fig. 1**).[11]

Thus, extremely preterm newborns experience the greatest challenge in achieving and maintaining homeostasis. Early fluid management practices have been associated with outcomes including patent ductus arteriosus (PDA), bronchopulmonary dysplasia (BPD), and necrotizing enterocolitis (NEC) in retrospective studies, though the directionality has varied.[2,3,12–15] Rigorously conducted studies examining optimal nutritional and fluid management for extremely preterm newborns are limited. As such, clinicians caring for most preterm newborns often rely on anecdotal experience and expert opinion to inform clinical decisions about fluid and nutritional management during the transitional period.

Although it has been increasingly evident that early enteral feeds with expressed human milk are critically important to optimize preterm newborn outcomes, a variety of other topics pertaining to early fluid and nutritional management during the fetal-to-neonatal transition remain poorly explored.

1. What are the expected weight loss patterns for preterm newborns, and what are the optimum physiologic weight loss window(s), if any?

2. Is serum sodium an adequate proxy for fluid status and/or weight loss among preterm infants during this transitional period?
3. What is the ideal timeline for extremely preterm newborns to regain birthweight, and how might time to regain birthweight influence outcomes?
4. What are optimal total fluid goals during the first few days after birth, noting the need to distinguish between *parenteral* versus *enteral* fluid contribution to overall fluid goals?

   Here, we will highlight existing evidence and future areas of research to determine the best management of small and sick newborns, especially those born extremely preterm, during the fetal-to-neonatal transitional period.

What is the Expected Weight Loss Pattern for Preterm Newborns, and is There an Optimal Degree of Physiologic Weight Loss for Preterm Infants?

Clinicians caring for term newborns commonly expect physiologic weight loss to occur up to 10% from birthweight, with higher weight loss anticipated for preterm newborns.[16–18] Excessive weight loss has been associated with adverse health conditions such as jaundice and kernicterus,[19–21] acute renal injury and renal failure,[22,23] shock,[24] and seizures,[25,26] among others.[27] However, most studies have focused on the term, breastfeeding newborns.[16,17] A relative paucity of data exists on whether preterm newborns, and especially extremely preterm newborns, have similar patterns of transitional weight loss.

One large UK cohort study of more than 5000 newborns born at <32 weeks' gestation reported that the majority of preterm infants experienced *no* weight loss.[28] Their results conflict with findings from other studies demonstrating weight loss of 3% to 12% is typical for preterm newborns born <1000 g at birth.[29,30] A recent secondary analysis of extremely preterm (24w0d–27w6d) newborns enrolled in the Premature Erythropoietin Neuroprotection Trial (PENUT) also sought to determine typical weight loss patterns.[12] Among the 842 extremely preterm newborns across 30 US centers, all gestational ages had similar weight loss patterns after birth, with a mean maximal weight loss (MWL) of 9% to 11% from birthweight and a nadir at day 3 after birth.[12] Interestingly, while decreasing gestational age at birth is well-known to be associated with increased insensible fluid losses, the percentage weight loss from birthweight appeared similar across the spectrum of newborns born extremely preterm in this study.[12] Overall, there is an amassing body of evidence supporting the concept of expected physiologic weight loss between 5 and 15% for extremely preterm newborns.

A related question to explore is whether extremes of MWL from birthweight are associated with adverse health outcomes. There have been several attempts to evaluate the association of early weight loss patterns with outcomes of preterm newborns. Several retrospective cohort studies have reported associations between BPD, intraventricular hemorrhage (IVH), and necrotizing enterocolitis (NEC) with minimal (or lack of) transitional weight loss.[12,13,31,32] Two large cohort studies found two-fold increased odds of death or BPD among extremely low birthweight newborns (ELBW) who had no physiologic weight loss within the first 10 days compared to newborns with weight loss.[13,31] A smaller study in Turkey evaluated weight loss in the first 72 hours after birth in 126 ELBW neonates and described that weight loss <3% or >12% from birthweight was associated with increased odds of mortality and IVH.[32] Similarly, the secondary analysis of extremely preterm newborns from PENUT also sought to assess whether there exists an optimal MWL percentage target for extremely preterm newborns.[12] Investigators evaluated newborns in three groups based on MWL percentage: (a) those in the lowest quartile (lost <5% MWL, inclusive of no weight loss); (b) those in the middle quartiles (5%–15% MWL); and (c) those in the highest quartile (>15% MWL).[12] Extremely preterm infants with MWL between 5% and 15% from birthweight had less risk of developing NEC compared to those in the highest quartile.[12] These results collectively demonstrate that extremes of weight loss from birthweight, especially <5% and >15% are associated with adverse health outcomes among extremely preterm newborns, even after adjusting for markers of severity of illness.

The only randomized prospective trial that evaluates targeting specific MWL ranges after birth was published in 1982 by Lorenz and colleagues[15] in which they randomized 88 infants <1500 g at birth to gradually achieve an MWL of 8% to 10% or MWL of 13% to 15% from birthweight. With the mean gestational age of participants being 29 weeks, they reported *no difference* in the incidence of PDA, BPD, IVH, or mortality despite confirmed differences in mean body weight lost, total fluid intake, and urine output within the first 5 days after birth.[15] Although Lorenz's study evaluated health outcomes of <1500 g newborns prescribed specific MWL goals, contemporary studies suggest their MWL goals within the two groups (8%–10% vs 13%–15%) likely were within the normal range of expected weight loss percentages. Additionally, management and outcomes of extremely preterm infants have changed significantly since 1982, including routine use of antenatal steroids and surfactant.

Overall, emerging data support that physiologic weight loss is an important milestone for short- and long-term health outcomes among extremely preterm newborns. Minimal (ie, <5%) or substantial (ie, >15%) weight loss from birthweight appears to be associated with adverse health outcomes in several modern cohort studies. To our knowledge, no contemporary, prospective, randomized trial has been conducted evaluating the impact of targeting specific MWL goals and evaluating the impact on short- and long-term health outcomes. The last clinical trial was published in the pre-surfactant era by Lorenz and colleagues' study, whose findings were limited by the small difference in MWL range between groups. Contemporary, prospective studies are necessary to determine if a prescriptive MWL goal, such as between 5% and 15% (vs >15% or <5%), can further improve health outcomes for extremely preterm newborns.

Can Sodium be Used as a Proxy for Overall Fluid Status During the Transitional Period?

Another common conundrum clinicians face is whether there are appropriate mechanisms or proxies for monitoring the overall fluid and hydration status of extremely preterm newborns. Anecdotally, clinicians have monitored sodium and daily weights closely over the first few days following birth. With increasing use of intraventricular prevention bundles to minimize handling, daily weights of extremely preterm newborns may be deferred in the first 72 hours after birth. Thus, clinicians must rely on proxies such as sodium values for hydration status, especially when daily weights are not obtained. However, there is a paucity of evidence that sodium is an accurate proxy for hydration and/or weight status during the transitional period in preterm infants with serum sodium poorly representing total body sodium.

Although hypernatremia is often attributed to dehydration and hyponatremia to fluid overload in older children and adults, extremely preterm infants' physiology is inherently affected by their immature organ function, increased insensible water losses, and expected intra- and extracellular fluid compartment shifts during the fetal-to-neonatal transition. Further complicating the reliance upon sodium as a biomarker for overall hydration status, preterm newborns have higher sodium requirements (mEq/kg) than term infants, children, or adults.[33] As preterm kidneys have limited ability to concentrate urine and reabsorb key electrolytes, including bicarbonate, they experience a transient, functional type II, proximal renal tubular acidosis.[6,34] Due to this renal tubular immaturity, preterm nephrons are unable to adequately retain sodium. Given these inherent differences in the preterm neonate, namely increased sodium excretion and alterations within the extracellular fluid compartment, a relative lack of steady-state exists making reliance on serum sodium challenging.

Furthermore, while sodium fluctuations are expected during the transitional period, high sodium variability has also been associated with adverse health outcomes.[35] In fact, sodium fluctuations have been associated with altered neural myelination within the central nervous system in animal models and with IVH risk in preterm newborns.[35,36] Although sodium and fluid status are integrally linked, the underlying changes occurring during the transitional period call into question the reliability of serum sodium values as a proxy for overall hydration status. Moreover, it remains unclear what the expected range of normal sodium variability may be (if any) during this transition and whether efforts seeking to reduce sodium variability may improve outcomes.

In summary, sodium and its variability may be better proxies of immaturity rather than overall hydration status for extremely preterm infants. Studies are needed exploring when, and if, sodium can be used as an accurate proxy for overall fluid management decisions in the transitional period of extremely preterm newborns. Studies are also needed to determine if reducing such sodium variability during the first few days after birth may translate to improved health outcomes.

When Should Extremely Preterm Newborns Regain Birthweight for Optimal Health Outcomes?

Guidelines surrounding the timeline to regain birthweight exist, though focus is on term infants. The American Academy of Pediatrics (AAP) and the American College of Obstetricians and Gynecologists *Guidelines for Perinatal Care* include a description that for term newborns, failure to regain birthweight by 2 weeks after birth requires "careful evaluation".[37] The AAP's publication *Bright Futures: Nutrition*, states that term newborns generally regain their birthweight by 7 days after birth.[38] However, a large cohort study of 143,889 newborns born at $\geq$ 36 weeks' gestation demonstrated that only approximately 50% "were at or above birthweight at 9 and 10 days after vaginal and cesarean delivery, respectively".[18] In fact, 14% of newborns born vaginally and 24% of newborns born via cesarean section were not back to birthweight by 14 days after birth.[18] Thus, a significant percentage of term newborns may take longer than 14 days to regain birthweight, with a high likelihood that an even greater percentage of preterm newborns may take even longer.

Time to regain birthweight is increasingly being acknowledged as a primary outcome of interest, associated with short- and long-term health outcomes for preterm newborns.[39–41] However, the influence of speed by which birthweight is regained remains controversial. Supporting a faster time to regain, Anvekar and colleagues[42] evaluated 137 newborns born at <27 weeks' gestation in a retrospective case-control study and association with type 1 retinopathy of prematurity (ROP). A longer time to regain birthweight was associated with increased risk of type 1 ROP, though was not statistically significant after adjusting for confounders (median day to regain 9 vs 7, aOR 1.08, 95% CI 1.00–1.17, P = 0.059).[42] Similarly, experts and dietitians from the Academy of Nutrition and Dietetics and the American Society for Parenteral and Enteral Nutrition have proposed guidance on what constitutes malnutrition among preterm newborns.[40] Time to regain birthweight of 15 to 18 days, 19 to 21 days, or >21 days is associated with diagnoses of mild, moderate, or severe malnutrition, respectively.[40] Notably, diagnosis of malnutrition requires an additional indicator to meet the definition of malnutrition such as a slow linear growth velocity or a decline in the length-for-age z score.[40] Collectively, these recommendations and data suggest that a longer time to regain birthweight is associated with malnutrition and adverse health outcomes (ie, ROP).

However, Ehrenkranz and colleagues[41] evaluated in-hospital growth velocity on neurodevelopmental outcomes at 18 to 22 months' corrected age among 600 newborns with birthweights between 501 and 1000 g The authors divided the cohort into quartiles based on in-hospital growth velocity rates, defined as "the period of time that the infant regained birthweight and discharge, transfer, death, age 120 days, or until a body weight of 2000 g was reached…".[41] Interestingly, the newborns with the highest overall in-hospital growth velocity rates had the *longest* time to regain birthweight while those with the slowest in-hospital growth velocity rates had the *shortest* time to regain birthweight (average 19.5 days vs 15.9 days, $P = 0.0031$). The study demonstrated a decreased incidence of cerebral palsy and severe neurodevelopmental delay in those newborns with the highest overall growth velocity rates.[41] These findings question whether earlier time to regain birthweight is associated with overall improved growth velocity past the transitional period. It is possible that *gradual* regain of birthweight, rather than either rapid or delayed, may be ideal, or there may exist an optimal "window" in which time to regain birthweight is associated with optimal short- and long-term outcomes.

In summary, a shorter time to regain birthweight does not equate nor guarantee improved growth velocities throughout the remainder of hospitalization. Moreover, it is possible that rapid regain of birthweight may be associated with higher severity of illness as newborns in life-threatening situations are more likely to receive transfusions, vasopressors, and increased total fluids; these infants may fail to lose birthweight and/or may regain birthweight quickly due to increased fluid intake required for severity of illness. Thus, time to regain birthweight may be a proxy for the severity of illness and overall well-being rather than a marker of nutritional status. Time to regain birthweight as an indicator for both short- and long-term health outcomes needs further investigation as there is no definitive evidence supporting which direction is optimal.

What is the Ideal Total Fluid Administration, and are Enteral and Parenteral Fluids Equivalent?

Provision of intravenous fluids in the first days after birth is ubiquitous among extremely preterm newborns, with ongoing questions as to the ideal volume to be administered and rate of advancement. Liberal fluid administration compared to more restrictive fluid administration has been associated with adverse health outcomes such as NEC, BPD, and PDA.[12,13,43] A 2014 Cochrane review analyzing "restricted" versus "liberal" fluid management, defined as usual care versus above-control volumes, concluded that careful restriction is warranted to meet preterm newborns' physiologic needs while avoiding the adverse consequences of dehydration (although a uniform definition for dehydration during the fetal-to-neonatal transitional period is currently undefined and unclear).[43] More recent analyses of total fluid administration have continued to find similar associations.[31,44] A retrospective analysis of 24w0d to 27w6d newborns enrolled in the PENUT study evaluated total fluid administration (TFA) and its relationship to health outcomes.[12] TFA included enteral feeds and parenteral fluids. After describing average TFA over the first week after birth in the cohort (lowest quartile [<120 mL/kg/day], middle quartiles [120–150 mL/kg/day], highest quartile [>150 mL/kg/day]), TFA of the highest quartile was associated with a three-fold increased odds of NEC and a two-fold increased odds of having a PDA requiring surgery (OR 2.14, 95% CI 1.10–4.15).[12] Another study by Soullane and colleagues[45] demonstrated that increased TFA over the first 10 days after birth was associated with increased risk of death or BPD among newborns born at 23 to 28 weeks. Yet, not all studies have reported associations between increasing fluid administration and adverse health outcomes.[46]

Although existing studies have evaluated overall TFA associations with outcomes, few, if any, have granularly distinguished *parenteral* versus *enteral* fluid contributions to the overall total fluid regimens. In an era acknowledging the benefits of early initiation of trophic human milk feeds and faster advancements,[47–49] it may be of increasing importance to investigate the role of the routine of fluid administration separated by the routine of administration with outcomes. Namely, are parenteral fluids and enteral feeds equivalent in associated risk of BPD, PDA, and NEC, among other outcomes?

Given the difference in content and biological activity of enteral human milk, it seems an oversimplification to assume parenteral versus enteral fluids would have the same implications on preterm newborn outcomes. Recent studies among preterm newborns in India have emerged exploring the use of early total enteral feeding (ETEF), minimizing parenteral fluid use, as compared to conventional enteral feeding (CEF) advancements with standard parenteral fluid administration.[47–49] One study evaluated 180 stable very low birthweight (defined as <1500 g, VLBW) newborns via an unblinded, individually-randomized controlled trial comparing ETEF (n = 91) to a CEF control group (n = 89).[47] VLBW newborns receiving ETEF had earlier attainment of full feeds, decreased duration of hospital stay, and no difference in risk of feeding intolerance or NEC.[47] Importantly, the mothers of babies receiving ETEF had significantly higher expression of breast milk by day 3 after birth compared to those who had babies in the CEF group.[47] A subsequent Cochrane review conducted in 2020 included six trials evaluating ETEF versus CEF.[50] The ETEF trials started enteral feeding at 60 to 80 mL/kg/day and the CEF started enteral feeding at 20 mL/kg/day, with feeding volumes advanced in both groups by 20 to 30 mL/kg/day with no evidence of effect on the risk of NEC in the meta-analysis (RR 0.98, 95% CI 0.38–2.56).[50] Nonetheless, further research is critically needed with the level of evidence low and context limited to India. Nonetheless, ETEF literature calls into question historical belief in the safety of slow advances in enteral feeds, especially with the overwhelming evidence of the benefits of expressed human milk.

Although increasing TFA is associated with adverse health outcomes among extremely preterm newborns, it is unclear whether that association pertains to all fluids (enteral and parenteral) or is driven primarily by parenteral fluids, especially acknowledging the historical norm of delayed and slow introduction of enteral fluids. The burgeoning evidence on the possible benefits of ETEF among preterm newborns throughout the world, with two large trials currently being conducted in the United Kingdom and the United States underway, demonstrate the equipoise that exists related to optimal enteral feeding regimens among extremely preterm newborns.

Specific Considerations for < 24-Week Gestational-Age Newborns

We conclude this review on the transitional period and evidence relating to the nutritional management of the periviable gestational ages, less than 24 weeks of gestation. With some centers providing resuscitation and care to newborns born as low as weeks' gestation,[51] evidence-based, optimal nutritional management remains uncertain for this population. With most of the literature surrounding optimizing early fluid and nutritional management including newborns 24 weeks' gestation at birth and higher, studies seeking to understand optimal fluid and electrolyte management for babies born <24 weeks' gestation are needed. Agren and colleagues[1] propose some specific recommendations for this age group pertaining to early fluid management: starting fluid intake at 100 to 170 mL/kg/day if using a humidified incubator or 130 to 220 mL/kg/day if utilizing a non-humidified warmer,[2,52] avoid sodium in maintenance fluids for the first 2 to 3 days following birth,[53] and monitor daily weights using a bed scale and targeting 2% to 3% weight loss per day with a goal of approximately 10% MWL.[1] Such recommendations are consistent with the findings presented throughout this review, though should be regarded as expert opinion until further trials can be conducted. Studies should include periviable newborns born at <24 weeks of gestation to better define whether specific considerations should be given to these newborns as compared to their more mature preterm counterparts 24 weeks and greater.

SUMMARY

Overall, the fetal-to-neonatal transitional period is a challenging, complex period for clinicians as they make fluid and electrolyte management decisions for extremely preterm newborns. A relative paucity of data exists related to optimal early fluid and nutritional practices for extremely preterm newborns in the first few days after birth. There is an urgent need for robust, prospective research studies exploring relationships between transitional nutritional practices and extremely preterm in-hospital and long-term health outcomes. Much of what has been understood as foundational principles for older infants may not correlate with extremely preterm newborns, especially those born at <24 weeks' gestation. Based on existing literature, we propose a renewed focus on MWL patterns rather than the prescribed total fluid regimens with a goal to maintain 5 to 15% MWL with a gradual regain. Finally, caution should be taken with interpreting serum sodium values as markers of fluid and hydration status with similar caution in early sodium supplementation during the transitional period. Inter-institutional collaborative, multi-center trials are needed to explore the questions proposed throughout this review that will lead to optimizing care for this vulnerable population.

CLINICS CARE POINTS

- Maximal weight loss from birthweight among extremely preterm newborns between 5-15% is associated with improved in-hospital outcomes.
- If possible, clinicians should consider starting enteral feeds early, without prolonged periods of fasting.
- Serum sodium may not be an ideal proxy for overall hydration status, and further studies are needed.

DISCLOSURE

All authors have no commercial or financial conflicts of interest to disclose.

Best Practices

What is the current practice for fluid and nutritional management of extremely preterm newborns during the fetal-to-neonatal transitional period?

Best Practice Objective(s):

- Determine optimal MWL (from birthweight) percentages for extremely preterm newborns))
- Evaluate the medical literature to determine optimal clinical practices in fluid and nutritional therapy for extremely preterm newborns during the fetal-to-neonatal transitional period

What changes in current practice are likely to improve outcomes?

- Early initiation of enteral feedings without prolonged periods of trophic feedings

- Promotion of physiologic MWL of 5% to 15% from birthweight

- Limited use of serum sodium as a proxy for overall hydration status

Pearls/pitfalls at the point-of-care:
- Limited use of serum sodium as a proxy for overall hydration status
- Limited use of time to regain birthweight as a proxy for overall growth status

Major Recommendations:
- Physiologic MWL from birthweight of 5% to 15% should be targeted for extremely preterm newborns
- Clinicians should use caution in interpreting serum sodium values to dictate the overall fluid status of extremely preterm infants
- Shorter time to regain birthweight does not equate to improved growth velocity during hospitalization. Further studies are needed to evaluate the optimal time to regain birthweight and its association with short- and long-term health outcomes.

Bibliographic source(s)

Valentine GC, Perez KM, Wood TR, et al. Postnatal MWL, fluid administration, and outcomes in extremely preterm newborns. J Perinatol. Mar 25 2022;doi:10.1038/s41372-022-01369-7.

Oh W, Poindexter BB, Perritt R, et al. Association between fluid intake and weight loss during the first ten days of life and risk of BPD in extremely low birth weight infants. J Pediatr. Dec 2005;147(6):786–90. doi:10.1016/j.jpeds.2005.06.039.

Ehrenkranz RA, Dusick AM, Vohr BR, Wright LL, Wrage LA, Poole WK. Growth in the neonatal intensive care unit influences neurodevelopmental and growth outcomes of extremely low birth weight infants. Pediatrics. Apr 2006;117(4):1253–1261. doi:10.1542/peds.2005-1368

REFERENCES

1. Agren J, Segar JL, Soderstrom F, et al. Fluid management considerations in extremely preterm infants born at 22-24 weeks of gestation. Semin Perinatol 2022;46(1):151541.
2. Bell EF, Weinstein MR, Oh W. Heat balance in premature infants: comparative effects of convectively heated incubator and radiant warmer, with without plastic heat shield. J Pediatr 1980;96(3 Pt 1):460–5.
3. Hammarl-nd K, Nilsson GE, Oberg PA, et al. Transepidermal water loss in newborn infants. I. Relation to ambient humidity and site of measurement and estimation of total transepidermal water loss. Acta Paediatr Scand 1977;66(5): 553–62.
4. Chiou YB, Blume-Peytavi U. Stratum corneum maturation. A review of neonatal skin function. Skin Pharmacol Physiol 2004;17(2):57–66.
5. Evans NJ, Rutter N. Development of the epidermis in the newborn. Biol Neonate 1986;49(2):74–80.
6. Gubhaju L, Sutherland MR, Horne RS, et al. Assessment of renal functional maturation and injury in preterm neonates during the first month of life. Am J Physiol Renal Physiol 2014;307(2):F149–58.
7. Jose PA, Fildes RD, Gomez RA, et al. Neonatal renal function and physiology. Curr Opin Pediatr 1994;6(2):172–7.

8. Valentine GC, Umoren RA, Perez KM. Early inadequate or excessive weight loss: a potential contributor to mortality in premature newborns in resource-scarce settings? Pediatr Neonatol 2021;62(3):237–9.

9. Hartnoll G, Betremieux P, Modi N. Body water content of extremely preterm infants at birth. Arch Dis Child Fetal Neonatal Ed 2000;83(1):F56–9.

10. Bauer K, Bovermann G, Roithmaier A, et al. Body composition, nutrition, and fluid balance during the first two weeks of life in preterm neonates weighing less than 1500 grams. J Pediatr 1991;118(4 Pt 1):615–20.

11. Agren J, Sjors G, Sedin G. Transepidermal water loss in infants born at 24 and 25 weeks of gestation. Acta Paediatr 1998;87(11):1185–90.

12. Valentine GC, Perez KM, Wood TR, et al. Postnatal maximal weight loss, fluid administration, and outcomes in extremely preterm newborns. J Perinatol 2022. https://doi.org/10.1038/s41372-022-01369-7.

13. Wadhawan R, Oh W, Perritt R, et al. Association between early postnatal weight loss and death or BPD in small and appropriate for gestational age extremely low-birth-weight infants. J Perinatol 2007;27(6):359–64.

14. Bell EF, Warburton D, Stonestreet BS, et al. High-volume fluid intake predisposes premature infants to necrotising enterocolitis. Lancet 1979;2(8133):90.

15. Lorenz JM, Kleinman LI, Kotagal UR, et al. Water balance in very low-birth-weight infants: relationship to water and sodium intake and effect on outcome. J Pediatr 1982;101(3):423–32.

16. Miyoshi Y, Suenaga H, Aoki M, et al. Determinants of excessive weight loss in breastfed full-term newborns at a baby-friendly hospital: a retrospective cohort study. Int Breastfeed J 2020;15(1):19.

17. Flaherman VJ, Schaefer EW, Kuzniewicz MW, et al. Early weight loss nomograms for exclusively breastfed newborns. Pediatrics 2015;135(1):e16–23.

18. Paul IM, Schaefer EW, Miller JR, et al. Weight change nomograms for the first month after birth. Pediatrics 2016;138(6). https://doi.org/10.1542/peds.2016-2625.

19. Huang A, Tai BC, Wong LY, et al. Differential risk for early breastfeeding jaundice in a multi-ethnic Asian cohort. Ann Acad Med Singap 2009;38(3):217–24.

20. Zuppa AA, Sindico P, Antichi E, et al. Weight loss and jaundice in healthy term newborns in partial and full rooming-in. J Matern Fetal Neonatal Med 2009;22(9):801–5.

21. Caglar MK, Ozer I, Altugan FS. Risk factors for excess weight loss and hypernatremia in exclusively breast-fed infants. Braz J Med Biol Res 2006;39(4):539–44.

22. Nada A, Bonachea EM, Askenazi DJ. Acute kidney injury in the fetus and neonate. Semin Fetal Neonatal Med 2017;22(2):90–7.

23. Pandey V, Kumar D, Vijayaraghavan P, et al. Non-dialytic management of acute kidney injury in newborns. J Ren Inj Prev 2017;6(1):1–11.

24. Seri I. Management of hypotension and low systemic blood flow in the very low birth weight neonate during the first postnatal week. J Perinatol 2006;26(Suppl 1):S8–13 [discussion: S22-3].

25. Trotman H, Antoine M, Barton M. Hypernatraemic dehydration in exclusively breastfed infants: a potentially fatal complication. West Indian Med J 2006;55(4):282–5.

26. Trotman H, Lord C, Barton M, et al. Hypernatraemic dehydration in Jamaican breastfed neonates: a 12-year review in a baby-friendly hospital. Ann Trop Paediatr 2004;24(4):295–300.

27. Clarke AJ, Sibert JR. Hypernatraemic dehydration and necrotizing enterocolitis. Postgrad Med J 1985;61(711):65–6.

28. Cole TJ, Statnikov Y, Santhakumaran S, et al. Birth weight and longitudinal growth in infants born below 32 weeks' gestation: a UK population study. Arch Dis Child Fetal Neonatal Ed 2014;99(1):F34–40.

29. Verma RP, Shibli S, Fang H, et al. Clinical determinants and utility of early post-natal maximum weight loss in fluid management of extremely low birth weight infants. Early Hum Dev 2009;85(1):59–64.

30. Verma RP, Shibli S, Komaroff E. Postnatal transitional weight loss and adverse outcomes in extremely premature neonates. Pediatr Rep 2017;9(1):6962.

31. Oh W, Poindexter BB, Perritt R, et al. Association between fluid intake and weight loss during the first ten days of life and risk of bronchopulmonary dysplasia in extremely low birth weight infants. J Pediatr 2005;147(6):786–90.

32. Aksoy HT, Guzoglu N, Eras Z, et al. The association of early postnatal weight loss with outcome in extremely low birth weight infants. Pediatr Neonatol 2019;60(2):192–6.

33. Segar DE, Segar EK, Harshman LA, et al. Physiological approach to sodium sup-plementation in preterm infants. Am J Perinatol 2018;35(10):994–1000.

34. Al-Dahhan J, Haycock GB, Chantler C, et al. Sodium homeostasis in term and preterm neonates. I. Renal aspects. Arch Dis Child 1983;58(5):335–42.

35. Lim WH, Lien R, Chiang MC, et al. Hypernatremia and grade III/IV intraventricular hemorrhage among extremely low birth weight infants. J Perinatol 2011;31(3):193–8.

36. Smith MR, Smith RD, Plummer NW, et al. Functional analysis of the mouse Scn8a sodium channel. J Neurosci 1998;18(16):6093–102.

37. Riley LS, A R. Guidelines for perinatal care. American Academy of Pediatrics and the American College of Obstetricians and Gynecologists 2012. 7th ed.

38. Holt KW, Wooldridge NH, Story M, et al. Bright Futures: Nutrition. 3rd Edition. Elk Grove Village, IL: American Academy of Pediatrics; 2011.

39. Gao C, Ehsan L, Jones M, et al. Time to regain birth weight predicts neonatal growth velocity: a single-center experience. Clin Nutr ESPEN 2020;38:165–71.

40. Goldberg DL, Becker PJ, Brigham K, et al. Identifying malnutrition in preterm and neonatal populations: recommended indicators. J Acad Nutr Diet 2018;118(9):1571–82.

41. Ehrenkranz RA, Dusick AM, Vohr BR, et al. Growth in the neonatal intensive care unit influences neurodevelopmental and growth outcomes of extremely low birth weight infants. Pediatrics 2006;117(4):1253–61.

42. Anvekar A, Athikarisamy S, Rao S, et al. Time to regain birth weight - a marker to predict the severity of retinopathy of prematurity? BMC Pediatr 2021;21(1):540.

43. Bell EF, Acarregui MJ. Restricted versus liberal water intake for preventing morbidity and mortality in preterm infants. Cochrane Database Syst Rev 2014;12:CD000503.

44. Stephens BE, Gargus RA, Walden RV, et al. Fluid regimens in the first week of life may increase risk of patent ductus arteriosus in extremely low birth weight infants. J Perinatol 2008;28(2):123–8.

45. Soullane S, Patel S, Claveau M, et al. Fluid status in the first 10 days of life and death/bronchopulmonary dysplasia among preterm infants. Pediatr Res 2021;90(2):353–8.

46. Diderholm B, Normann E, Ahlsson F, et al. The impact of restricted versus liberal early fluid volumes on plasma sodium, weight change, and short-term outcomes in extremely preterm infants. Nutrients 2022;14(4). https://doi.org/10.3390/nu14040795.

47. Nangia S, Vadivel V, Thukral A, et al. Early total enteral feeding versus conventional enteral feeding in stable very-low-birth-weight infants: a randomised controlled trial. Neonatology 2019;115(3):256–62.
48. Bora R, Murthy NB. In resource limited areas complete enteral feed in stable very low birth weight infants (1000-1500 g) started within 24 h of life can improve nutritional outcome. J Matern Fetal Neonatal Med 2017;30(21):2572–7.
49. Sanghvi KP, Joshi P, Nabi F, et al. Feasibility of exclusive enteral feeds from birth in VLBW infants >1200 g--an RCT. Acta Paediatr 2013;102(7):e299–304.
50. Walsh V, Brown JVE, Copperthwaite BR, et al. Early full enteral feeding for preterm or low birth weight infants. Cochrane Database Syst Rev 2020;12: CD013542.
51. Ahmad KA, Frey CS, Fierro MA, et al. Two-year neurodevelopmental outcome of an infant born at 21 weeks' 4 days' gestation. Pediatrics 2017;140(6). https://doi.org/10.1542/peds.2017-0103.
52. Kjartansson S, Arsan S, Hammarlund K, et al. Water loss from the skin of term and preterm infants nursed under a radiant heater. Pediatr Res 1995;37(2):233–8.
53. Spath C, Sjostrom ES, Ahlsson F, et al. Sodium supply influences plasma sodium concentration and the risks of hyper- and hyponatremia in extremely preterm infants. Pediatr Res 2017;81(3):455–60.

Administering Parenteral Nutrition in the Neonatal Intensive Care Unit
Logistics, Existing Challenges, and a Few Conundrums

Anne L. Smazal, MD, MS[a,b], Imran M. Ilahi, DO[a,b],
Janice Raucci, PharmD, BCPPS[b], Daniel T. Robinson, MD, MSc[a,b,*]

KEYWORDS

• Parenteral nutrition • Drug compatibility • Neonatal nutrition • Preterm • Infant

KEY POINTS

- Anticipated prolonged duration of parenteral nutrition (PN), high osmolality, and drug incompatibility should prompt the consideration of central venous catheter placement.
- Patients receiving PN are at risk of aluminum, manganese, and oxidative peroxide exposures, as well as refeeding syndrome.
- The transition from PN to full enteral nutrition can be complicated by inadvertent suboptimal nutrition delivery.
- Opportunities to reduce risks of PN administration would be maximized by developing a multidisciplinary team that performs the daily assessment of all logistical aspects of PN administration.

INTRODUCTION

Parenteral nutrition (PN) including lipid injectable emulsions (ILEs) provides essential nutrients to neonates and infants hospitalized in the neonatal intensive care unit (NICU) during times in which enteral feedings contribute no or inadequate energy and nutrients. While copious research identifies risks and benefits of parenteral nutrient doses and composition, additional practicalities must be considered in decision making when prescribing PN, such as neonatal populations most likely to receive benefit, catheter utilization and admixture stability. Additional considerations are the

[a] Department of Pediatrics, Northwestern University Feinberg School of Medicine; [b] Ann & Robert H. Lurie Children's Hospital of Chicago, Chicago, IL, USA
* Corresponding author. Lurie Children's Hospital, 225 East Chicago Avenue, Box 45, Chicago, IL 60611.
E-mail address: daniel-robinson@northwestern.edu

Clin Perinatol 50 (2023) 557–573
https://doi.org/10.1016/j.clp.2023.04.004
0095-5108/23/© 2023 Elsevier Inc. All rights reserved.
perinatology.theclinics.com

inherent risks of PN administration including central line-associated bloodstream infection (CLABSI), photooxidative stress, and inadvertent exposures. The goal of this article is to discuss practical considerations when administering PN to neonates and infants in NICUs, considerations that are influenced by but still separate from deciding specific doses of nutrients.

LOGISTICS

Identifying Neonatal Populations Expected to Benefit from Parenteral Nutrition

Decisions to utilize PN in neonatal populations stem from considering the metabolic consequences of utilizing dextrose-only intravenous fluids when nutrient goals cannot be met via enteral feedings. One consideration is the duration over which parenteral infusions would be expected to provide most of the energy and nutrient needs. Inherent to that consideration is the expectation that energy and nutrient deficits are expected to accrue rapidly without parenteral sources of nutrients during minimal enteral nutrition intake.[1] Another practical consideration is the cost of custom PN. While studies suggest cost savings from using 3-chamber bags, higher calcium doses used in neonatal PN increase precipitation risk which would be hard to identify visually with the ILE mixed in solution.[2,3] There are no specific definitions of acceptable durations during which PN should not be provided. In a recent survey of neonatologists' opinions on initiating PN in neonates born full-term or late preterm (34–36 weeks of gestation), the ideal time to initiate amino acids and lipids was within the first day of admission for just over 40% of the clinicians, whereas one-third suggested the ideal time was after admission for 72 hours.[4] Three percent of respondents suggested no PN was indicated for such neonates who, in the case scenarios, were specified as unable to receive enteral nutrition.[4] In contrast, it is generally accepted that neonates born under 32 weeks or 1500 g and surgical neonates such as those with gastroschisis or surgical necrotizing enterocolitis (NEC) would benefit given extended durations before which these neonates may tolerate full enteral nutrition (FEN), indicating goal energy and nutrient intake through enteral feedings. While FEN may be achieved more quickly in neonates born 1500g-2500 g, a short duration of PN may help with earlier regain of birthweight in the smaller neonates in that birthweight range.[5] Long-term follow-up studies are needed in those low birthweight populations.

Recent data identified concern about earlier initiation for neonatal populations managed in pediatric intensive care units (PICUs). In a randomized control trial of 1440 term infants and children up to age 17 years admitted to participating PICUs in Belgium, Canada, and the Netherlands, children received either early PN (started within 24 hours of admission) or late PN (started after 7 days of hospitalization if enteral feedings supplied <80% of recommended energy intake).[6] Participating children were admitted to the PICU for either medical diagnoses, such as respiratory infections or oncologic treatment, and surgical indications including abdominal or cardiac surgeries. However, most neonates <4 weeks old were admitted for surgical indications. Late PN was associated with lower rates of new infection, decreased length of stay, higher likelihood of survival to discharge, shorter duration of mechanical ventilation, and decreased inflammatory markers.[6] Further subgroup analyses demonstrated no worsening of weight deterioration or long-term neurodevelopmental outcomes in the late PN group.[7,8] In a subgroup analysis of term neonates ages 28 days and younger, late PN was associated with increased likelihood of earlier discharge but was not associated with infection.[9] In neonates admitted 7 days and younger, late PN was associated with lower risk of infection. However, late PN was associated with higher risk of hypoglycemia, raising concern for long-term neurodevelopmental outcomes in this population. Results from this group of term neonates, the majority admitted primarily for surgical reasons, must be interpreted cautiously for the broader NICU population. These findings contradict evidence for improved neurodevelopmental outcomes in preterm neonates who receive early PN with enhanced nutrient composition.[10,11]

Identifying Appropriate Catheter Use

A necessary logistical decision is whether to infuse PN via a peripherally versus centrally inserted venous catheter. Infusing a higher osmolarity solution in a peripheral vein may cause infiltration and phlebitis. Therefore, higher osmolarity solutions require administration via central venous catheters (CVC) which terminate in larger vessels.

While the totality of the admixture's nutrient content determines the final osmolarity, amino acids and dextrose contribute most to total osmolarity. Studies in neonatal and pediatric patients suggest a maximum solution concentration of 900-1000 mOsm/L is appropriate for peripheral infusion, though one study demonstrated safety up to 1250 mOsm/L.[12,13] Without the consideration of other nutrients, a common practice is to limit the dextrose concentration administered peripherally to 12.5 g/dL (approximately 700 mOsm/L) for concern of phlebitis.[14] Maximum osmolarity of centrally administered PN has not been well defined. Many electronic medical record systems (EMR) utilize automated osmolarity calculations as a safety measure to prevent the ordering of hyperosmolar fluids. When the desired volume cannot safely contain the desired nutrient concentrations, pharmacists can help prioritize each component within safe osmolarity limits.

While calcium-containing PN can be administered peripherally, this carries the risk of extravasation.[15] Calcium extravasation injuries can be severe, causing localized skin inflammation and necrosis with resulting functional and cosmetic complications.[16,17] Although extravasation injury causing skin necrosis are relatively uncommon, the risk is increased in low birth weight and premature infants.[17–19] The need to supply adequate calcium and phosphorus to avoid osteopenia is another consideration for using CVC.

CVC utilization requires monitoring for known complications. While the hypertonicity and pH of most PN solutions prohibit bacterial growth, duration of PN exposure is associated with CLABSI risk.[18] Furthermore, malpositioned CVC can result in inadvertent administration of PN into peritoneal, pericardial, and pleural spaces.[20–22] One study showed improved growth of moderately preterm neonates who received PN via CVC without increased risk of CLABSI; average catheter dwell time was 8 days, indicating benefits of optimized nutrition can supersede risk of CLABSI.[23] For context, nearly 80% of neonates who need CVCs have a dwell time ≥8 days.[24] When utilizing a CVC, best practice is the daily assessment of catheter need to avoid prolonged dwell times. These assessments are a key part of infection control bundles which demonstrate efficacy in reducing CLABSI.[25,26]

Umbilical artery catheters (UACs) can be used for PN administration. Recently, one trial evaluated the impact of administering an additional 1 g/dL of amino acids to very low birth weight (VLBW) neonates by replacing the typical nonnutritive fluids used in UACs with an amino acid solution (TrophAmine).[27] Safety of PN administration via UAC is likely comparable to administration via CVC, but this is not a common practice.[28]

Compatibility of Parenteral Nutrition with Other Infusions

For critically ill infants, PN is likely just one admixture needing parenteral infusion, and the compatibility of PN with other medications must be considered. To accommodate multiple infusions, stopcocks can be used to administer 2 or more drugs via a single catheter. This practice, called Y-site administration, results in a mixture of medications within the catheter and vessel. Alternatively, single catheters with multiple lumens may be utilized so that medications do not mix within a single lumen, but double-lumen catheters are a known risk factor for CLABSIs.[29]

While Y-site administration is a practical choice for delivering multiple medications, drug incompatibility (DI) may occur, a scenario of visible precipitation in the mixture, or loss of >10% of drug dose.[30] Incompatibility can destabilize ILE and increase fat globule size, increasing risk of vascular occlusion by large droplets.[31,32] Definitive physical compatibility data are available for only an estimated 25% of commonly co-administered drugs used in the NICU.[33] It is vital to understand that the testing leading to reported compatibilities have only evaluated very limited scenarios as compared to the complexities that emerge during routine clinical care (ie, compatibility was tested after short exposures while clinical practice often involves continuous mixing via Y-site for 24 hours; only one amino acid solution was tested when others may be utilized in different NICUs; continuous infusion medications may be mixed in fluids different than those tested).[34] Neonates are at higher risk of DI given the utilization of higher concentrations of some medications to avoid fluid overload, slower fluid administration rates allowing for longer mixing time, and small catheters which are more easily occluded by physical precipitation.

Many commonly used medications, including ceftazidime, dexamethasone, levetiracetam, ibuprofen, and morphine can be safely administered via Y-site with PN.[35] Given the paucity of data on compatibility with neonatal PN, pharmacists may rely on clinical experience to guide decision making. **Table 1** summarizes known compatibilities to consider for the co-administration of commonly used neonatal medications with PN.

Increasing Safety Through Photoprotection

With the exposure of vitamins, amino acids, ILE, and minerals in PN to light and oxygen, photooxidation reactions produce hydrogen peroxide and other cytotoxic organic peroxides.[41] Vitamins and ILE are most susceptible to these reactions. Sunlight, ambient light, and phototherapy lights trigger the production of oxygen radicals. Phototherapy caused a 60-fold increase in hydroperoxides in 100% soybean oil ILE after a 24-h exposure compared to an approximately 8-fold increase after 24 hours of ambient light exposure.[42] In animal models and in vitro studies, these oxidation products disrupt lipid metabolism, induce hepatic steatosis, promote hemolysis, and induce oxidative damage in the lungs.[43-45] In clinical studies, photooxidation products were associated with increased risk of chronic lung disease, higher blood glucose concentration, and hypertriglyceridemia, although not all clinical trials showed increased risk of lung disease.[46,47] Retrospective studies suggest that photoprotecting PN is associated with decreased risk of bronchopulmonary dysplasia (BPD), increased enteral feeding tolerance, and decreased mortality.[48-50] A reduced risk of mortality with photoprotection was identified through combined analysis of clinical trials in preterm neonates.[48] Preterm neonates are considered especially susceptible to oxidative stress given limited endogenous antioxidants and exposure to other triggers of oxidative stress, such as supplemental oxygen, transfusions, and medications.

Photoprotection, or light shielding, with the use of commercially available photoprotective bags, amber-colored tubing, or aluminum foil reduces concentrations of hydroxy radicals.[41,51] The optimal scenario is to achieve complete photoprotection, meaning that all nutrients are photoprotected at every step of PN manufacturing, distribution, and compounding.[52] This includes protecting storage containers for the individual nutrients during production, storage, and transport, the admixture during

Table 1
Compatibility of parenteral nutrition and lipid injectable emulsions in admixture with select neonatal medications[a]

	2 in 1 PN[b]	100% SO ILE	100% FO ILE	SO,MCT,OO,FO ILE
Gastrointestinal				
Famotidine		N	N	
Famotidine 0.25 mg/mL[3]				C
Famotidine 2 mg/mL	C			
Famotidine 2.5 mg/mL				I
Pantoprazole sodium	N	N	N	N
Cardiopulmonary				
Atropine sulfate	N	N	N	N
Dobutamine hydrochloride		N	N	N
Dobutamine hydrochloride 1 and 4 mg/mL	C			
Dopamine hydrochloride		N	N	
Dopamine hydrochloride 1.6 and 3.2 mg/mL	C			I[c]
Epinephrine		N	N	N
Epinephrine 0.0096 and 0.2 mg/mL	C			
Hydralazine hydrochloride	N	N	N	N
Ibuprofen lysine	I		N	N
Ibuprofen lysine 10 mg/mL		U[d]		
Norepinephrine bitartrate		N	N	N
Norepinephrine bitartrate 0.016 mg/mL	C			
Phenylephrine hydrochloride	N	N	N	N
Prostaglandin E1			N	
Prostaglandin E1 0.015 mg/mL	C			
Prostaglandin E1 0.02 mg/mL		C		U[e]
Sildenafil citrate	N		N	
Sildenafil citrate 0.8 mg/mL		C		C
Neurologic				
Acetaminophen	N	N	N	N
Caffeine citrate		N	N	N
Caffeine citrate 20 mg/mL	C			
Dexmedetomidine hydrochloride			N	
Dexmedetomidine hydrochloride 4 mcg/mL	C	C		C
Hydromorphone hydrochloride			N	
Hydromorphone hydrochloride 0.5 mg/mL	C			
Hydromorphone hydrochloride 2.5 mg/mL		C		C
Fentanyl citrate		N	N	
Fentanyl citrate 0.0125 mg/mL	C			
Fentanyl citrate 0.05 mg/mL	C			C
Fosphenytoin sodium		N	N	N
Fosphenytoin sodium 50 mgPE/mL	C			
Indomethacin sodium		N	N	N

(continued on next page)

Table 1 *(continued)*				
	2 in 1 PN[b]	100% SO ILE	100% FO ILE	SO,MCT,OO,FO ILE
Indomethacin sodium 1 mg/mL	I			
Levetiracetam	N	N	N	N
Lorazepam		N	N	N
Lorazepam 0.1 mg/mL	C			
Methadone hydrochloride	N	N	N	N
Midazolam hydrochloride		N	N	
Midazolam hydrochloride 0.5 mg/mL				C
Midazolam hydrochloride 2 and 5 mg/mL	I			
Morphine sulfate		N	N	
Morphine sulfate 1 mg/mL	C			C
Phenobarbital		N	N	N
Phenobarbital 5 mg/mL	C			
Rocuronium bromide	N		N	
Rocuronium bromide 10 mg/mL		U[e]		U[e]
Vecuronium bromide		N	N	N
Renal				
Bumetanide			N	
Bumetanide 0.04 mg/mL	C			
Bumetanide 0.25 mg/mL		C		C
Chlorothiazide sodium		N	N	N
Chlorothiazide sodium 28 mg/mL	I			
Enalaprilat		N	N	N
Enalaprilat 0.08 and 0.1 mg/mL	C			
Furosemide			N	
Furosemide 1 mg/mL	C			
Furosemide 2 mg/mL				C
Furosemide 3 mg/mL	I			
Furosemide 10 mg/mL		C		C
Vasopressin	N	N	N	N
Infectious Disease				
Acyclovir		N	N	N
Acyclovir 7 mg/mL	I			
Ampicillin sodium			N	
Ampicillin sodium 20 mg/mL	C			
Ampicillin sodium 30 mg/mL		C		C
Ampicillin sodium 100 and 200 mg/mL	I			
Cefotaxime		N	N	N
Cefotaxime 20, 60, and 200 mg/mL	C			
Ceftazidime			N	N
Ceftazidime 10 mg/mL		C		
Ceftazidime 40, 50, 60, and 200 mg/mL	C			

(continued on next page)

Table 1 *(continued)*	2 in 1 PNb	100% SO ILE	100% FO ILE	SO,MCT,OO,FO ILE
Ceftriaxone sodium			N	N
Ceftriaxone sodium 10 mg/mL		C		
Ceftriaxone sodium 20 mg/mL	I			
Metronidazole			N	N
Metronidazole 5 mg/mL	C	I		
Fluconazole			N	N
Fluconazole 1 mg/mL		I		
Fluconazole 0.5, 1.75, and 2 mg/mL	C			
Gentamicin sulfate			N	
Gentamicin sulfate 0.4 mg/mL		I		
Gentamicin sulfate 2 mg/mL		Ue		I
Gentamicin sulfate 1, 5, and 10 mg/mL	C			
Linezolid		N	N	N
Linezolid 2 mg/mL	C			
Meropenem	N		N	N
Meropenem 5 mg/mL		C		
Oxacillin sodium		N	N	N
Oxacillin sodium 100 mg/mL	C			
Penicillin G sodium		N	N	N
Penicillin G sodium 200,000, 320,000, and 500,000 units/mL	C			
Piperacillin sodium-tazobactam sodium		N	N	N
Piperacillin sodium-tazobactam sodium 45 mg/mL	C			
Vancomycin hydrochloride			N	N
Vancomycin hydrochloride 5 mg/mL	C	I		
Zidovudine		N	N	N
Zidovudine 4 mg/mL	C			
Endocrine				
Dexamethasone sodium phosphate	Uf	N	N	N
Hydrocortisone sodium succinate		N	N	N
Hydrocortisone sodium succinate 1 mg/mL	C			
Insulin regular		N	N	N
Insulin regular 0.5 unit/mL	C			
Levothyroxine sodium	N	N	N	N

Abbreviations: C, compatible; FO, fish oil; I, incompatible; ILE, lipid injectable emulsions; MCT, medium chain triglyceride; N, no data; OO, olive oil; PN, parenteral nutrition; SO, soybean oil; U, uncertain or variable results.

[a] Data on compatibilities from Lexicomp Online.[36] Drug concentrations are indicated if they were specifically reported and only concentrations relevant to neonatal/young infant populations (eg, weight <10 kg) are included. However, not all concentrations tested would be expected to be administered without dilution. This table should not be utilized in place of independent clinical decision making as the intricacies of each specific clinical scenario in which PN is administered have not been tested, including the specific concentrations and composition of dextrose, amino acids, ILE, and medication concentrations and/or dilutions.

^b Indicates a solution containing dextrose, amino acids and other nutrients/electrolytes without ILE contained in the solution.
^c Only tested for 3.2 mg/mL.[37]
^d The authors indicate that simulated Y-site compatibility between ibuprofen lysine and 100% SO ILE (10% concentration) could not be evaluated; complicating factors included an opacity and "milky white appearance" that can be attributable to the ILE as well as concerns regarding turbidity.[38]
^e Mixture approached incompatibility threshold and should be coadministered with increased caution.[37]
^f Variable compatibility results have been reported for this drug with PN admixtures depending on drug concentrations and PN composition.[39,40]

compounding, the solution during delivery to the patient's bedside as well as during infusion. Complete photoprotection is challenging to achieve given the current materials available, costs associated with obtaining materials, and the complexity of PN production inclusive of manufacturing through administration.[52] However, partial protection using products such as photoprotective bags and amber-colored tubing can be implemented and is expected to reduce the oxidant load infused.

CHALLENGES
Unintended Exposures: Aluminum and Manganese

Aluminum is a natural contaminant of some parenteral products. Contamination occurs in sodium phosphate, potassium phosphate, and calcium gluconate, essential components for preterm infants at risk of metabolic bone disease. Concentrations in PN range 50-150 mcg in 100 mL.[53–55] A clinical trial randomized preterm neonates to receive standard or aluminum-depleted PN, with aluminum depletion achieved by the substitution of calcium chloride for calcium gluconate and exclusion of potassium phosphate. However, in clinical practice, this change would be challenging to ensure solubility as published references on solubility tested calcium gluconate. Neonates receiving the standard solution demonstrated lower Bayley Mental Development Index scores at 18 months, estimating a drop of one point on the Mental Development Index per day of standard aluminum-containing PN.[56] This trial did not assess bone mineralization. Substituting sodium phosphate for potassium phosphate and calcium chloride for calcium gluconate allows appropriate calcium and phosphorus provision in neonates receiving >120 mL/kg/day while limiting aluminum exposure to approximately 6.3 mcg/dL.[57] An analysis measuring aluminum content of standard neonatal PN formulations found that while measured aluminum content was lower than that calculated and labeled, all exceeded FDA safe limits (5mcg/kg/day) by at least 10 mcg/kg/day[55] In a review of pediatric patients receiving PN, meeting the FDA safe limit was only achievable for patients weighing over 50 kg, suggesting that this limit is not feasible for neonatal patients.[58] This conundrum of natural contamination remains and affirms the priority of reducing PN duration by advancing enteral nutrition when possible.

Manganese is an essential metal for growth and development, functioning as a cofactor for several enzymes and contributing to hormone production and hemostasis.[59] At high levels, manganese can accumulate in the central nervous system (CNS), with resulting neurotoxic effects that manifest similarly to Parkinson's disease as observed in adults on long term PN.[60] PN provides substantially higher concentrations of manganese (up to eight times the recommended provision of 1 mcg/kg/d) due to natural contamination and bypasses the enteric system's protective mechanisms. Infants receiving PN have increased plasma concentration of manganese and increased manganese deposition in the basal ganglia.[61,62] The clinical manifestations of manganese toxicity and its CNS deposition are reversible with the cessation of manganese exposure.[60,63] Because most manganese (approximately 0.9 mcg/kg/d) supplied by PN comes from the natural contamination of other components, specifically magnesium sulfate and calcium gluconate, PN formulations without added manganese still meet recommended intake (1 mcg/kg/d).[59,64]

Achieving euglycemia: avoiding the highs and lows

Neonatal glucose metabolism can be affected by prematurity-related insulin resistance, physiologic stressors including sepsis, and medications including corticosteroids; frequent adjustments of the glucose infusion rate (GIR, mg/kg/min) in these specific clinical scenarios can occur.[65–67] Up to 80% of VLBW neonates develop hyperglycemia, typically defined as serum glucose >150 mg/dL, in the first week.[68] Hyperglycemia has been associated with higher morbidity and mortality through undefined mechanisms.[69] Insulin infusion has been proposed as a strategy to mitigate hyperglycemia, achieve higher energy provisions and thus improve growth.[70,71] However, early insulin infusion has been associated with increased risk of hypoglycemia and mortality.[72] Using the euglycemia hyperinsulinemic clamp technique, exogenous hyperinsulinism was associated with significant lactic acidosis without achieving an anabolic state for protein.[73] In a randomized trial comparing outcomes of preterm neonates assigned to tight glucose control (<155 mg/dL) or standard (<180 mg/dL), tight glycemic control did not improve survival without neurodevelopmental impairment.[74] Near school age, the tight glycemic control group was shorter but had greater height-adjusted lean mass and lower fasting blood glucose concentration.[74] Currently, routine insulin use to preempt hyperglycemia and increase total energy delivery is not advised. Of note, early amino acid delivery increases endogenous insulin production as tested in VLBW neonates.[75]

Aside from insulin, hyperglycemia may be ameliorated by lowering the GIR. A conundrum exists that a common clinical belief is that the GIR cannot be lower than 4 mg/kg/min, often stated in the context of concerns of brain glucose supply. What is not a conundrum is the fact that glucose supply across endothelial cells, the blood-brain barrier, and into neurons is concentration-dependent, not GIR-dependent.[76] It can be anticipated that treating sepsis and, if/when physiologically safe, reducing corticosteroid doses will contribute to lower blood glucose concentrations. ILEs contribute to gluconeogenesis.[77] While lowering or discontinuing the ILE dose might be considered to lower the blood glucose concentration, energy provisions will also be reduced. Regardless of these considerations, severe hyperglycemia, or serum glucose >300 mg/dL, increases the osmolality of the blood and induces osmolar diuresis, which can lead to severe dehydration.[78,79] If multiple measures fail to reduce serum glucose, insulin infusion can be considered for neonates with serum glucose persistently >300 mg/dL. Importantly, and in relevant consideration of hyperglycemia, endogenous glucose production occurs even in extremely preterm neonates.[80]

While the definitions of neonatal hypoglycemia vary, adverse outcomes identified with its occurrence include apnea, respiratory distress, lethargy, and seizure, while prolonged or repeated episodes are associated with epilepsy, cognitive impairment, cerebral palsy, and motor delay.[81,82] Hypoglycemia will likely be avoided in most patients by maintaining a GIR above endogenous glucose production rates, in the range of 4-7 mg/kg/min.[78]

Opportunities for reduced blood testing during parenteral nutrition administration

Many clinicians perform blood tests while neonates receive PN in efforts to optimize its composition. This practice may induce iatrogenic anemia. Intermittent tests of liver function often called hepatic panels are utilized to monitor direct bilirubin as a marker of cholestasis and alkaline phosphatase as a marker of metabolic bone disease. A cohort study of preterm neonates born $</= 34$ weeks of gestation evaluated the frequency with which weekly hepatic panels resulted in changes in clinical management. Less than 5% of hepatic panels (n = 147 panels) in neonates born <32 weeks resulted in the initiation of ursodiol, vitamin D, or change in dosing of either medication.[83] None of four hepatic panels drawn in neonates born 32-34 weeks resulted in clinical intervention. Comparing neonates receiving customized PN to neonates receiving standard PN formulas, both groups demonstrated similar weight gain, yet the group received standardized PN had higher incidence of hypernatremia and hyperchloremia, suggesting some benefit to electrolyte monitoring to titrate PN components.[84] If a multidisciplinary team routinely reviews the potential value of blood testing in each neonate exposed to PN, lab frequency and costs associated with PN utilization may be reduced.[85]

Avoiding refeeding syndrome

Preterm neonates with fetal growth restriction (FGR), and even those born appropriate for gestational age, benefit from careful titration of early PN to avoid refeeding syndrome (RS), a constellation of electrolyte derangements that occurs with in-utero nutrient deprivation most commonly attributed to placental insufficiency, followed by a postnatal relative abundance of nutrients that occurs when PN is administered.[86] Increased intracellular uptake of phosphate, magnesium, and potassium for anabolic processes triggers hypophosphatemia, the hallmark finding in RS, as well as possible hypokalemia, hypomagnesemia, hyperglycemia, hypercalcemia, and hypernatremia.[86] Such electrolyte imbalances can trigger hypertonic dehydration and worsen myocardial function. Increased risk of mortality was identified in a secondary analysis of preterm infants with RS and some but not all cohorts reveal risk of BPD, jaundice, and sepsis.[87,88]

Biochemical abnormalities typically develop within 5-7 days but can be seen as early as the second postnatal day. A conundrum exists resulting from the broad expectation that neonates have no physiologic electrolyte requirements during the first 2-3 postnatal days.[89,90] In addition, withholding sodium in the first days is thought to promote diuresis which is expected to decrease the risk of chronic lung disease.[91] However, these expectations and the practice of providing electrolyte-free PN in the first days were established prior to and not updated since the emphasis on the earlier introduction of amino acids and higher energy provision in the first days.[92,93] As RS usually develops within the first 5 days, maintaining amino acid doses without advancement while monitoring electrolyte and mineral levels may be safer than an automatic daily advancement of amino acids and total energy.[86] Early provision of calcium and phosphate has been shown to decrease the risk of refeeding syndrome.[87]

Transitioning from parenteral nutrition to enteral nutrition

PN is typically weaned gradually as enteral feeding volumes advance. However, this practice has been shown to provide significantly less protein and energy while the infant is nearing FEN.[94] Growth velocity in preterm infants may falter during this transitional period.[95] Discontinuation of PN when enteral feeds reached 100 mL/kg/day was associated with reduced early linear growth of VLBW neonates compared to later discontinuation at enteral feeds of 140 mL/kg/day[95] Diligent monitoring of daily energy and protein intake while transitioning to FEN can minimize inadvertent suboptimal provision. Such monitoring would be facilitated with clinical decision support, i.e., EMR systems calculating details accurately and in real time for clinicians. Such support is surprisingly unavailable despite the universal presence of EMR.[96]

SUMMARY

Opportunities for risk-reduction exist during neonatal PN administration. A common theme for many elements in PN utilization is that daily assessments of the risks and benefits of the PN-related intervention (eg, continuing CVC utilization, repeated blood testing in the context of past and anticipated results) can be expected to reduce risk. The highest yield of such assessments will stem from multidisciplinary input, including pharmacists and dieticians. Examples of research gaps include further delineation of ideal times for PN initiation in select neonatal populations, especially those born late preterm and full-term, cost-effective materials to achieve complete photoprotection, and mechanisms by which suboptimal energy and nutrient delivery may be mitigated during transitions from PN to FEN. Still, early initiation and transition to FEN for patients without contraindications to enteral nutrition should remain a priority for neonates receiving PN.

CLINICS CARE POINTS

- Photoprotective materials such as photoprotective bags and amber tubing can be used for parenteral nutrition solutions whenever possible to reduce concentrations of hydroxy radicals.
- The need for high osmolarity or calcium-containing parenteral nutrition should prompt consideration of central venous catheter placement for support of optimal nutrition.
- Calculate daily energy and protein intake from both enteral and parenteral sources during transitions to enteral nutrition to maintain appropriate nutrient delivery.
- Consider a stable amino acid dose with early provision of calcium and phosphate, balanced with electrolytes as indicated, and careful laboratory monitoring in infants born after fetal growth restriction to reduce risk of refeeding syndrome.

DISCLOSURE

D.T. Robinson received compensation for serving as a member of the Data Safety Monitoring Board for a clinical investigation sponsored by Fresenius Kabi during the past 12 months; he no longer serves in that role. D.T. Robinson serves as institutional principal investigator, with no salary funding, for a consortium database sponsored by Mead Johnson Nutrition, United States. The other authors have nothing to disclose.

REFERENCES

1. Embleton NE, Pang N, Cooke RJ. Postnatal malnutrition and growth retardation: an inevitable consequence of current recommendations in preterm infants? Pediatrics 2001;107(2):270–3.
2. Cogle Sv, Martindale RG, Ramos M, et al. Multicenter prospective evaluation of parenteral nutrition preparation time and resource utilization: 3-chamber bags compared with hospital pharmacy–compounded bags. J Parenter Enteral Nutr 2021;45(7):1552–8.
3. Kriz A, Wright A, Paulsson M, et al. Cost-consequences analysis of increased utilization of triple-chamber-bag parenteral nutrition in preterm neonates in seven European countries. Nutrients 2020;12(9):1–17.
4. Moon K, Rao S, Patole S, et al. Use of parenteral nutrition in term and late preterm infants: an Australian and New Zealand survey. Br J Nutr 2022;128(1):131–8.

5. Robinson DT, Shah S, Murthy K. Parenteral nutrition use and associated out-comes in a select cohort of low birth weight neonates. Am J Perinatol 2014; 31(11):933–8.

6. Eulmesekian P. Early versus late parenteral nutrition in critically ill children. Arch Argent Pediatr 2016;114(4):e274–5.

7. Jacobs A, Dulfer K, Eveleens RD, et al. Long-term developmental effect of with-holding parenteral nutrition in paediatric intensive care units: a 4-year follow-up of the PEPaNIC randomised controlled trial. Lancet Child Adolesc Health 2020;4(7): 503–14.

8. van Puffelen E, Hulst JM, Vanhorebeek I, et al. Effect of late versus early initiation of parenteral nutrition on weight deterioration during PICU stay: secondary anal-ysis of the PEPaNIC randomised controlled trial. Clinical Nutrition 2020;39(1): 104–9.

9. van Puffelen E, Vanhorebeek I, Joosten KFM, et al. Early versus late parenteral nutrition in critically ill, term neonates: a preplanned secondary subgroup analysis of the PEPaNIC multicentre, randomised controlled trial. Lancet Child Adolesc Health 2018;2(7):505–15.

10. Wilson DC, Cairns P, Halliday HL, et al. Randomised controlled trial of an aggres-sive nutritional regimen in sick very low birthweight infants. Arch Dis Child Fetal Neonatal Ed 1997;77(1):F4–11.

11. Trivedi A, Sinn JKH. Early versus late administration of amino acids in preterm in-fants receiving parenteral nutrition. Cochrane Database Syst Rev 2013;2013(7): CD008771.

12. Dugan S, Le J, Jew RK. Maximum tolerated osmolarity for peripheral administra-tion of parenteral nutrition in pediatric patients. J Parenter Enteral Nutr 2014; 38(7):847–51.

13. Fessler AG, Rejrat CE. Re-evaluating safe osmolarity for peripheral parenteral nutrition in neonatal intensive care patients. J Pediatr Pharmacol Ther 2021; 26(6):632–7.

14. Boullata JI, Gilbert K, Sacks G, et al. A.S.P.E.N. Clinical guidelines: parenteral nutrition ordering, order review, compounding, labeling, and dispensing. J Parenter Enteral Nutr 2014;38(3):334–77.

15. Ainsworth S, Mcguire W. Percutaneous central venous catheters versus periph-eral cannulae for delivery of parenteral nutrition in neonates. Cochrane Database Syst Rev 2015;2015(10):CD004219.

16. Yosowitz P, Ekland DA, Shaw RC, et al. Peripheral intravenous infiltration necrosis. Ann Surg 1975;182(5):553–6.

17. Kostogloudis N, Demiri E, Tsimponis A, et al. Severe extravasation injuries in ne-onates: a report of 34 cases. Pediatr Dermatol 2015;32(6):830–5.

18. McCullen KL, Pieper B. A retrospective chart review of risk factors for extravasa-tion among neonates receiving peripheral intravascular Ffluids. J Wound Ostomy Continence Nurs 2006;33(2):133–9.

19. Wilkins CE, Emmerson AJB. Extravasation injuries on regional neonatal units. Arch Dis Child Fetal Neonatal Ed 2004;89(3).

20. Mabee R, Kazi S, Yim D, et al. Intraperitoneal extravasation of TPN and associ-ated hepatic hemorrhage as a complication of a malpositioned UVC in a preterm neonate. S D Med 2021;74(12):554–8.

21. Kumar J, Sudeep KC, Mukhopadhyay K, et al. A misplaced peripherally inserted central catheter presenting as contralateral pleural effusion. BMJ Case Rep 2018; 2018.

22. Hartley M, Ruppa Mohanram G, Ahmed I. TPNoma: an unusual complication of umbilical venous catheter malposition. Arch Dis Child Fetal Neonatal Ed 2019; 104(3):F326.

23. Smazal AL, Kavars AB, Carlson SJ, et al. Peripherally inserted central catheters optimize nutrient intake in moderately preterm infants. Pediatr Res 2016;80(2): 185–9.

24. Milstone AM, Reich NG, Advani S, et al. Catheter dwell time and clabsis in neonates with piccs: a multicenter cohort study. Pediatrics 2013;132(6):e1609.

25. Payne V, Hall M, Prieto J, et al. Care bundles to reduce central line-associated bloodstream infections in the neonatal unit: a systematic review and meta-analysis. Arch Dis Child Fetal Neonatal Ed 2018;103(5):F422–9.

26. Pitiriga V, Bakalis J, Kampos E, et al. Duration of central venous catheter placement and central line-associated bloodstream infections after the adoption of prevention bundles: a two-year retrospective study. Antimicrob Resist Infect Control 2022;11(1):96.

27. Bloomfield FH, Crowther CA, Harding JE, et al. The ProVIDe study: the impact of protein intravenous nutrition on development in extremely low birthweight babies. BMC Pediatr 2015;15(1):100.

28. Smith L, Dills R. Survey of medication administration through umbilical arterial and venous catheters. Am J Health Syst Pharm 2003;60(15):1569–72.

29. Khieosanuk K, Fupinwong S, Tosilakul A, et al. Incidence rate and risk factors of central line-associated bloodstream infections among neonates and children admitted to a tertiary care university hospital. Am J Infect Control 2022;50(1): 105–7.

30. Trissel LA. Handbook on injectable drugs. 15th edition. Bethesda, MD: American Society of Health System Pharmacists; 2009.

31. Hardy G, Puzovic M. Formulation, stability, and administration of parenteral nutrition with new lipid emulsions. Nutr Clin Pract 2009;24(5):616–25.

32. Bettner FS, Stennett DJ. Effects of pH, temperature, concentration, and time on particle counts in lipid-containing total parenteral nutrition admixtures. J Parenter Enteral Nutr 1986;10(4):375–80.

33. Fernández-Peña A, Katsumiti A, de Basagoiti A, et al. Drug compatibility in neonatal intensive care units: gaps in knowledge and discordances. Eur J Pediatr 2021;180(7):2305–13.

34. Boullata JI, Mirtallo JM, Sacks GS, et al. Parenteral nutrition compatibility and stability: a comprehensive review. J Parenter Enteral Nutr 2022;46(2):273–99.

35. Aeberhard C, Steuer C, Saxer C, et al. Physicochemical stability and compatibility testing of levetiracetam in all-in-one parenteral nutrition admixtures in daily practice. Eur J Pharm Sci 2017;96:449–55.

36. Lexicomp online: pediatric and neonatal lexi-drugs online. Wolters Kluwer; 2022. Available at: https://online.lexi.com. Accessed November 14, 2022.

37. Ross EL, Salinas A, Petty K, et al. Compatibility of medications with intravenous lipid emulsions: effects of simulated Y-site mixing. Am J Health Syst Pharm 2020;77(23):1980–5.

38. Holt RJ, Siegert SWK, Krishna A. Physical compatibility of ibuprofen lysine injection with selected drugs during simulated Y-site injection. J Pediatr Pharmacol Therapeut 2008;13(3):156–61.

39. Johnson GE, Jacobson PA, Chan E. Stability of ganciclovir sodium and amino acids in parenteral nutrient solutions. Am J Hosp Pharm 1994;51(4):503–8.

40. Puzovic M, Kukec-Jerkovic M. Compatibility of selected drugs with pediatric parenteral nutrition solutions during simulated Y-site administration. Paediatr Croat 2006;50(4):179–85.
41. Silvers KM, Darlow BA, Winterbourn CC. Lipid peroxide and hydrogen peroxide formation in parenteral nutrition solutions containing multivitamins. J Parenter Enteral Nutr 2001;25(1):14–7.
42. Neuzil J, Darlow BA, Inder TE, et al. Oxidation of parenteral lipid emulsion by ambient and phototherapy lights: potential toxicity of routine parenteral feeding. J Pediatr 1995;126(5):785–90.
43. Lavoie JC, Laborie S, Rouleau T, et al. Peroxide-like oxidant response in lungs of newborn Guinea pigs following the parenteral infusion of a multivitamin preparation. Biochem Pharmacol 2000;60(9):1297–303.
44. Chessex P, Lavoie JC, Rouleau T, et al. Photooxidation of parenteral multivitamins induces hepatic steatosis in a neonatal Guinea pig model of intravenous nutrition. Pediatr Res 2002;52(6):958–63.
45. Elremaly W, Mohamed I, Mialet-Marty T, et al. Ascorbylperoxide from parenteral nutrition induces an increase of redox potential of glutathione and loss of alveoli in newborn Guinea pig lungs. Redox Biol 2014;2(1):725–31.
46. Hoff DS, Michaelson AS. Effects of light exposure on total parenteral nutrition and its implications in the neonatal population. J Pediatr Pharmacol Therapeut 2009; 14(3):132–43.
47. Bassiouny MR, Almarsafawy H, Abdel-Hady H, et al. A randomized controlled trial on parenteral nutrition, oxidative stress, and chronic lung diseases in preterm infants. J Pediatr Gastroenterol Nutr 2009;48(3):363–9.
48. Chessex P, Laborie S, Nasef N, et al. Shielding parenteral nutrition from light improves survival rate in premature infants. J Parenter Enteral Nutr 2017;41(3): 378–83.
49. Khashu M, Harrison A, Lalari V, et al. Photoprotection of parenteral nutrition enhances advancement of minimal enteral nutrition in preterm infants. Semin Perinatol 2006;30(3):139–45.
50. Chessex P, Harrison A, Khashu M, et al. In preterm neonates, is the risk of developing bronchopulmonary dysplasia influenced by the failure to protect total parenteral nutrition from exposure to ambient light? J Pediatr 2007;151(2):213–4.
51. Khashu M, Harrison A, Lalari V, et al. Impact of shielding parenteral nutrition from light on routine monitoring of blood glucose and triglyceride levels in preterm neonates. Arch Dis Child Fetal Neonatal Ed 2009;94(2):F111–5.
52. Robinson DT, Ayers P, Fleming B, et al. Recommendations for photoprotection of parenteral nutrition for premature infants: an ASPEN position paper. Nutr Clin Pract 2021;36(5):927–41.
53. Klein GL, Leichtner AM, Heyman MB. Aluminum in large and small volume parenterals used in total parenteral nutrition: response to the Food and Drug Administration notice of proposed rule by the North American Society for Pediatric Gastroenterology and Nutrition. J Pediatr Gastroenterol Nutr 1998 Oct;27(4): 457–60.
54. Driscoll MB, Driscoll DF. Calculating aluminum content in total parenteral nutrition admixtures. Am J Health Syst Pharm 2005;62(3):312–5.
55. Poole RL, Schiff L, Hintz SR, et al. Aluminum content of parenteral nutrition in neonates: measured versus calculated levels. J Pediatr Gastroenterol Nutr 2010; 50(2):208–11.
56. Bishop NJ, Morley R, Day JP, et al. Aluminum neurotoxicity in preterm infants receiving intravenous-feeding solutions. N Engl J Med 1997;336(22):1557–62.

57. Migaki EA, Melhart BJ, Dewar CJ, et al. Calcium chloride and sodium phosphate in neonatal parenteral nutrition containing TrophAmine: precipitation studies and aluminum content. J Parenter Enteral Nutr 2012;36(4):470–5.

58. Poole RL, Hintz SR, Mackenzie NI, et al. Aluminum exposure from pediatric parenteral nutrition: meeting the new FDA regulation. J Parenter Enteral Nutr 2008;32(3):242–6.

59. Institute of Medicine (US) Panel on Micronutrients Washington (DC): National Academies Press (US); 2001.

60. Ono J, Harada K, Sakurai K, et al. Manganese deposition in the brain during long-term total parenteral nutrition. J Parenter Enteral Nutr 1995;19(4):310–2.

61. Hambidge KM, Sokol RJ, Fidanza SJ, et al. Plasma manganese concentrations in infants and children receiving parenteral nutrition. J Parenter Enteral Nutr 1989; 13(2):168–71.

62. Aschner JL, Anderson A, Slaughter JC, et al. Neuroimaging identifies increased manganese deposition in infants receiving parenteral nutrition. AJCN 2015; 102(6):1482–9.

63. Khan A, Hingre J, Dhamoon AS. Manganese neurotoxicity as a complication of chronic total parenteral nutrition. Case Rep Neurol Med 2020;2020:1–6.

64. Sauberan J, Mercier M, Katheria A. Sources of unintentional manganese delivery in neonatal parenteral nutrition. J Parenter Enteral Nutr 2022;46(6):1283–9.

65. Ahmad S, Khalid R. Blood glucose levels in neonatal sepsis and probable sepsis and its association with mortality. Journal of the College of Physicians and Surgeons Pakistan 2012;22(1):15–8.

66. Yeh TF, Lin YJ, Hsieh WS, et al. Early postnatal dexamethasone therapy for the prevention of chronic lung disease in preterm infants with respiratory distress syndrome: a multicenter clinical trial. Pediatrics 1997;100(4):E3.

67. Salis ER, Reith DM, Wheeler BJ, et al. Insulin resistance, glucagon-like peptide-1 and factors influencing glucose homeostasis in neonates. Arch Dis Child Fetal Neonatal Ed 2017;102(2):F162–6.

68. Beardsall K, Vanhaesebrouck S, Ogilvy-Stuart AL, et al. Prevalence and determinants of hyperglycemia in very low birth weight infants: cohort analyses of the NIRTURE study. J Pediatr 2010;157(5):715–9, e1-3.

69. Hays SP, Smith EOB, Sunehag AL. Hyperglycemia is a risk factor for early death and morbidity in extremely low birth-weight infants. Pediatrics 2006;118(5): 1811–8.

70. Binder ND, Raschko PK, Benda GI, et al. Insulin infusion with parenteral nutrition in extremely low birth weight infants with hyperglycemia. J Pediatr 1989;114(2): 273–80.

71. Thabet F, Bourgeois J, Guy B, et al. Continuous insulin infusion in hyperglycaemic very-low-birth-weight infants receiving parenteral nutrition. Clinical Nutrition 2003; 22(6):545–7.

72. Beardsall K, Vanhaesebrouck S, Ogilvy-Stuart AL, et al. Early insulin therapy in very-low-birth-weight infants. N Engl J Med 2008;359(18):1873–84.

73. Poindexter BB, Karn CA, Denne SC. Exogenous insulin reduces proteolysis and protein synthesis in extremely low birth weight infants. J Pediatr 1998;132(6): 948–53.

74. Tottman AC, Alsweiler JM, Bloomfield FH, et al. Long-term outcomes of hyperglycemic preterm infants randomized to tight glycemic control. J Pediatr 2018;193: 68–75.

75. Thureen PJ, Melara D, Fennessey Pv, et al. Effect of low versus high intravenous amino acid intake on very low birth weight infants in the early neonatal period. Pediatr Res 2003;53(1):24–32.
76. Sprague JE, Arbeláez AM. Glucose counterregulatory responses to hypoglycemia. Pediatr Endocrinol Rev 2011;9(1):463–73.
77. Sunehag AL. The role of parenteral lipids in supporting gluconeogenesis in very premature infants. Pediatr Res 2003;54(4):480–6.
78. Arsenault D, Brenn M, Kim S, et al. A.S.P.E.N. Clinical guidelines: hyperglycemia and hypoglycemia in the neonate receiving parenteral nutrition. J Parenter Enteral Nutr 2012;36(1):81–95.
79. Gökşen Şimşek D, Ecevit A, Hatipoğlu N, et al. Neonatal Hyperglycemia, which threshold value, diagnostic approach and treatment?: Turkish neonatal and pediatric endocrinology and diabetes societies consensus report. Turk Pediatri Ars 2018;53(Suppl 1):S234–8.
80. Sunehag A, Ewald U, Larsson A, et al. Glucose production rate in extremely immature neonates (<28 weeks) studied by use of deuterated glucose. Pediatr Res 1993;33(2):97–100.
81. Duvanel CB, Fawer CL, Colling J, et al. Long-term effects of neonatal hypoglycemia on brain growth and psychomotor development in small-for-gestational-age preterm infants. J Pediatr 1999;134(4):492–8.
82. Boardman JP, Wusthoff CJ, Cowan FM. Hypoglycaemia and neonatal brain injury. Arch Dis Child Educ Pract Ed 2013;98(1):2–6.
83. Kazmi SH, Caprio M, Boolchandani H, et al. The value of routine laboratory screening in the neonatal intensive care unit. J Neonatal Perinatal Med 2020; 13(2):247–51.
84. Evering VHM, Andriessen P, Duijsters CEPM, et al. The effect of individualized versus standardized parenteral nutrition on body weight in very preterm infants. Original Article J Clin Med Res 2017;9(4):339–44.
85. Smith A, Feuling MB, Larson-Nath C, et al. Laboratory monitoring of children on home parenteral nutrition: a prospective study. J Parenter Enteral Nutr 2018; 42(1):148–55.
86. da Silva JSV, Seres DS, Sabino K, et al. ASPEN consensus recommendations for refeeding syndrome. Nutr Clin Pract 2020;35(2):178–95.
87. Cormack BE, Jiang Y, Harding JE, et al. Neonatal refeeding syndrome and clinical outcome in extremely low-birth-weight babies: secondary cohort analysis from the ProVIDe trial. J Parenter Enteral Nutr 2021;45(1):65–78.
88. Ross JR, Finch C, Ebeling M, et al. Refeeding syndrome in very-low-birth-weight intrauterine growth-restricted neonates. J Perinatol 2013;33(9):717–20.
89. Hartnoll G, Bétrémieux P, Modi N. Randomised controlled trial of postnatal sodium supplementation on body composition in 25 to 30 week gestational age infants. Arch Dis Child Fetal Neonatal Ed 2000;82(1):F24–8.
90. Baumgart S, Langman CB, Sosulski R, et al. Fluid, electrolyte, and glucose maintenance in the very low birth weight infant. Clin Pediatr (Phila) 1982;21(4):199–206.
91. Oh W, Poindexter BB, Perritt R, et al. Association between fluid intake and weight loss during the first ten days of life and risk of bronchopulmonary dysplasia in extremely low birth weight infants. J Pediatr 2005;147(6):786–90.
92. Bloomfield FH, Jiang Y, Harding JE, et al. Early amino acids in extremely preterm infants and neurodisability at 2 years. N Engl J Med 2022;387(18):1661–72.
93. Senterre T, Zahirah IA, Pieltain C, et al. Electrolyte and mineral homeostasis after optimizing early macronutrient intakes in VLBW infants on parenteral nutrition. J Pediatr Gastroenterol Nutr 2015;61(4):491–8.

94. Falciglia GH, Murthy K, Holl JL, et al. Energy and protein intake during the transition from parenteral to enteral nutrition in infants of very low birth weight. J Pediatr 2018;202:38–43.e1.
95. Perrem L, Semberova J, O'Sullivan A, et al. Effect of early parenteral nutrition discontinuation on time to regain birth weight in very low birth weight infants: a randomized controlled trial. J Parenter Enteral Nutr 2019;43(7):883–90.
96. Falciglia GH, Murthy K, Holl JL, et al. Low prevalence of clinical decision support to calculate caloric and fluid intake for infants in the neonatal intensive care unit. J Perinatol 2020;40:497–503.

Parenteral Nutrition in the Neonatal Intensive Care Unit

Intravenous Lipid Emulsions

Alvin P. Chan, MD, MPH[a], Sara Rostas, PharmD, BCPPS[b],
Samantha Rogers, RD, CDN, CNSC[c], Camilia R. Martin, MD, MS[d],
Kara L. Calkins, MD, MS[e],*

KEYWORDS

- Neonates • Premature • Parenteral nutrition • Lipids • Fatty acids
- Intestinal failure–associated liver disease

KEY POINTS

- An intravenous lipid emulsion (ILE) oil composition determines its triglyceride, fatty acid (FA), phytosterol, and antioxidant content.
- FAs play a critical role in regulating inflammation, immunity, organ development and disease, and growth.
- Previously, the only ILE available in most neonatal intensive care units was 100% soybean oil; however, newer ILEs have replaced soybean oil with medium-chain triglycerides, olive oil, and fish oil.
- Intravenous fish oil monotherapy helps biochemically reverse intestinal failure–associated liver disease (IFALD).
- Prescribers should be mindful of an ILE's dose and FA and phytosterol content; these factors influence an infant's growth and risk for an essential fatty acid deficiency and IFALD.

[a] Division of Gastroenterology, Department of Pediatrics, David Geffen School of Medicine UCLA, 10833 Le Conte Avenue, MDCC 12-383, Los Angeles, CA 90095, USA; [b] New York-Presbyterian Department of Pharmacy, New York-Presbyterian Hospital/Komansky Children's Hospital, 1283 York Avenue, FL15, New York, NY 10065, USA; [c] New York-Presbyterian Food & Nutrition Services, New York-Presbyterian Hospital/Weill Cornell Medical Center, 1283 York Avenue, FL15, New York, NY 10065, USA; [d] Division of Neonatology, Department of Pediatrics, Weill Cornell Medicine, 1283 York Avenue, FL15, New York, NY 10065, USA; [e] Division of Neonatology & Developmental Biology, Department of Pediatrics, Neonatal Research Center of the UCLA Children's Discovery and Innovation Institute, David Geffen School of Medicine UCLA, 1088 Le Conte Avenue, Room B2-375 MDCC, Los Angeles, CA 90095, USA
* Corresponding author.
E-mail address: KCalkins@mednet.ucla.edu

Clin Perinatol 50 (2023) 575–589
https://doi.org/10.1016/j.clp.2023.04.012
0095-5108/23/© 2023 Elsevier Inc. All rights reserved.

INTRODUCTION

Intravenous lipid emulsions (ILEs) are a vital component of parenteral nutrition (PN) for premature infants and infants with intestinal failure (IF). ILEs provide a concentrated energy source and fatty acids (FAs) until enteral nutrition is established. FAs are the building blocks of complex membrane lipids and are responsible for cell tissue structure, function, and metabolism. However, infants who require prolonged PN are at risk for an essential fatty acid deficiency (EFAD) and intestinal failure–associated liver disease (IFALD).[1–3] This article provides an overview of different ILEs and the role ILEs play in infant health.

INTRAVENOUS LIPID EMULSION COMPONENTS AND SOLUTIONS

ILEs consist of oil-in-water solutions. To ensure solubility, phospholipids are added and surround triglycerides (TGs) to emulsify the solution and create chylomicron-like particles that are safe for intravenous injection. TGs in ILEs are derived from various oil sources and are plant-derived (soybean oil [SO], coconut oil, or olive oil [OO]) or animal-derived (fish oil [FO]). The ILE oil source determines the ILE TG, FA, phytosterol, and vitamin E content, which in turn impacts inflammation, immune function, oxidative stress, and hepatic disease risk. When selecting an ILE, clinicians should consider the oil source and dose because these factors mediate an infant's risk for an EFAD and IFALD.[4–6]

Pure soybean oil (SO ILE) was the standard ILE option in most neonatal intensive care units (NICUs) before the availability of other ILEs. Alternative, dual-oil ILEs combine SO with coconut oil, a source of medium-chain TGs (MCTs) (SO,MCT ILE) or OO (SO,OO ILE). A multi-oil ILE consists of 30% SO mixed with 30% MCTs, 25% OO, and 15% FO (SO,MCT,OO,FO ILE). Pure FO (FO ILE) is devoid of plant-derived oils and prescribed to manage pediatric IFALD (**Table 1**).[7,8] FO ILE was originally designed to be a supplement to soybean-derived ILEs. Because FO ILE is dosed at 1 g/kg/d and safety data are lacking on its use as a maintenance ILE, FO ILE should not be prescribed to patients without IFALD.

Triglycerides and Fatty Acids

FAs are carbon chains attached to hydrogen atoms with a terminal carboxyl group and methyl end (**Fig. 1**). Three FAs are attached to a glycerol backbone to form a TG. When ingested, lingual, gastric, and pancreatic lipases hydrolyze TGs for intestinal absorption. In contrast, chylomicrons in ILEs must acquire apoprotein C-II. Once activated by apoprotein C-II, the TGs are hydrolyzed by lipoprotein lipase in the blood and tissues (**Fig. 2**).

SO is a rich source of long-chain TGs and the essential FAs, linoleic acid (LA) (ϖ-6) and α-linolenic acid (ALA) (ϖ-3). These long-chain polyunsaturated FAs (PUFAs) are considered to be essential because mammals lack the Δ 12 and Δ 15 desaturases to insert a double bond at the n-3 and n-6 positions. As a result, these FAs must be obtained from the diet. Coconut oil is a source of MCTs. Compared with soy-derived long-chain TGs, MCTs are more efficiently metabolized, do not accumulate in the liver, and are resistant to lipid peroxidation. The primary FA in OO is oleic acid, a ϖ-9 monounsaturated FA that has anti-inflammatory and immune-regulating properties. Lastly, FO contains a negligible amount of the essential FAs and arachidonic acid (ARA) but is a rich source of the very-long-chain ϖ-3 PUFAs, docosahexaenoic acid (DHA) and eicosapentaenoic acid (EPA) (see **Table 1**).

LA and ALA are elongated and desaturated to produce ARA, EPA, and DHA. These PUFAs generate bioactive lipid molecules known as eicosanoids (see **Fig. 2**). When

Table 1
Composition of intravenous lipid emulsions

	SO ILE	Multi-oil ILE	FO ILE	SO,MCT ILE	SO,OO ILE
Oil source (%)					
Soybean oil	100	30	0	50	20
Coconut oil	0	30	0	50	0
Olive oil	0	25	0	0	80
Fish oil	0	15	100	0	0
Fatty acid (% by weight, mean value, or range)					
Caprylic acid	0	17	0	29	0
Capric acid	0	12	0	20	0
Linoleic acid, 18:2ω-6	44–62	14-25	1.5	27	13-22
α-Linolenic acid, 18:3ω-3	4–11	1.5-3.5	1.1	4	0.5-4
Arachidonic acid, 20:4ω-6	0	0.5	0.2–2.0	0.2	ND
Docosahexaenoic acid, 22:6ω-6	0	1.0–3.5	14.0–27.1	0	0
Eicosapentaenoic acid, 20:5ω-3	0	1.0–3.5	13.0–26.0	0	0
ω-6:ω-3 ratio	7:1	2.5:1	1:8	7:1	9:1
Oleic acid, 18:1ω-9	19-30	23–35	4–11	11	40-80
Phospholipid (g/100 mL)	1.2	1.2	1.2	12	1.2
Phytosterol (mg/L)					
β-sitosterol	243±4	131±7	ND	191.6	198±5
Campesterol	37±0.5	20±1	0.95±0.08	30.9	11±0.3
Stigmasterol	50±0.6	19±1	1.4±0.4	46	11±0.5
α-Tocopherol (mg/L)	ND	163-225	150-300	169-171	32
FDA-approved in the United States for children	Yes	Yes	Yes	No	No

Abbreviations: FDA, Food and Drug Administration; Mixed ILE, SO, MCTs, OO, and FO intravenous lipid emulsion; ND, not determined.

activated, phospholipase A_2 releases PUFAs from the plasma membrane. These freed PUFAs are then oxygenated to generate eicosanoid families. The ARA-derived eicosanoids are more potent inducers of acute inflammation, vasoconstriction, and thrombosis compared with the EPA-derived eicosanoids and ARA-derived lipoxins. ARA-derived lipoxins play a role counteracting inflammation and, together with prostaglandins, are important for central nervous system, gut, lung, and muscle development.[9] EPA and DHA give rise to the resolvins, protectins, and maresins. These eicosanoids, along with the ARA-derived lipoxins, are known as special pro-resolving mediators and help resolve inflammation by inhibiting the production of reactive oxygen species and cytokine expression.

Vitamin E

An ILE oil source also determines the ILE provision of vitamin E, an antioxidant that prevents lipid peroxidation (see **Table 1**). Vitamin E exists as eight isoforms (α, β, δ, and γ); each isoform exists as a tocopherol or tocotrienol. Lipid peroxidation occurs when free radicals attack carbon-carbon double bonds in PUFAs. This results in a cascade of free radicals, leading to cell death and tissue damage. The oxidation

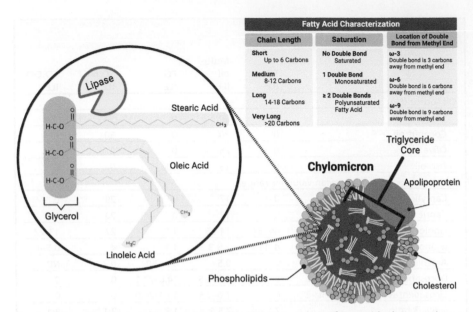

Fig. 1. Fatty acids. Triglycerides are cleaved by lipases to release fatty acids that are characterized by their chain length, saturation, and presence and location of double bonds.

rate correlates with the number of double bonds in the PUFA. α-Tocopherol, the most potent vitamin E isoform, is added to mult-ioil, PUFA-rich ILEs. In contrast, γ-tocopherol possesses approximately 10% to 30% of the activity of α-tocopherol and is mainly derived from SO.

Phytosterols

Phytosterols (campesterol, stigmasterol, and sitosterol) are plant-based sterols compared with cholesterols, which are animal-based sterols. Although humans digest and synthesize cholesterol, humans cannot make phytosterols. SO and OO are rich phytosterol sources (300 mg/100 mL of oil and 200 mg/100 mL of oil, respectively). In contrast, coconut oil provides less phytosterols (70 mg/100 mL of oil). Because FO is animal-based, it is essentially devoid of phytosterols (see **Table 1**).

Dietary phytosterols are poorly absorbed (<5%) compared with cholesterol (~50%). At the intestinal level, phytosterols interfere with the dietary cholesterol absorption, reducing serum cholesterol concentrations and cardiovascular disease risk. When given intravenously, phytosterols are directly absorbed into the circulation and accumulate in the liver.[10,11] Infants and young children who receive SO ILE and who have IFALD have higher serum phytosterol concentrations compared with infants and young children who receive SO,MCT,OO,FO ILE or FO ILE and those without IFALD.[12–14]

Experiments prove that intravenous phytosterols disrupt bile acid homeostasis and farnesoid X receptor (FXR) signaling, causing IFALD.[10,11,15] In IFALD mouse models, stigmasterol antagonizes FXR and suppresses the expression of canalicular bile transporters (*Abcb11*/BSEP, *Abcc2*/MRP2) and hepatic sterol exporters (*Abcg5/g8*/ABCG5/8), causing hepatic inflammation and cholestasis.[10] Parenteral phytosterols also displace cell membrane cholesterol, altering liver plasma membrane fluidity and membrane-bound enzyme activity. Lastly, phytosterols promote hepatic

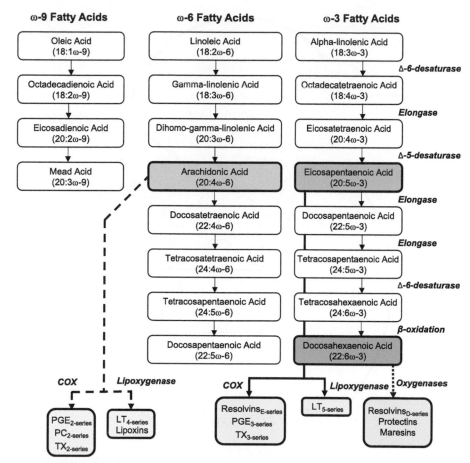

Fig. 2. Metabolism of polyunsaturated fatty acids. Polyunsaturated fatty acids are metabolized to generate eicosanoids. LT, leukotrienes; PC, prostacyclins; PG, prostaglandins; TX, thromboxanes.

macrophage activation and inflammatory cytokine production, further contributing to hepatocyte destruction (**Fig. 3**).[10]

In summary, there are concerns about SO ILE's insufficient antioxidant protection and high phytosterol load. New ILEs have replaced SO with different types of oils to help decrease inflammation, oxidative stress, and IFALD risk, and potentially improve other outcomes in adults and children.[1,2,7,8,13,16–23]

LIPID AND FATTY ACID REQUIREMENTS FOR NEONATES
Intravenous Lipid Emulsion Dose

The early initiation of ILEs is well tolerated by most infants in the NICU.[3,5,6,24] Current recommendations from the European Society of Pediatric Gastroenterology, Hepatology, and Nutrition (ESPGHAN) advise prescribing ILEs immediately after birth. Although this recommendation does not endorse a specific starting dose, randomized controlled trials (RCTs) demonstrate improved growth with the early initiation and swift advancement of ILEs.[3] A large meta-analysis evaluated 520 very low birth weight infants (VLBW; birth weight <1.5 kg). ILEs dosed at approximately 1.5 g/kg/d in the first

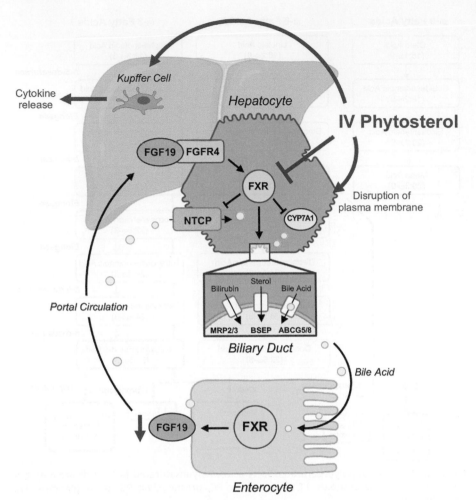

Fig. 3. The role of intravenous lipids in IFALD. FXR-FGF19-CYP7A1 signaling in IFALD. Intravenous phytosterols disrupts FXR-FGF19-CYP7A1 signaling, causing IFALD. Phytosterols inhibit FXR, suppressing hepatobiliary flow. Phytosterols also promote plasma membrane damage, Kupffer cell activation, and inflammatory cytokine production. ABCG6/8, ATP-binding cassette, subfamily G5/G8; BSEP, bile salt export pump; FGF19, fibroblast growth factor 19; FGFR4, fibroblast growth factor receptor 4; MRP2/3, multidrug resistance protein 2/3; NTCP, sodium taurocholate cotransporting polypeptide.

24 hours of age were associated with less postnatal growth failure (odds ratio, 0.27; 95% confidence interval [CI], 0.15–0.48) and a higher mean term equivalent head circumference (mean difference, 0.67 cm; 95% CI, 0.25–1.09) and body weight (mean difference, 70.27 g; 95% CI, 4.73–135.81). ILE intake has also been correlated with increased cerebellar, brainstem, and total brain volume at term equivalent age.[25]

Specific neonatal populations may be unable to tolerate ILE infusions. Extremely low birth weight infants (birth weight <1 kg) are susceptible to hypertriglyceridemia because they are unable store and metabolize TGs efficiently because of a lack of adipose tissue and reduced lipoprotein lipase activity. Additional risk factors for hypertriglyceridemia include the ILE type and dose, fetal growth restriction, sepsis, liver and renal disease, corticosteroids, and excessive glucose infusion rates.[26] Soy-derived long-chain TGs, compared with long-chain TGs in FO and MCTs in coconut oil, tend to clear from systemic circulation at a slower rate. Compared with SO ILE, FO ILE is associated with lower TG concentrations.[7] FO reduces lipolysis and the hepatic synthetic rate of very-low-density lipoproteins and upregulates tissue expression of lipoprotein lipase. Although one retrospective study of 672 VLBWs demonstrated a decreased incidence of hypertriglyceridemia with SO,MCT,OO,FO ILE, RCTs have reported comparable TG concentrations for VLBWs who received either SO ILE or SO,MCT,OO,FO ILE.[13,17,20,21]

The American Society of Pediatric Enteral and Parenteral Nutrition and ESPGHAN recommend that TG concentrations not exceed 200 mg/dL and 265 mg/dL, respectively.[3] Despite these recommendations, more data are needed to demonstrate that outcomes are improved by adhering to specific TG thresholds and surveillance strategies. It is important to remember that withholding ILEs or suboptimal ILE dosing can cause an EFAD, which can, in turn, exacerbate hypertriglyceridemia.[4]

Essential Fatty Acid Deficiency

The total body fat stores of a premature infant weighing 1 kg are only 20 g and are almost entirely contained in structural lipids. PN-dependent infants who receive ILE-free regimens or an inadequate ILE dose are at risk for an EFAD. EFADs are diagnosed by an increase in the triene/tetraene (Mead acid/ARA) ratio. When LA stores are depleted, there is a decrease in the production of ARA (a tetraene). As a result, oleic acid is converted to Mead acid (a trienoic ϖ-9 FA). Traditionally, a triene/tetraene ratio greater than 0.2 was considered diagnostic of an EFAD. However, lower thresholds are sometimes used for infants.[4,27] The FA profile of an infant reflects the ILE FA composition. As a result, patients who receive SO,OO ILE have high concentrations of oleic acid and Mead acid, which may erroneously lead to the diagnosis of an EFAD. However, because an increase in Mead acid is not accompanied by a decrease in ARA, these patients do not have a biochemical EFAD.[4]

EFADs are generally silent. Therefore, clinicians must have a high index of suspicion for an EFAD. In cases of severe EFADs, patients may develop dry, scaly skin. LA and ARA form waxy lipid molecules known as ceramides that maintain the epidermal skin barrier. LA and ARA are used to treat EFAD-induced dermatologic conditions. In contrast, ALA is less effective in reversing EFAD symptoms. Other signs of an EFAD include poor growth, increased susceptibility to infections, platelet dysfunction, thrombocytopenia, hepatitis, and hypertriglyceridemia.[8] When the provision of SO is reduced in alternative ILEs, a higher dose is required to prevent an EFAD. LA must reach a daily intake of approximately 0.25 g/kg in premature infants and at least 0.1 g/kg in term infants to prevent an EFAD.[4,28] Hence, the minimum dose for SO ILE and SO,MCT,OO,FO ILE to prevent an EFAD is approximately 0.25 to 1 g/kg/d and 2.2 to 3 g/kg/d, respectively.

Previously, there were concerns that FO ILE would cause an EFAD. However, one of the original case reports of FO ILE use was in a 17 year old who developed IF and was soy-allergic, which precluded the use of SO ILE. After several weeks of fat-free PN, the patient was diagnosed with an EFAD, which was characterized by a triene/tetraene ratio greater than 0.23 and a skin rash. The patient's EFAD was treated with FO ILE.[29] Since then, several studies in animals and children with IFALD provide support that 1 g/kg/d of FO ILE does not cause an EFAD and can be used to treat an EFAD.[7,30,31] This is most likely because FO ILE contains a small amount of the essential FAs and substantially more ARA than SO ILE (see **Table 1**). Also, ARA and DHA can be retroconverted into upstream FAs. Most importantly, ARA, EPA, and DHA are precursors to the eicosanoids that are responsible for regulating critical biologic processes (see **Fig. 2**).

Arachidonic Acid and Docosahexaenoic Acid

ARA and DHA play an important role in neurodevelopment. The placenta preferentially transfers ARA and DHA over other FA. This process is referred to as "biomagnification" and is accelerated during the third trimester of pregnancy and is disrupted by preterm birth.[32] Estimated ARA and DHA placental accretion rates are 212 mg/kg/d and 45 mg/kg/d, respectively.[32] Despite enteral nutrition and SO ILE's high LA and ALA content and SO,MCT,OO,FO ILE's provision of 30% SO and 15% FO, premature infants who receive these two ILEs exhibit declining levels of ARA and DHA.[33–35] There are several potential explanations.[34] First, the capacity to store and mobilize ϖ-6 and ϖ-3 FAs is reduced in VLBWs. Second, the ability to synthesize ARA and DHA from the essential FAs is limited and unpredictable. Single-nucleotide polymorphisms in the FA desaturase genes (FADS1/FADS2) may explain this variability. Third, SO ILE's high concentration of LA inhibits the metabolization of ALA to EPA and DHA, whereas SO,MCT,OO,FO ILE's high concentration of EPA inhibits the conversion of LA to ARA. This occurs because the ϖ-6 and ϖ-3 PUFAs compete for the same enzymes (see **Fig. 2**). Some studies have demonstrated a more pronounced ARA deficit with SO,MCT,OO,FO ILE compared with SO ILE.[36–38] It remains to be determined what the parenteral and enteral ARA, DHA, and EPA requirements for infants in the NICU are, and if remedying these deficits will improve outcomes.

INTRAVENOUS LIPID EMULSIONS AND PRETERM INFANTS

In the United States, the Food and Drug Administration (FDA)-approved ILEs for pediatric use include SO ILE, SO,MCT,OO,FO ILE, and FO ILE. SO,OO ILE is FDA-approved for adult use only, and SO,MCT ILE is available outside the United States (see **Table 1**). Because SO consists primarily of ϖ-6 FAs, SO ILE has a higher ϖ-6:ϖ-3 compared with most other ILEs (7:1). SO,MCT,OO,FO ILE has been prescribed in Europe, Canada, and other countries prior to FDA approval in the United States. The FDA approved SO,MCT,OO,FO ILE for adult use in 2016 and pediatric use in 2022. Compared with SO ILE, SO,MCT,OO,FO ILE contains a reduced dose of LA and ALA. This four-oil ILE also contains coconut-derived MCTs, monounsaturated FA-rich OO, and FO-derived EPA and DHA. Consequently, the ϖ-6:ϖ-3 is approximately 2.5:1. At equivalent doses, SO,MCT,OO,FO ILE provides less phytosterols and more vitamin E in the form α-tocopherol compared with SO ILE (see **Table 1**).

Published studies and meta-analyses have failed to provide evidence that one specific ILE (SO ILE vs SO,MCT,OO,FO ILE) is superior for premature infants without IF.[17–23,39] In an RCT, VLBWs were prescribed either SO ILE or SO,MCT,OO,FO ILE. Infants who received the multi-oil ILE compared with the control ILE had a higher weight gain (27.6 ± 6.5 g/kg/d vs 24.5 ± 6.0 g/kg/d) and smaller change in their weight z scores (discharge–birth) (0.2 ± 1.1 vs −0.5 ± 1.3).[13] Although these changes were significant, the average weight velocity and z score changes would be considered appropriate for both groups.[40] Despite these findings, meta-analyses and RCTs have failed to replicate these results. In general, VLBWs without underlying gastrointestinal disorders who receive either SO ILE or SO,MCT,OO,FO ILE have similar growth trajectories and rates for cholestasis, chronic lung disease, retinopathy of prematurity, sepsis, and necrotizing enterocolitis.[13,17–22,41,42] Additionally, an RCT reported no difference in neurodevelopment.[43]

Although preterm infants without intestinal disorders who receive SO ILE have higher concentrations of phytosterols and LA and lower vitamin E concentrations compared with preterm infants who receive SO,MCT,OO,FO ILE, rates for liver dysfunction in most studies and meta-analyses are similar.[13,17–21,33,38,42,44] In one study of 60 infants with a gestational age less than 34 weeks, serum γ-glutamyltransferase was lower in the group who received SO,MCT,OO,FO ILE compared with the group who received SO ILE. However, other liver function tests were similar.[21] Contrary to this study, a meta-analysis of 152 preterm infants concluded that recipients of SO,MCT,OO,FO ILE had a similar odds of developing cholestasis compared with recipients of SO ILE (odds ratio, 0.81; 95% CI, 0.29–2.22).[1] Another meta-analysis of 673 preterm infants with a gestational age less than 37 weeks, some of who had surgical conditions, demonstrated that the mean difference for serum conjugated bilirubin was similar (mean difference, 0.48 μmol/L) when these two ILEs were compared.[18] These results are most likely because PN duration was short, and these studies did not exclusively target infants with IF.[13,18,20,23,41–43]

INTRAVENOUS LIPID EMULSIONS AND INFANTS WITH INTESTINAL FAILURE–ASSOCIATED LIVER DISEASE
Intestinal Failure–Associated Liver Disease

IFALD is a progressive, multifactorial liver disease caused by intestinal dysfunction requiring prolonged PN (**Box 1**). IF is defined as a significant functional intestinal deficit that requires PN for hydration and nutrition for a minimum of 60 days within a 74-day period.[45] The most common cause of IF is short bowel syndrome (SBS), which is defined as a loss of small bowel because of surgical resection or a congenital disorder. Common causes of SBS include necrotizing enterocolitis, intestinal atresia, and malrotation with volvulus. Although rare, other causes of IF include mucosal enteropathies and dysmotility disorders.

Hepatic biochemical and histologic abnormalities associated with IF in the absence of other causes of liver dysfunction are the hallmark of IFALD. The histologic features of IFALD range from cholestasis and steatosis to fibrosis and cirrhosis, with a predominant cholestatic pattern in infants. IFALD can progress from cholestasis to fulminant liver failure. The traditional definition of IFALD is a serum conjugated bilirubin greater

---

Box 1
Risk factors for intestinal failure–associated liver disease in infants

Patient-specific risk factors
    Prematurity
    Fetal growth restriction
    Genetics
    Sepsis
    Gastrointestinal disorder
    Intestinal anatomy (small bowel length and dilation, intestinal continuity, presence of ileocecal valve)
    Small bowel bacterial overgrowth

Parenteral nutrition–specific risk factors
    Lack of enteral nutrition
    Parenteral nutrition duration
    Intravenous lipid composition and dose
    Dextrose and amino acid dose

than or equal to 2.0 mg/dL in the setting of prolonged PN. However, this threshold is not universal, and many experts have argued that a lower threshold is warranted.

Enteral Nutrition and Intestinal Failure–Associated Liver Disease

IFALD is caused by physiologic abnormalities that underpin the cause of the IF. The risk for IFALD is proportional to PN duration[46] (see **Box 1**). A premature infant with an immature liver is more susceptible to the insults caused by sepsis, disrupted enterohepatic circulation, PN, and lipid peroxidation.[47] Immature bile secretory mechanisms lead to the hepatotoxic accumulation of bile acids, bilirubin, and sterols.[48] A lack of enteral feeding induces bacterial dysbiosis and intestinal permeability, further aggravating systemic and hepatic proinflammatory signaling cascades.[49]

The most important intervention for preventing IFALD is enteral nutrition.[47] The presence of nutrients in the intestinal lumen stimulates gut hormone secretion, intestinal motility, gallbladder contractility, and bile flow to promote structural and functional intestinal adaptations.[50,51] In animal models of SBS, enteral feeding induces crypt cell proliferation and intestinal mass and length following resection.[52] The protective role of enteral feeding is mediated through the FXR/fibroblast growth factor (FGF)19 signaling pathway.[53–55]

FXR is a bile acid sensor and master transcriptional regulator, whereas FGF19 is a gut-derived hormone produced in response to food intake. Under normal feeding conditions, the liver secretes bile acids into the small intestine to enhance the digestion and absorption of lipids and lipid-soluble nutrients. The bile acids are primarily reabsorbed in the distal small intestine, where they activate intestinal FXR to induce the secretion of FGF19 into the portal circulation. FGF19 then binds to fibroblast growth factor receptor 4 in the liver to downregulate cholesterol 7α-hydroxylase (*CYP7A1*/ CYP7A1) to suppress bile acid synthesis, completing a negative feedback loop. Simultaneously, the bile acids that return to the liver via the enterohepatic circulation activate hepatic FXR in a second suppressive feedback pathway.[56] Hepatic FXR further downregulates *CYP7A1* to inhibit bile acid synthesis, but also induces bile acid transporters (*ABCB11*/BSEP, *ABCC3*/MRP3, *SLC10A1*/NTCP) to promote bile acid and bilirubin efflux and inhibit hepatic reuptake. Thus, feeding promotes bile acid, bilirubin, and sterol secretion from the hepatocyte into the bile canaliculi. Conversely, the absence of enteral stimulation disrupts FXR-FGF19-CYP7A1 signaling, leading to the retention of toxic bile acids, bilirubin, and sterols in the liver (see **Fig. 3**).

Fish Oil and Intestinal Failure–Associated Liver Disease

The ILE type has an important effect on the development and progression of IFALD. The ideal ILE to prevent IFALD would contain minimal or no phytosterols and sufficient antioxidant protection while meeting the nutritional requirements of the infant. Before the advent of mixed ILEs and FO ILE, SO ILE dose reduction was a common strategy to prevent and treat IFALD.[57] RCTs in infants with gastrointestinal disorders have demonstrated a slower serum conjugated bilirubin rise with SO ILE minimization compared with 2 to 3 g/kg/d of SO ILE.[58] Nonetheless, given the potential concerns with growth, neurodevelopment, and EFADs, long-term, low-dose SO ILE provision should be used cautiously with close monitoring.

A multicenter study was conducted and enrolled infants with a birth weight greater than 750 g and a gastrointestinal disorder, who were predicted to require greater than 28 days of PN, and had a serum conjugated bilirubin less than or equal to 0.6 mg/dL. Subjects were randomized to either SO ILE or SO,MCT,OO,FO ILE at the same dose. Fifty-four percent (87 out 161 subjects) weaned from PN before 28 days. There was no difference in cholestasis rates (3.8% in SO ILE group vs 2.4% in SO,MCT,OO,FO ILE group).[44] In contrast, in a small, multisite RCT in Canada, infants with gastrointestinal disorders with an average age of 5 to 6 weeks, gestational age of 34 to 35 weeks, and mild cholestasis were randomized to either SO ILE or SO,MCT,OO,FO ILE. All infants required approximately 4 to 5 weeks of PN before enrollment and remained on PN for approximately 2 months. After excluding an outlier in the mixed ILE group, the mean difference in conjugated bilirubin was 2.75 mg/dL, favoring the SO,MCT,OO,FO ILE group.[16] Although we lack large RCTs in patients with IF and IFALD comparing SO ILE to SO,MCT,OO,FO ILE, ESPGHAN recommends the use of SO,MCT,OO,FO ILE in patients who require prolonged PN and who are at high risk for IFALD.[3]

In contrast to SO ILE and SO,MCT,OO,FO ILE, FO ILE provides a higher amount of anti-inflammatory ϖ-3 FAs and α-tocopherol and a negligible amount of phytosterols. When dosed at 1 g/kg/d, FO ILE biochemically reverses IFALD in most infants and young children.[7,8,30,31] In a multicenter integrated analysis, infants with IFALD who received FO ILE were pair-matched to historical control subjects who received SO ILE. When compared with the SO ILE group, the FO ILE group was more likely to experience cholestasis resolution (65% vs 16%; $P<.0001$), less likely to require a liver transplant (4% vs 12%; $P = .03$), and had a lower aspartate aminotransferase platelet ratio index at the end of treatment. Aspartate aminotransferase platelet ratio index is a noninvasive biomarker for liver fibrosis.[8]

Once a patient with IF crosses the threshold for cholestasis, FO ILE should be considered to normalize hepatic function. Serum conjugated bilirubin concentrations are positively correlated with mortality, and delayed FO ILE treatment is associated with treatment failures and slower response times.[59] FO ILE when combined with a multidisciplinary approach is associated with improved mortality and morbidity for infants and young children with IF.[7,8,18,30,31]

SUMMARY

Clinicians should consider each patient's nutritional goal and underlying risk for prolonged PN and IFALD when prescribing an ILE in the NICU. Specifically, the clinician should account for the ILE dose, TG, FA, phytosterol, and vitamin E content. FAs and antioxidants play a vital role in mediating inflammation, immunity, organogenesis, and development. The initiation of ILEs after birth at doses of 1 to 2 g/kg/d with target doses of 3 g/kg/d promotes growth in most preterm infants. Clinicians should ensure that they are dosing ILEs appropriately to prevent an EFAD, which can have long-term consequences.

IFALD is a multifactorial disease that occurs in patients with gastrointestinal disorders who require prolonged PN. In contrast to the nonsurgical preterm infant, infants with IF are at high risk for IFALD. Delaying the onset and severity of the IFALD by considering the prescription of PN and ILEs is essential to improving mortality and morbidity. Intravenous phytosterols play an important role in IFALD. Although multioil ILEs may delay the onset of cholestasis by reducing the dose of SO and replacing SO with MCTs, OO, and FO, a multidisciplinary approach to IF is vital to promote intestinal rehabilitation and complications associated with IF. FO ILE helps reverse biochemical cholestasis and prevents liver failure and the need for transplant.

The optimal ILE does not exist. There is currently no ILE that satisfies the FA requirements of the preterm infant. It also remains unclear if an ILE can be developed that will contribute to the reduction in diseases related to prematurity, such as sepsis, retinopathy of prematurity, and chronic lung disease. Lastly, considering the complexity of IFALD, it is doubtful that a specific ILE product will eradicate IFALD. Continued research and scientific collaboration is warranted to help solve some of these gaps.

DISCLOSURE

K.L. Calkins serves as an advisor for Fresenius Kabi, Mead Johnson Nutrition, Baxter, and Prolacta; and serves as institutional principal investigator, with no salary funding, for a consortium database sponsored by Mead Johnson Nutrition. C.R. Martin serves as institutional principal investigator, with no salary funding, for a consortium database sponsored by Mead Johnson Nutrition; and serves on the scientific advisory board of Lactalogics, Inc, Plakous Therapeutics, and Vitara Biomedical, Inc.

REFERENCES

1. Hojsak I, Colomb V, Braegger C, et al. ESPGHAN Committee on Nutrition position paper. Intravenous lipid emulsions and risk of hepatotoxicity in infants and children: a systematic review and meta-analysis. J Pediatr Gastroenterol Nutr 2016;62(5):776–92.

2. Cober MP, Gura KM, Mirtallo JM, et al. ASPEN lipid injectable emulsion safety recommendations part 2: neonate and pediatric considerations. Nutr Clin Pract 2021;36(6):1106–25.

3. Lapillonne A, Fidler Mis N, Goulet O, et al. ESPGHAN/ESPEN/ESPR/CSPEN guidelines on pediatric parenteral nutrition: lipids. Clin Nutr 2018;37(6 Pt B):2324–36.

4. Gramlich L, Ireton-Jones C, Miles JM, et al. Essential fatty acid requirements and intravenous lipid emulsions. JPEN J Parenter Enteral Nutr 2019;43(6):697–707.

5. Vlaardingerbroek H, Vermeulen MJ, Rook D, et al. Safety and efficacy of early parenteral lipid and high-dose amino acid administration to very low birth weight infants. J Pediatr 2013;163(3):638–44.e1-5.

6. Alburaki W, Yusuf K, Dobry J, et al. High early parenteral lipid in very preterm infants: a randomized-controlled trial. J Pediatr 2021;228:16–23.e1.

7. Gura K, Premkumar MH, Calkins KL, et al. Intravenous fish oil monotherapy as a source of calories and fatty acids promotes age-appropriate growth in pediatric patients with intestinal failure-associated liver disease. J Pediatr 2020;219:98–105.e4.

8. Gura KM, Premkumar MH, Calkins KL, et al. Fish oil emulsion reduces liver injury and liver transplantation in children with intestinal failure-associated liver disease: a multicenter integrated study. J Pediatr 2021;230:46–54.e2.

9. Martin CR, Zaman MM, Gilkey C, et al. Resolvin D1 and lipoxin A4 improve alveolarization and normalize septal wall thickness in a neonatal murine model of hyperoxia-induced lung injury. PLoS One 2014;9(6):e98773.

10. El Kasmi KC, Anderson AL, Devereaux MW, et al. Phytosterols promote liver injury and Kupffer cell activation in parenteral nutrition-associated liver disease. Sci Transl Med 2013;5(206):206ra137.

11. Hukkinen M, Mutanen A, Nissinen M, et al. Parenteral plant sterols accumulate in the liver reflecting their increased serum levels and portal inflammation in children with intestinal failure. JPEN J Parenter Enteral Nutr 2017;41(6):1014–22.

12. Calkins KL, DeBarber A, Steiner RD, et al. Intravenous fish oil and pediatric intestinal failure-associated liver disease: changes in plasma phytosterols, cytokines, and bile acids and erythrocyte fatty acids. JPEN J Parenter Enteral Nutr 2018; 42(3):633–41.

13. Vlaardingerbroek H, Vermeulen MJ, Carnielli VP, et al. Growth and fatty acid profiles of VLBW infants receiving a multicomponent lipid emulsion from birth. J Pediatr Gastroenterol Nutr 2014;58(4):417–27.

14. Nghiem-Rao TH, Tunc I, Mavis AM, et al. Kinetics of phytosterol metabolism in neonates receiving parenteral nutrition. Pediatr Res 2015;78(2):181–9.

15. Clayton PT, Bowron A, Mills KA, et al. Phytosterolemia in children with parenteral nutrition-associated cholestatic liver disease. Gastroenterology 1993;105(6): 1806–13.

16. Diamond IR, Grant RC, Pencharz PB, et al. Preventing the progression of intestinal failure-associated liver disease in infants using a composite lipid emulsion: a pilot randomized controlled trial of SMOFlipid. JPEN J Parenter Enteral Nutr 2017; 41(5):866–77.

17. Repa A, Binder C, Thanhaeuser M, et al. A mixed lipid emulsion for prevention of parenteral nutrition associated cholestasis in extremely low birth weight infants: a randomized clinical trial. J Pediatr 2018;194:87–93.e1.

18. Kapoor V, Malviya MN, Soll R. Lipid emulsions for parenterally fed preterm infants. Cochrane Database Syst Rev 2019;6:CD013163.

19. Skouroliakou M, Konstantinou D, Koutri K, et al. A double-blind, randomized clinical trial of the effect of omega-3 fatty acids on the oxidative stress of preterm neonates fed through parenteral nutrition. Eur J Clin Nutr 2010;64(9):940–7.

20. Skouroliakou M, Konstantinou D, Agakidis C, et al. Parenteral MCT/ω-3 polyunsaturated fatty acid-enriched intravenous fat emulsion is associated with cytokine and fatty acid profiles consistent with attenuated inflammatory response in preterm neonates: a randomized, double-blind clinical trial. Nutr Clin Pract 2016; 31(2):235–44.

21. Tomsits E, Pataki M, Tölgyesi A, et al. Safety and efficacy of a lipid emulsion containing a mixture of soybean oil, medium-chain triglycerides, olive oil, and fish oil: a randomised, double-blind clinical trial in premature infants requiring parenteral nutrition. J Pediatr Gastroenterol Nutr 2010;51(4):514–21.

22. Rayyan M, Devlieger H, Jochum F, et al. Short-term use of parenteral nutrition with a lipid emulsion containing a mixture of soybean oil, olive oil, medium-chain triglycerides, and fish oil: a randomized double-blind study in preterm infants. JPEN J Parenter Enteral Nutr 2012;36(1 Suppl):81S–94S.

23. Beken S, Dilli D, Fettah ND, et al. The influence of fish-oil lipid emulsions on retinopathy of prematurity in very low birth weight infants: a randomized controlled trial. Early Hum Dev 2014;90(1):27–31.

24. Kim K, Kim NJ, Kim SY. Safety and efficacy of early high parenteral lipid supplementation in preterm infants: a systematic review and meta-analysis. Nutrients 2021;13(5). https://doi.org/10.3390/nu13051535.

25. Ottolini KM, Andescavage N, Kapse K, et al. Early lipid intake improves cerebellar growth in very low-birth-weight preterm infants. JPEN J Parenter Enteral Nutr 2021;45(3):587–95.

26. Chan AP, Robinson DT, Calkins KL. Hypertriglyceridemia in preterm infants. NeoReviews 2022;23(8):e528–40.

27. Lagerstedt SA, Hinrichs DR, Batt SM, et al. Quantitative determination of plasma c8-c26 total fatty acids for the biochemical diagnosis of nutritional and metabolic disorders. Mol Genet Metab 2001;73(1):38–45.

28. Koletzko B, Goulet O, Hunt J, et al. 1. Guidelines on paediatric parenteral nutrition of the European Society of Paediatric Gastroenterology, Hepatology and Nutrition (ESPGHAN) and the European Society for Clinical Nutrition and Metabolism (ESPEN), supported by the European Society of Paediatric Research (ESPR). J Pediatr Gastroenterol Nutr 2005;41(Suppl 2):S1–87.

29. Gura KM, Parsons SK, Bechard LJ, et al. Use of a fish oil-based lipid emulsion to treat essential fatty acid deficiency in a soy allergic patient receiving parenteral nutrition. Clin Nutr 2005;24(5):839–47.

30. Calkins KL, Dunn JC, Shew SB, et al. Pediatric intestinal failure-associated liver disease is reversed with 6 months of intravenous fish oil. JPEN J Parenter Enteral Nutr 2014;38(6):682–92.

31. Gura KM, Lee S, Valim C, et al. Safety and efficacy of a fish-oil-based fat emulsion in the treatment of parenteral nutrition-associated liver disease. Pediatrics 2008; 121(3):e678–86.

32. Hadley KB, Ryan AS, Forsyth S, et al. The essentiality of arachidonic acid in infant development. Nutrients 2016;8(4):216.

33. Kim ES, Lee LJ, Romero T, et al. Outcomes in preterm infants who received a lipid emulsion with fish oil: an observational study. JPEN J Parenter Enteral Nutr 2023; 47(3):354–63.

34. Martin CR, Dasilva DA, Cluette-Brown JE, et al. Decreased postnatal docosahexaenoic and arachidonic acid blood levels in premature infants are associated with neonatal morbidities. J Pediatr 2011;159(5):743–9.e1-2.

35. Robinson DT, Carlson SE, Murthy K, et al. Docosahexaenoic and arachidonic acid levels in extremely low birth weight infants with prolonged exposure to intravenous lipids. J Pediatr 2013;162(1):56–61.

36. Rubin D, Laposata M. Cellular interactions between n-6 and n-3 fatty acids: a mass analysis of fatty acid elongation/desaturation, distribution among complex lipids, and conversion to eicosanoids. J Lipid Res 1992;33(10):1431–40.

37. Najm S, Löfqvist C, Hellgren G, et al. Effects of a lipid emulsion containing fish oil on polyunsaturated fatty acid profiles, growth and morbidities in extremely premature infants: a randomized controlled trial. Clin Nutr ESPEN 2017;20:17–23.

38. D'Ascenzo R, Savini S, Biagetti C, et al. Higher docosahexaenoic acid, lower arachidonic acid and reduced lipid tolerance with high doses of a lipid emulsion containing 15% fish oil: a randomized clinical trial. Clin Nutr 2014;33(6):1002–9.

39. Papandreou P, Gioxari A, Ntountaniotis D, et al. Administration of an intravenous fat emulsion enriched with medium-chain triglyceride/ω-3 fatty acids is beneficial towards anti-inflammatory related fatty acid profile in preterm neonates: a randomized, double-blind clinical trial. Nutrients 2020;12(11). https://doi.org/10.3390/nu12113526.

40. Costa S, Cocca C, Barone G, et al. Growth of head circumference and body length in preterm infants receiving a multicomponent vs a soybean-based lipid emulsion: a randomized controlled trial. JPEN J Parenter Enteral Nutr 2021;45(1):94–101.

41. Uthaya S, Liu X, Babalis D, et al. Nutritional evaluation and optimisation in neonates: a randomized, double-blind controlled trial of amino acid regimen and intravenous lipid composition in preterm parenteral nutrition. Am J Clin Nutr 2016;103(6):1443–52.

42. Savini S, D'Ascenzo R, Biagetti C, et al. The effect of 5 intravenous lipid emulsions on plasma phytosterols in preterm infants receiving parenteral nutrition: a randomized clinical trial. Am J Clin Nutr 2013;98(2):312–8.

43. Thanhaeuser M, Fuiko R, Oberleitner-Leeb C, et al. A randomized trial of parenteral nutrition using a mixed lipid emulsion containing fish oil in infants of extremely low birth weight: neurodevelopmental outcome at 12 and 24 Months Corrected age, a secondary outcome analysis. J Pediatr 2020;226:142–8.e5.

44. Abrams S. Phase 3 study to Compare safety and Efficacy of Smoflipid 20% to Intralipid 20% in Hospitalized Neonates and infants. Fresenius Kabi; 2022. Available at: https://clinicaltrials.gov/ct2/show/NCT02579265.

45. Modi BP, Galloway DP, Gura K, et al. ASPEN definitions in pediatric intestinal failure. JPEN J Parenter Enteral Nutr 2022;46(1):42–59.

46. Diamond IR, de Silva NT, Tomlinson GA, et al. The role of parenteral lipids in the development of advanced intestinal failure-associated liver disease in infants: a multiple-variable analysis. JPEN J Parenter Enteral Nutr 2011;35(5):596–602.
47. Lacaille F, Gupte G, Colomb V, et al. Intestinal failure-associated liver disease: a position paper of the ESPGHAN Working group of intestinal failure and intestinal transplantation. J Pediatr Gastroenterol Nutr 2015;60(2):272–83.
48. Sokol RJ, Straka MS, Dahl R, et al. Role of oxidant stress in the permeability transition induced in rat hepatic mitochondria by hydrophobic bile acids. Pediatr Res 2001;49(4):519–31.
49. El Kasmi KC, Anderson AL, Devereaux MW, et al. Toll-like receptor 4-dependent Kupffer cell activation and liver injury in a novel mouse model of parenteral nutrition and intestinal injury. Hepatology 2012;55(5):1518–28.
50. Greenberg GR, Wolman SL, Christofides ND, et al. Effect of total parenteral nutrition on gut hormone release in humans. Gastroenterology 1981;80(5 pt 1):988–93.
51. Lucas A, Bloom SR, Aynsley-Green A. Metabolic and endocrine consequences of depriving preterm infants of enteral nutrition. Acta Paediatr Scand 1983;72(2): 245–9.
52. Turner JM, Wales PW, Nation PN, et al. Novel neonatal piglet models of surgical short bowel syndrome with intestinal failure. J Pediatr Gastroenterol Nutr 2011; 52(1):9–16.
53. Mutanen A, Lohi J, Heikkilä P, et al. Loss of ileum decreases serum fibroblast growth factor 19 in relation to liver inflammation and fibrosis in pediatric onset intestinal failure. J Hepatol 2015;62(6):1391–7.
54. Jain AK, Stoll B, Burrin DG, et al. Enteral bile acid treatment improves parenteral nutrition-related liver disease and intestinal mucosal atrophy in neonatal pigs. Am J Physiol Gastrointest Liver Physiol 2012;302(2):G218–24.
55. Xiao YT, Cao Y, Zhou KJ, et al. Altered systemic bile acid homeostasis contributes to liver disease in pediatric patients with intestinal failure. Sci Rep 2016;6:39264.
56. Kim I, Ahn SH, Inagaki T, et al. Differential regulation of bile acid homeostasis by the farnesoid X receptor in liver and intestine. J Lipid Res 2007;48(12):2664–72.
57. Wales PW, Allen N, Worthington P, et al. A.S.P.E.N. clinical guidelines: support of pediatric patients with intestinal failure at risk of parenteral nutrition-associated liver disease. JPEN J Parenter Enteral Nutr 2014;38(5):538–57.
58. Calkins KL, Havranek T, Kelley-Quon LI, et al. Low-dose parenteral soybean oil for the prevention of parenteral nutrition-associated liver disease in neonates with gastrointestinal disorders. JPEN J Parenter Enteral Nutr 2017;41(3):404–11.
59. Wang C, Venick RS, Shew SB, et al. Long-term outcomes in children with intestinal failure-associated liver disease treated with 6 months of intravenous fish oil followed by resumption of intravenous soybean oil. JPEN J Parenter Enteral Nutr 2019;43(6):708–16.

Calcium and Phosphorus
All You Need to Know but Were Afraid to Ask

Katerina Kellar, MD[a], Nisha Reddy Pandillapalli, MBBS[a],
Alvaro G. Moreira, MD, MSc[a],*

KEYWORDS

- Calcium • Phosphorus • Prematurity • Metabolic bone disease
- Very low birth weight neonate

KEY POINTS

- Preterm neonates are at increased risk for hypocalcemia and hypophosphatemia because of limited mineral stores and immature regulatory mechanisms.
- Metabolic bone disease (MBD) is a condition in premature newborns characterized by bone demineralization and impaired skeletal growth caused by inadequate mineral intake, absorption, and immature growth of bone structure.
- Adequate supplementation of calcium and phosphorus, and careful monitoring of chronically ill neonates, can help prevent and treat MBD.

INTRODUCTION
Calcium

Calcium is a vital mineral in the body that plays a role in muscle contraction, nerve conduction, energy metabolism, and cell proliferation. Its most important function is skeletal mineralization, which provides bony integrity and acts as a dynamic store to maintain the intracellular and extracellular calcium pools.[1]

Most calcium in the human body is found in bones and exists in combination with phosphate to form hydroxyapatite crystals (**Fig. 1**). The ratio of calcium stored in bone versus that found circulating in the serum is approximately 99:1. In the serum, calcium is found in inactive and active forms. Its active form, ionized calcium, accounts for approximately 45% of the serum composition and is under tight hormonal control.

Hypocalcemia in premature infants is defined by a total serum calcium less than 7.0 mg/dL (<1.75 mmol/L) or ionized calcium less than 1.10 mmol/L (<4.4 mg/dL), and is most commonly caused by inadequate calcium stores and poor parathyroid gland function (**Table 1**).[2,3] Symptoms of hypocalcemia can mimic those of hypoglycemia

[a] Pediatrics, University of Texas Health San Antonio, San Antonio, TX, USA
* Corresponding author.
E-mail address: moreiraa@uthscsa.edu

Clin Perinatol 50 (2023) 591–606
https://doi.org/10.1016/j.clp.2023.04.013
0095-5108/23/© 2023 Elsevier Inc. All rights reserved.

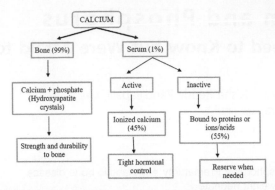

Fig. 1. Calcium distribution in the body.

and opioid withdrawal, with primarily neurologic manifestations, such as apnea, hypotonia, seizures, tetany, poor feeding, and prolonged QT interval tachyarrhythmias.[4]

Early onset hypocalcemia usually occurs within the first few days of life, and is caused by prematurity, intrauterine growth restriction, maternal diabetes, perinatal asphyxia, and congenital syndromes.[5] Late-onset hypocalcemia occurs around 1 week of life and is caused by phosphate loading and resistance to parathyroid hormone (PTH) by the immature kidney, among other factors.[5]

Hypercalcemia in premature infants is defined by a total serum calcium greater than 11.0 mg/dL (>2.75 mmol/L) or ionized calcium greater than 1.35 mmol/L (>5.4 mg/dL), and is most commonly iatrogenic by excessive supplementation of calcium or vitamin D.[6,7] Other causes include congenital hyperparathyroidism; subcutaneous fat necrosis after therapeutic hypothermia; and genetic causes, such as Williams syndrome (**Table 2**).[8]

In states of hypocalcemia, a decrease in free circulating calcium within the blood is sensed by a calcium-sensing receptor, which triggers the synthesis and secretion of PTH from the parathyroid glands (**Fig. 2**).[9] PTH then acts on the intestines, bone, and kidneys to create a rise in serum calcium levels.[10] Calcitriol also acts to increase calcium reabsorption and resorption from the bony matrix. In states of hypercalcemia, calcitonin acts in opposition to PTH to decrease the absorption of calcium from the intestines and kidneys while decreasing bony resorption (**Fig. 3**).[11]

Phosphorus

Phosphorus is important for energy metabolism, membrane composition, enzyme activation/inactivation via phosphorylation, and bone mineralization. Unlike calcium, phosphorus is not as strictly regulated and is primarily regulated secondarily to the

Table 1		
Normal calcium ranges in term neonates		
	Form	**Range**
Total serum calcium[a]	Active + inactive	9–10.6 mg/dL (2.25–2.65 mmol/L)
Ionized calcium[b]	Active (free form)	4.84–5.12 mg/dL (1.21–1.28 mmol/L)

[a] The measurement often is misleading because it is under the influence of other protein level derangements, such as hypoalbuminemia/hyperalbuminemia.
[b] Considered to be the most physiologically relevant measurement.

Table 2	
Signs and symptoms of calcium dysregulation	
Hypocalcemia	**Hypercalcemia**
Poor feeding	Feeding intolerance (reflux/emesis)
QT interval tachyarrhythmias	Bradycardia with QT interval
Tetany	Nephrocalcinosis
Apnea	Lethargy
Hypotonia	Hypotonia
Seizures	Seizures

body's regulation of calcium levels. Approximately 85% of the body's phosphate content is found in bone **(Table 3)**.

Normal serum phosphorus values for term infants range from 5.0 to 9.5 mg/dL and for preterm infants range from 6.0 to 8.0 mg/dL.[12] Hypophosphatemia is generally defined by a serum phosphorus level less than 4.0 mg/dL in premature infants and is typically caused by nutritional issues or defects in renal tubular phosphate reabsorption. Hyperphosphatemia is caused **(Table 4)** by excessive infusion of phosphorus or abnormal delivery of calcium and phosphorus with parenteral nutrition (PN). **Table 5** provides a summary of signs of hypophosphatemia.

Calcitriol acts on the gastrointestinal tract and kidney to increase phosphorus levels in states of hypophosphatemia. PTH and FGF23 play a major role in reestablishing homeostasis in states of hyperphosphatemia, with PTH secretion increased directly and indirectly by elevated phosphorus levels.

Fetal Physiology of Calcium and Phosphorus

During fetal development, the kidneys are less important for mineral regulation compared with the active transport of calcium and phosphorus from the maternal

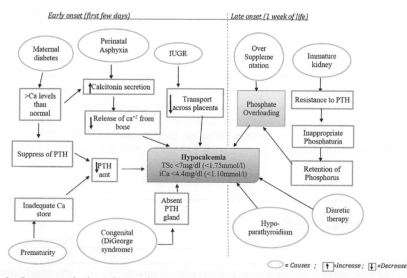

Fig. 2. Causes and physiology of hypocalcemia. Ca, calcium; iCa, ionized calcium; IUGR, intra-uterine growth retardation; TSc, total serum calcium.

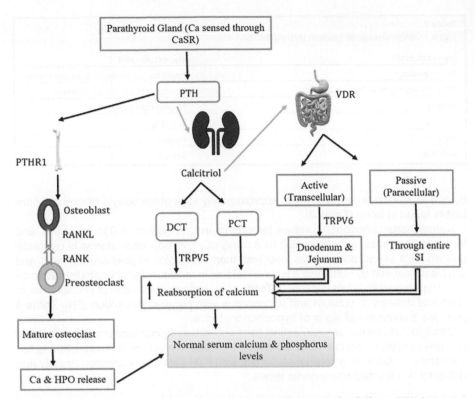

Fig. 3. Response to states of hypocalcemia/hypercalcemia. In the kidney, PTH increases resorption of calcium at the distal convoluted tubule (DCT) via the TRPV5 ion channel. Calcitriol binds to vitamin D receptors (VDR) in the small intestine and stimulates active and passive transport across the membrane. In the bones, PTH binds to a PTH receptor (PTHR1) causing the expression of rank ligand (RANKL) on osteoblasts. RANKL then binds to rank receptors on osteoclast precursors. Green arrow indicates activate. Ca, calcium; CaSR, calcium sensing receptor; HPO, hydroxyapatite crystals; PCT, proximal convoluted tubule; SI, small intestine.

circulation across the placenta.[13] The fetal system responds to this by downregulating the synthesis and release of PTH and calcitriol from the fetal parathyroid glands and kidneys.[14] The elevated levels of both minerals in utero is beneficial at the time of birth when there is an abrupt stop in maternal supply with the cutting of the umbilical cord preventing a devastating drop in levels. Although the formation of bone occurs early, it is not until the third trimester that most of the mineral is deposited into the bone (**Table 6**).

Table 3 Forms of existence of phosphorus	
Site	**Percentage**
Bone (major)	85
Adenosine triphosphate, nucleic acid, and within cell membranes	15 (intracellular)
Plasma (inorganic phosphate)	<1 (extracellular)

Table 4 Causes of hyperphosphatemia	
Nutritional (More Common)	**Nonnutritional (Less Common)**
Excess infusion of phosphorus	Perinatal asphyxia
Abnormal calcium or phosphorus delivered with parenteral nutrition	Disorder in which PTH is absent or inadequate
	Iatrogenic
	Diuretics therapy

Perinatal Changes to Mineral Regulation

After birth, the regulation of calcium and phosphorus changes abruptly because of the cutting of the umbilical cord and the newborn taking its first breath, which leads to a fall in serum and ionized calcium levels. This triggers the neonate's intestine, kidneys, and bones to begin regulating these minerals.[15] In preterm infants, the rise in PTH may be delayed and may not reach normal values until the third week of life. To compensate for the derangement in calcium, stores of calcium from the bone are accessed under control of increasing PTH resulting in increasing levels of calcium and decreasing levels of phosphorus.[16] This process leads to demineralization of the bone. The formation of bone occurs only when there is an optimal proportion of calcium and phosphorus in the body.[17]

METABOLIC BONE DISEASE

Metabolic bone disease of prematurity (MBD), historically referred to as osteopenia of prematurity, has become a recent topic of interest for many neonatal intensive care units. Osteopenia in premature infants was first observed by Von Sydow in 1946.[18] Currently, no concise definition for diagnosing MBD has been established. The disease itself is multifactorial and characterized by a reduction of bone mineral content specifically with respect to calcium and phosphorus.[19,20] The resulting low bone mineral density puts infants at risk for pathologic fractures, failure to achieve optimum growth during childhood/adolescence, and may subject them to an increased risk for osteoporosis later in life. The exact incidence of MBD is unclear, although it is thought to occur in up to 30% to 40% of infants who fall into the category of very low birth weight (VLBW; <1500 g).[17,21] Infants born prematurely, specifically those with VLBW, are at highest risk for mineral deficiencies and development of MBD.[19,22]

Risk Factors

Despite lack of defining the diagnosis, there has been widespread agreement on the antenatal and postnatal risk factors.[20,23] The most important antenatal risk factor

Table 5 Signs of hypophosphatemia	
System	**Sign**
Musculoskeletal	Osteopenia, pathologic fractures, most common finding because of chronic low phosphorous levels
Respiratory	Respiratory muscle dysfunction; decreased oxygen supply
Cardiac	Decreased contractility; arrhythmias
Hematologic	Hemolysis; leukocyte and platelet dysfunction
Neuromuscular	Myopathy; seizures; altered mental status

Table 6
Fetal accretion of bone-forming minerals

Gestation	% Accretion	Calcium	Phosphorus
Until 3rd trimester	20	6 g	4 g
Final week	80	90–120 mg/kg	60–75 mg/kg
At term	Total	28–30 g	16–20 g

involves states in which placental transfer of nutrients to the fetus is impaired, such as chorioamnionitis or preeclampsia. Premature infants have a shortened period of gestation and consequently do not undergo the rapid accumulation of mineral accretion that occurs during the final gestational weeks. Postnatal risk factors include prematurity, prolonged duration of total PN (>4 weeks), and various comorbidities that accompany prematurity. **Table 7** and **Fig. 4** highlight risk factors for MBD.

After birth, these infants still undergo rapid growth but do so in the absence of the high rates of transplacental delivery of minerals. This period of rapid growth requires a higher-than-normal availability of calcium and phosphorus to ensure adequate bone growth and development.[2,24] Calcium and phosphorus are primarily absorbed via passive diffusion in the small intestines relative to the amount of calcium that is nutritionally provided.[25] Preterm infants ultimately have reduced nutritional intake and poor absorption of minerals from their gut. Because of this, many preterm infants are placed on PN. Infants requiring longer than predicted use of total PN are limited on the amount of mineral supplementation that can be provided.[26] Although the aim of mineral supplementation from PN is to provide high concentrations of calcium and phosphorus, there are limitations that ultimately prohibit optimum amounts of supplementation for adequate bony growth.[26,27]

Furthermore, premature infants with comorbidities are at even greater risk for inadequate mineral intake. The use of medications in disease states, such as apnea of prematurity (caffeine) and chronic lung disease (diuretics), disturbs absorption and retention of minerals. Gastrointestinal tract abnormalities seen in the preterm population, such as necrotizing enterocolitis, disrupt absorption processes and the ability to provide enteral nutrition leading to prolonged use of PN. This is discussed in additional detail later in the treatment section.

Diagnosis

No specific criteria have been identified for the diagnosis of MBD. Clinically, these infants may show no signs until bone mineral content has been substantially reduced

Table 7
Risk factors for MBD

Antenatal	Postnatal
Impaired placental transfusion of nutrients	Prolonged duration of TPN (>4 wk)
Chorioamnionitis	Metabolic or endocrine disorders
Preeclampsia	Morbidities of prematurity
Premature delivery	• Apnea of prematurity • Bronchopulmonary dysplasia • Necrotizing enterocolitis

Abbreviation: TPN, total parenteral nutrition.

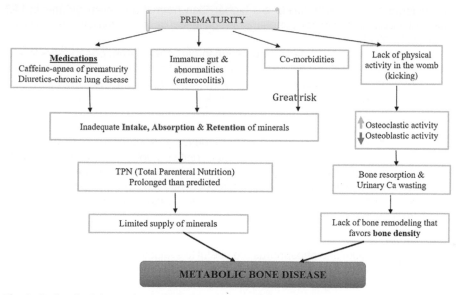

Fig. 4. Pathophysiology of metabolic bone disease of prematurity.

and signs may not be present until they have reached 11 weeks of life.[18,23] To detect the early stages of suboptimal or impaired bone mineralization, routine laboratory monitoring protocols have been implemented but these vary greatly between institutions. Various biochemical markers and imaging modalities have been proposed for screening but interpretation of these is dependent on an understanding of the complex physiology involved in calcium and phosphorus homeostasis (**Table 8**).[17] Unfortunately, no single marker exists as a specific marker for predicting or diagnosing MBD.[28] There are no screening tests that are sensitive and specific.

Serum markers
Although serum markers are easily obtained, there are limitations to their interpretation. Serum calcium levels are not reliable because they are subject to the influence of factors that do not involve osteopenia.[2] Additionally, calcium levels can remain within normal ranges at the expense of bone breakdown. However, serum phosphorus can more adequately reflect the state of the bone especially when interpreted in conjunction with alkaline phosphatase (ALP).[23] ALP is a marker of bone turnover but is expressed in other tissues, such as the liver, kidney, and brain. ALP typically rises during the first few weeks of life in normal physiologic states.[29,30] In premature infants

Table 8		
Markers/imaging techniques to assess bone development		
Serum	**Urine**	**Radiologic**
Calcium	Calcium	Skeletal x-ray
Phosphorus	Phosphorus	Dual-energy x-ray absorptiometry
Alkaline phosphatase	Tubular resorption of phosphorus	Quantitative ultrasound
Parathyroid hormone		
25-(OH) vitamin D		

who undergo rapid growth, levels are higher than normal and even greater in the setting of insufficient mineral supplementation because bone turnover is used to compensate (**Table 9**).[16,26]

A strong association has been found between persistent serum phosphorus levels less than 5.6 mg/dL (1.8 mmol/L) and the presence of radiologic findings consistent with osteopenia. Additional studies have found that ALP level greater than 900 IU/L in combination with serum phosphorus levels less than 5.6 mg/dL have a sensitivity of 70% and a specificity of 100% in infants who are premature.[20] PTH levels are useful for detecting secondary hyperparathyroidism, which places infants at risk of MBD.[31] It can also be useful when evaluating for the underlying cause of hypophosphatemia when used in combination with the tubular reabsorption of phosphorus (TRP) (**Table 10**) as discussed later. 25-Hydroxy-vitamin D is not reliable because levels fluctuate in response to calcium and phosphorus concentrations but may be of use when evaluating malabsorptive disorders. Overall, the most widely used screening markers in the serum are phosphorus and ALP.

Urine markers

Urine levels of calcium and phosphorus are useful to evaluate the adequacy of supplementation for an individual infant. Unfortunately, a major drawback to urine studies is the difficulty of collecting proper samples and the influence of certain medications. Urine calcium levels greater than 1.2 mmol/L and urine phosphorus levels greater than 0.4 mmol/L have been shown to be present in infants who have high bone mineral content, because the excess is excreted into the urine indicating a slight surplus of supplementation. When a neonate has a prolonged cause of hypophosphatemia, the TRP is calculated with urine and serum samples as follows:

$$\{1 - [\, (UPh/UCr) \times (SCr/SPh) \,] \} \times 100.$$

(where UPh is urine phosphate, UCr is urine creatinine, SCr is serum creatinine, and SPh is serum phosphate).

Normal ranges for TRP have been weakly established as 78% to 91%. Levels greater than 95% are an indication of inadequate phosphorus supplementation. When used in conjunction with PTH, TRP can help to determine the underlying cause of low phosphate levels. A low TRP and high PTH is likely to be an indication of hypocalcemia-induced hypophosphatemia. A high TRP and low-normal PTH is likely to be an indicator of phosphate deficiency. A major pitfall is that inadequate intake of calcium leads to increase of PTH and the increased excretion of phosphorus.

Radiologic markers

Another tool in the monitoring of impaired bone mineralization is the use of imaging studies.[32] Skeletal x-ray imaging is low cost and portable. Images may show cortical thinning of bone and/or fractures; however, this is a late fining of MBD and does not become apparent until bone mineral content is reduced by 40%. Dual-energy x-ray absorptiometry is the gold standard for assessing bone mineral content in adult counterparts; however, the interpretation of results for infants is still being investigated. A

Table 9	
Alkaline phosphatase levels and MBD	
ALP Level	**Clinical Concern**
>500 IU/L	Impaired bone homeostasis
>700 IU/L	Demineralization

Table 10 Interpretation of TRP	
TRP	Normal range, 78%–91%
>95%	Inadequate supplementation
PTH + TRP	Underlying cause of low phosphate levels
Low TRP and high PTH	Hypocalcemia-induced hypophosphatemia
High TRP and low-normal PTH	Phosphate deficiency

more recent development is quantitative ultrasound.[33] It uses the speed of sound and bone transmission time to measure bone mineral density. **Table 11** provides a list of strengths and weaknesses for each imaging modality.

In 2013 the American Academy of Pediatrics released a statement with a guideline for implementing screening for MBD for infants at 4 to 6 weeks of life. Despite the release of this consensus statement, there are many varieties between neonatal units for the timing, frequency, and use of different biochemical markers and imaging used for screening. The variation seen is likely because of the lack of evidence-based guidelines for diagnosis.[26]

Treatment

Research that brought to light the physiology of mineral accretion rates in utero has brought awareness to the importance of providing supplementation during the early postnatal period. Initially, bone mineral content is appropriate for gestational age in the preterm infant but will not continue to increase appropriately if left unsupplemented.[24,34,35] If the need for serum minerals is not met, bone mineralization will be reduced, and resorption of the developing skeleton will be used to support serum mineral concentration requirements.[36] Therefore, treatment should be aimed at preventing resorption and focus on meeting the mineral requirements necessary to optimize skeletal mineralization.[21,37]

Many guidelines regarding calcium and phosphorus supplementation are aimed at achieving rates similar to that of in utero accretion rates.[38] The major determinant of the amount of mineral required is based on fetal growth.[21] Although some studies estimate average fetal weight gain and mineral accretion rates, the biggest challenge is that the estimated accretion for calcium and phosphorus are unable to be determined for each individual infant.[26] It is also important to consider that phosphorus is needed for protein accretion and the supplementation of amino acids increases the cellular uptake of phosphorus. Accordingly, one should consider providing a slight surplus of calcium and phosphorus especially when amino acids are provided to ensure adequate bone development in this vulnerable population.[34,39] Many centers are now fortifying the nutrition of VLBW neonates earlier and longer to reach a bone-forming homeostatic state. Although VLBW neonates may have steady weight gain, in our center we continue to recommend fortified preterm formula until at least 6 to 9 months of age to optimize calcium and phosphorus supplementation. For the preterm infant, mineral requirements for skeletal development exceed that of what the immature intestines are capable of absorbing.[40]

Parenteral Optimization

To optimize bone formation in VLBW infants, PN supplementation for calcium and phosphorus should aim for high concentrations and for an optimal ratio of calcium phosphorus ratios while preventing precipitation.[34] Multiple studies have shown that increasing amounts provide more optimal bone uptake; however, these studies are

Table 11
Imaging modalities to assess bone health

Imaging	Skeletal X-ray	DXA	QUS
Assesses	Cortical thinning of bone and fractures	Bone mineral content	Bone mineral density
Advantages	Low cost and portable	Costly, long time required for imaging; artifacts caused by movements	No exposure of radiation, noninvasive, portable, inexpensive
Disadvantages	Radiation	Small dose of radiation	Cortical bone thickness can only be assessed qualitatively
Notes	Late finding of MBD not apparent until bone mineral content <40%	Gold standard	Uses speed of sound and bone transmission time

Abbreviations: DXA, dual energy x-ray absorptiometry; QUS, quantitative ultrasound.

Table 12
Parenteral and enteral goals to improve bone mineralization

Optimization	Parenteral	Enteral
Early initiation	Traditionally relied on PN during the first few weeks of life.[a]	Early initiation of enteral feedings should be prioritized because it can lead to improved endocrine adaptation to mineral levels and more rapid maturation of the gut resulting in improved absorption of minerals.[35,42]
Functions	The goal of early PN is to provide energy, protein, and minerals to prevent catabolism immediately after birth.	Calcium absorption from the gut ranges between 40% for formula and 70% for breast milk. Phosphate absorption ranges between 65% and 90%.[36,40]
Availability for accretion	Mineral supplementation provided via PN is directly available for tissue and bone accretion.[24,43]	Enteral supplementation where absorption plays a factor in the amount available for accretion. Absorption rates that may depend on source and ratio.
Limitations[b]	Temperature, pH, order of ingredient mixing, type of Ca/Phos used for delivery, amino acid concentrations, and so forth.[44]	Although it may provide adequate amounts of minerals for the term infant, unfortified breast milk provides inadequate mineral content for the rapidly growing premature infant.
Provide higher mineral content	Use of organic compounds for calcium and phosphorus instead of inorganic compounds, increasing the acidity of the solution by adding cysteine, increasing glucose and amino acid concentration, preventing warming of the solution, and use of the preparation in <24 h from the time of formulation.	Human milk fortifiers or special preterm formulas should be used. As time passes, skeletal development, and the need for high amounts of mineral[45] accretion declines, the transition to unfortified human breast milk or formula can be made.
Forms	Calcium: calcium gluconate (organic), calcium chloride (inorganic). Phosphorus: sodium glycerophosphate (organic), K Phos and Na Phos (inorganic).	Human milk contains approximately 260 mg Ca/L and 140 mg P/L. Even when infants are feeding as much as 200 mL/kg/d, with the assumption that 70% Ca and 90% P are absorbed. Human milk has been shown to be higher than that of formula but little difference in absorption exists for phosphorus from either source.[36,41]
Recommended amounts[c]	40–120 mg/kg/d of calcium and 31–80 mg/kg/d for phosphorus.[21,44,46]	120–220 mg/kg/d for calcium and 60–140 mg/kg/d for phosphorus.[27,42,47]
Ca/P ratio	1.7:1 mass ratio (1.3:1 M ratio) according to the American Society for Parenteral and Enteral Nutrition. 1.1:1(mg/mg) up to 2:1(mg/mg)-other institutions.[12,18]	1.5:1–2:1 (mass ratio, mg/mg). Absorption is also affected by the ratio of Ca and Phos in the diet.[37,47]

[a] Although this sounds ideal, it is important to realize that delay in reaching full enteral feeds poses a risk for developing MBD because there are many difficulties encountered when relying solely on PN.

[b] These limitations make it difficult to provide the same amount of minerals to a growing fetus as expected in utero.

[c] The potential for calcium cations and phosphorus anions to precipitate is also more likely with increasing amounts.

Table 13		
Medications that affect bone mineralization		
Disease State	Drugs	Limitation Cause
Apnea of prematurity	Caffeine, theophylline	Increase calcium excretion
BPD	Glucocorticoids	Inhibits bone growth and remodeling via osteoblast impairment and inhibits intestinal transfer
BPD	Loop diuretics	Increases renal calcium excretion

Abbreviation: BPD, bronchopulmonary dysplasia.

also dependent on the ratio of their concentrations.[34] Moreover, one must consider that during initiation of PN, protein supplementation is optimized to prevent catabolism while calcium and phosphorus supplementation remain low (**Table 12**).

It may be of benefit during this time to provide lower calcium/phosphorus mass ratios (0.8–1) to provide sufficient phosphorus and avoid severe postnatal hypophosphatemia in the setting of high amino acid intake. Inadequate phosphorus supplementation in this setting can trigger a hypophosphatemic response where the available phosphorus is directed to cellular uptake.[27] This leads to low phosphorus, which is unable to provide an adequate state for calcium fixation to bone and in turn induces hypercalciuria because of the relative excess of calcium.[39] This potentially puts infants at risk for nephrocalcinosis.

Limiting Drug Use

Preterm infants are subjected to other disease states where medications are used, such as apnea of prematurity and bronchopulmonary dysplasia.[1,41] Unfortunately, multiple medications used for treatment affect mineral levels and play a role in the development of MBD. When able to, one should try to limit use of medications that may further increase the risk of developing MBD or consider use of alternative agents (**Table 13**).[2]

Additional Supplementation

Despite maximizing PN and enteral supplementation, some VLBW neonates may continue to have abnormal serum mineral levels or evidence of MBD. These infants may require additional supplementation from intravenous potassium phosphate and calcium gluconate or oral forms of potassium phosphate and calcium carbonate.[35]

SUMMARY

Premature infants, specifically VLBW neonates, are at high risk for developing MBD because they fail to establish adequate in utero accretion of minerals that play a vital role in skeletal maturation. Postnatally, it is difficult to achieve the same intake of minerals in comparison with that during fetal development. There has been consensus on the risk factors for developing osteopenia; however, a wide range of guidelines exist for diagnosis and treatment. There have been many expert opinions regarding the provision of mineral intake in spite of a lack of randomized controlled trials with statistical power. There is general agreement on ranges of adequate provision, but the optimal regimen remains uncertain. The varying viewpoints make apparent the lack of data on the matter. We conclude by providing a list of pressing questions that still remain.

1. Establish normal serum level values for calcium and phosphorus in the preterm/VLBW infant. Establishment of MBD definition and specific diagnostic criteria.

2. Development of a standardized screening and monitoring protocol for MBD, specifically one that can detect early suboptimal mineralization.
3. Lack of consensus of optimal parenteral and enteral daily intake.
4. Lack of consensus on optimal ratio for parenteral and enteral intake.
5. Lack of studies on safety of calcium and phosphorus supplementation.
6. Lack of studies on long-term outcomes for bone health in for VLBW infants.

Although advancements have been made there remain several conundrums worthy of improvement.

Best practices

1. Implementing routine screening protocols: Early detection of MBD is crucial in preventing long-term consequences. Neonatal units should develop and implement screening protocols that incorporate biochemical markers and imaging modalities to detect the early stages of impaired bone mineralization.

2. Providing adequate mineral supplementation: To prevent MBD, clinicians should tailor mineral supplementation according to gestational age, morbidities, medications, and postnatal growth to meet the needs of each individual neonate.

3. Limiting drug use: Medications used to treat common comorbidities in preterm infants can negatively affect mineral levels and contribute to the development of MBD. Providers should limit the use of such medications when possible and consider alternative agents to minimize the risk of MBD.

CLINICS CARE POINTS

- Regular monitoring of bone mineral content: Infants at risk for MBD, particularly those with very low birth weight (VLBW), should undergo regular monitoring (e.g., imaging, serum markers) of bone mineral content to identify early signs of bone demineralization.

- Adequate calcium and phosphorus supplementation: Premature infants often require additional calcium and phosphorus supplementation to support bone mineralization.: Adequate nutrition, including proper caloric intake and appropriate protein levels, is essential for promoting bone growth and preventing MBD in premature infants.

- Consideration of vitamin D status: Vitamin D plays a crucial role in calcium absorption and bone health. Evaluating and optimizing vitamin D status (25-OH vitamin D) in premature infants can help reduce the risk of MBD.

- Collaboration with a multidisciplinary team: Managing MBD requires a collaborative approach involving neonatologists, pediatricians, dietitians, and other healthcare professionals. In cases where MBD is suspected or diagnosed, involving a pediatric endocrinologist can provide specialized expertise in managing bone health and optimizing treatment strategies.

- Assessing for underlying conditions: Premature infants with MBD may have associated conditions or comorbidities that contribute to bone mineralization issues. Evaluating for underlying causes, such as genetic disorders or chronic illnesses, can guide treatment decisions.

- Long-term follow-up: Infants with a history of MBD should receive long-term follow-up to assess bone health during childhood and monitor for potential complications, such as delayed growth or osteoporosis.

- Parent education and support: Providing parents with information about MBD, its management, and preventive measures can empower them to actively participate in their child's care and promote optimal bone health.

DISCLOSURE

The authors have nothing to disclose.

REFERENCES

1. Taylor JG, Bushinsky DA. Calcium and phosphorus homeostasis. Blood Purif 2009;27(4):387–94.
2. Dokos C, Tsakalidis C, Tragiannidis A, et al. Inside the "fragile" infant: pathophysiology, molecular background, risk factors and investigation of neonatal osteopenia. Clin Cases Miner Bone Metab 2013;10(2):86–90.
3. Vuralli D. Clinical approach to hypocalcemia in newborn period and infancy: who should be treated? Int J Pediatr 2019;2019:4318075.
4. Bringhurst FR, Demay MB, Kronenberg HM. Chapter 28 - hormones and disorders of mineral metabolism. In: Melmed S, Polonsky KS, Larsen PR, et al, editors. Williams textbook of endocrinology. 13th edition. Philadelphia, PA: Elsevier; 2016. p. 1253–322.
5. Neonatal hypocalcemia: to treat or not to treat? (A review) Available at: https://www.tandfonline.com/doi/epdf/10.1080/07315724.1994.10718429?needAccess=true&role=button. Accessed 3 March, 2023.
6. Rodríguez Soriano J. Neonatal hypercalcemia. J Nephrol 2003;16(4):606–8.
7. Gorvin CM. Genetic causes of neonatal and infantile hypercalcaemia. Pediatr Nephrol Berl Ger 2022;37(2):289–301.
8. Stokes VJ, Nielsen MF, Hannan FM, et al. Hypercalcemic disorders in children. J Bone Miner Res 2017;32(11):2157–70.
9. Kumar R, Thompson JR. The regulation of parathyroid hormone secretion and synthesis. J Am Soc Nephrol JASN 2011;22(2):216–24.
10. Roy CC, O'Brien D. Calcium and phosphorus: current concepts of metabolism. Clin Pediatr (Phila) 1967;6(1):19–28.
11. Copp DH. Calcium and phosphorus metabolism. Am J Med 1957;22(2):275–85.
12. Pohlandt F, Mihatsch WA. Reference values for urinary calcium and phosphorus to prevent osteopenia of prematurity. Pediatr Nephrol Berl Ger 2004;19(11):1192–3.
13. Ziegler EE, O'Donnell AM, Nelson SE, et al. Body composition of the reference fetus. Growth 1976;40(4):329–41.
14. Abrams SA. In utero physiology: role in nutrient delivery and fetal development for calcium, phosphorus, and vitamin D. Am J Clin Nutr 2007;85(2):604S–7S.
15. Ellis KJ, Shypailo RJ, Schanler RJ. Body composition of the preterm infant. Ann Hum Biol 1994;21(6):533–45.
16. Harrison CM, Gibson AT. Osteopenia in preterm infants. Arch Dis Child Fetal Neonatal Ed 2013;98(3):F272–5.
17. Rustico SE, Calabria AC, Garber SJ. Metabolic bone disease of prematurity. J Clin Transl Endocrinol 2014;1(3):85–91.
18. Perrone M, Casirati A, Stagi S, et al. Don't forget the bones: incidence and risk factors of metabolic bone disease in a cohort of preterm infants. Int J Mol Sci 2022;23(18):10666.
19. Rayannavar A, Calabria AC. Screening for metabolic bone disease of prematurity. Semin Fetal Neonatal Med 2020;25(1). https://doi.org/10.1016/j.siny.2020.101086.
20. Chen W, Yang C, Chen H, et al. Risk factors analysis and prevention of metabolic bone disease of prematurity. Medicine (Baltim) 2018;97(42):e12861.

21. Motokura K, Tomotaki S, Hanaoka S, et al. Appropriate phosphorus intake by parenteral nutrition prevents metabolic bone disease of prematurity in extremely low-birth-weight infants. JPEN J Parenter Enteral Nutr 2021;45(6):1319–26.

22. Steichen JJ, Gratton TL, Tsang RC. Osteopenia of prematurity: the cause and possible treatment. J Pediatr 1980;96(3 Pt 2):528–34.

23. Faienza MF, D'Amato E, Natale MP, et al. Metabolic bone disease of prematurity: diagnosis and management. Front Pediatr 2019;7:143.

24. Senterre T, Abu Zahirah I, Pieltain C, et al. Electrolyte and mineral homeostasis after optimizing early macronutrient intakes in VLBW infants on parenteral nutrition. J Pediatr Gastroenterol Nutr 2015;61(4):491–8.

25. Mitchell DM, Jüppner H. Regulation of calcium homeostasis and bone metabolism in the fetus and neonate. Curr Opin Endocrinol Diabetes Obes 2010; 17(1):25–30.

26. Chacham S, Pasi R, Chegondi M, et al. Metabolic bone disease in premature neonates: an unmet challenge. J Clin Res Pediatr Endocrinol 2020;12(4):332–9.

27. Mu RHN. Metabolic bone disease in the preterm infant: current state and future directions. World J Methodol 2015;5(3). https://doi.org/10.5662/wjm.v5.i3.115.

28. Figueras-Aloy J, Álvarez-Domínguez E, Pérez-Fernández JM, et al. Metabolic bone disease and bone mineral density in very preterm infants. J Pediatr 2014; 164(3):499–504.

29. Backström M, Kouri T, Kuusela AL, et al. Bone isoenzyme of serum alkaline phosphatase and serum inorganic phosphate in metabolic bone disease of prematurity. Acta Paediatr 2000;89(7):867–73.

30. Abdallah EAA, Said RN, Mosallam DS, et al. Serial serum alkaline phosphatase as an early biomarker for osteopenia of prematurity. Medicine (Baltim) 2016; 95(37):e4837.

31. Moreira A, Swischuk L, Malloy M, et al. Parathyroid hormone as a marker for metabolic bone disease of prematurity. J Perinatol 2014;34(10):787–91.

32. Lucas-Herald A, Butler S, Mactier H, et al. Prevalence and characteristics of rib fractures in ex-preterm infants. Pediatrics 2012;130(6):1116–9.

33. Tong L, Gopal-Kothandapani JS, Offiah AC. Feasibility of quantitative ultrasonography for the detection of metabolic bone disease in preterm infants: systematic review. Pediatr Radiol 2018;48(11):1537–49.

34. Early High Calcium and Phosphorus Intake by Parenteral Nutri : Journal of Pediatric Gastroenterology and Nutrition. Available at: https://journals.lww.com/jpgn/Fulltext/2011/02000/Early_High_Calcium_and_Phosphorus_Intake_by.18.aspx. Accessed 9 February, 2023.

35. Bozzetti V, Tagliabue P. Metabolic bone disease in preterm newborn: an update on nutritional issues. Ital J Pediatr 2009;35(1):20.

36. Schanler RJ, Rifka M. Calcium, phosphorus and magnesium needs for the low-birth-weight infant. Acta Paediatr Oslo Nor 1994;405:111–6.

37. Loughrill E, Wray D, Christides T, et al. Calcium to phosphorus ratio, essential elements and vitamin D content of infant foods in the UK: possible implications for bone health. Matern Child Nutr 2017;13(3):e12368.

38. Chinoy A, Mughal MZ, Padidela R. Metabolic bone disease of prematurity: national survey of current neonatal and paediatric endocrine approaches. Acta Paediatr Oslo Nor 2021;110(6):1855–62.

39. Christmann V, Gradussen CJW, Körnmann MN, et al. Changes in biochemical parameters of the calcium-phosphorus homeostasis in relation to nutritional intake in very-low-birth-weight infants. Nutrients 2016;8(12):764.

40. Bronner F, Salle BL, Putet G, et al. Net calcium absorption in premature infants: results of 103 metabolic balance studies. Am J Clin Nutr 1992;56(6):1037–44.
41. Hicks PD, Rogers SP, Hawthorne KM, et al. Calcium absorption in very low birth weight infants with and without bronchopulmonary dysplasia. J Pediatr 2011; 158(6):885–90.e1.
42. Corpeleijn WE, Vermeulen MJ, van den Akker CH, et al. Feeding very-low-birth-weight infants: our aspirations versus the reality in practice. Ann Nutr Metab 2011;58(Suppl 1):20–9.
43. Wiechers C, Bernhard W, Goelz R, et al. Optimizing early neonatal nutrition and dietary pattern in premature infants. Int J Environ Res Public Health 2021; 18(14):7544.
44. Fusch C, Bauer K, Böhles HJ, et al. Neonatology/paediatrics: guidelines on parenteral nutrition, chapter 13. GMS Ger Med Sci 2009;7:Doc15.
45. Schanler RJ, Abrams SA. Postnatal attainment of intrauterine macromineral accretion rates in low birth weight infants fed fortified human milk. J Pediatr 1995; 126(3):441–7.
46. Mihatsch W, Fewtrell M, Goulet O, et al. ESPGHAN/ESPEN/ESPR/CSPEN guidelines on pediatric parenteral nutrition: calcium, phosphorus and magnesium. Clin Nutr Edinb Scotl 2018;37(6 Pt B):2360–5.
47. Agostoni C, Buonocore G, Carnielli VP, et al. Enteral nutrient supply for preterm infants: commentary from the European Society of Paediatric Gastroenterology, Hepatology and Nutrition Committee on Nutrition. J Pediatr Gastroenterol Nutr 2010;50(1):85.

The Practice of Enteral Nutrition
Clinical Evidence for Feeding Protocols

Ariel A. Salas, MD, MSPH*, Colm P. Travers, MD

KEYWORDS

- Randomized trials • Enteral feeding • Premature infants • Preterm • Newborn
- Infant • Nutrition • Growth

KEY POINTS

- Some feeding protocols advance enteral nutrition very slowly in preterm infants.
- Emerging evidence from randomized clinical trials indicates that slower and later progression of enteral nutrition does not mitigate the risk of necrotizing enterocolitis.
- Promoting the early establishment of full enteral nutrition reduces the risk of invasive infections.
- Feeding protocols can improve short- and long-term outcomes by decreasing practice variability and incorporating new clinical evidence favoring the early establishment of full enteral nutrition.

Abbreviations	
NEC	Necrotizing enterocolitis
SIP	Spontaneous intestinal perforation

INTRODUCTION

Most of the cumulative nutritional deficits in preterm infants occur in the first 2 weeks after birth. Limited enteral nutrition during the first 2 weeks is one of the critical barriers to solving the problem of postnatal growth faltering at term equivalent age among preterm infants. Observational data reveal that critically ill preterm infants rarely receive adequate nutritional intakes during early postnatal life.[1] Observational data also indicate that the cumulative nutritional deficits in energy and protein intake that occur

Division of Neonatology, Department of Pediatrics, Heersink School of Medicine, University of Alabama at Birmingham, 1700 6th Avenue South Women & Infants Center Suite 9380, Birmingham, AL 35233, USA
* Corresponding author.
E-mail address: asalas@uab.edu
Twitter: @ArielSalasMD (A.A.S.)

Clin Perinatol 50 (2023) 607–623
https://doi.org/10.1016/j.clp.2023.04.005
0095-5108/23/© 2023 Elsevier Inc. All rights reserved.
perinatology.theclinics.com

soon after birth account for approximately 50% of the decline in weight-for-age observed from birth to hospital discharge[2] and may explain the slow growth and increased risk of adverse outcomes observed in preterm infants.[1]

Meta-analyses of randomized trials designed to establish full enteral nutrition during the first 2 weeks after birth consistently show that early (before or on postnatal day 4)[3] and faster (30–40 mL/kg/d) progression of enteral feeding volumes[4] increases growth velocity rates from birth to hospital discharge and increases weight-for-age z scores at term equivalent age. In addition, higher volume feedings may allow for catch-up growth beyond the initial postnatal period. Observational data also suggest that enteral nutrition effectively prevents cumulative nutritional deficits in critically ill preterm infants, which may mitigate the risk of late-onset sepsis, bronchopulmonary dysplasia (BPD), neurodevelopmental impairment, and death.[1]

Despite this collective evidence that early full enteral nutrition reduces the risk of growth faltering and may lower the risk of adverse outcomes, there is marked variability across neonatal units in enteral nutrition practices during the acute phase of illness after birth in preterm infants. The severity of illness and concern for related complications, including spontaneous intestinal perforation (SIP) and necrotizing enterocolitis (NEC), are often cited as the main indications to limit enteral nutrition in these infants.

ENTERAL NUTRITION AND NECROTIZING ENTEROCOLITIS: AN EPIDEMIOLOGIC PERSPECTIVE

Establishing full enteral nutrition soon after birth in preterm infants is difficult without an epidemiologic perspective. Countless reports that enteral feeding is the final event before an infant is diagnosed with NEC are often interpreted as evidence that not offering enteral feeding can prevent NEC. This interpretation may reflect circular reasoning and highlights the importance of establishing differences between association and causation.[5] Enteral feeding occurs in 90% of infants diagnosed with NEC, but this report is not proof that exposure to enteral feeding explains 90% of all NEC cases. This finding is evidence that exposure to enteral feeding—which occurs every 2 to 3 h in neonatal units—is common among preterm infants. High exposure to enteral feeding is also observed in infants who never develop NEC. With these high exposure rates to enteral feeding, the occurrence of NEC in proximity to enteral feeding is predictable.

Furthermore, observing that enteral feeding precedes the diagnosis of NEC only establishes temporality in the association. Other criteria such as specificity (ie, enteral feeding is not exclusively associated with NEC), consistency (ie, not all experimental evidence suggests an increased risk of NEC with enteral feeding), or strength (ie, not all infants that receive enteral feeding develop NEC) are needed to establish a causal association.[5]

Defining the causes of NEC requires a new framework around the principle of multicausality. Like many other complications of prematurity, such as BPD, NEC has multiple causes. Decades of research have proven that enteral feeding is not the only risk factor for NEC. Other risk factors include fetal growth restriction,[6] persistent hypoxemia,[7] severe anemia,[8] and dysbiosis due to frequent exposure to broad-spectrum antibiotics.[9] Because these events play a role in the occurrence of NEC, enteral feeding should be considered a component cause along with several others (**Fig. 1**).

Multicausality implies that only certain NEC cases can be attributed to enteral feeding, even in clinical scenarios where enteral feeding is the final event before the diagnosis of NEC. With more clinical trials reporting on specific elements of enteral feeding that mitigate the risk of NEC (human milk feeding, arginine, probiotics, and

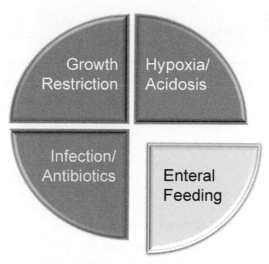

Fig. 1. Multicausality in necrotizing enterocolitis.

others), the proportion of NEC cases attributed to enteral feeding is decreasing. If this trend continues in subsequent decades, the prevalence of NEC will likely decline, and the proportion of NEC cases attributed to non-feeding factors will likely increase.

As NEC cases decrease, SIP is set to become the most common major intestinal morbidity among preterm infants.[10] SIP typically occurs in the first postnatal week when clinicians are initiating enteral feeding. However, early enteral feeding is rarely implicated in the pathogenesis of SIP. The etiology of SIP is also multifactorial and shares some risk factors with NEC including growth restriction and perinatal asphyxia. Bowel ischemia in vulnerable watershed areas, which may occur prenatally or postnatally, is usually the final common pathway leading to bowel perforation. In addition, certain medications are associated with SIP such as the early administration of steroids.[10]

ENTERAL NUTRITION AND FEEDING INTOLERANCE IN PRETERM INFANTS

The transition from parenteral to enteral nutrition often begins with minimal enteral feeding or trophic feeding (≤24 mL/kg/d), then changes to progressive feeding (increments of feeding volumes usually by 10–35 mL/kg/d each day), and concludes with full enteral feeding (≥120–150 mL/kg/d)[11–14] (**Fig. 2**).

Development of feeding intolerance is a common symptom of NEC. However, during the transition to full enteral feeding up to 50% of infants experience feeding intolerance.[3] Although the inability to absorb and digest human milk or formula in preterm infants is often cited as one of the primary causes,[3,15] dysmotility is the most common

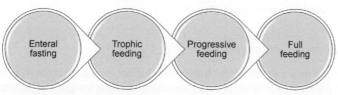

Fig. 2. Enteral nutrition in preterm infants.

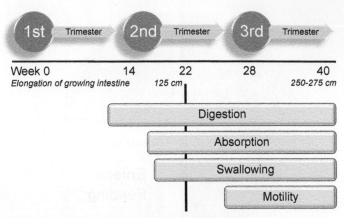

Fig. 3. Functional development of the gastrointestinal tract.

cause of feeding intolerance. Unlike digestion and absorption, gastrointestinal motility is underdeveloped in most infants born before 28 weeks of gestation[16] (**Fig. 3**).

High pre-feed gastric residual volume is a common indication to withhold enteral feeding in preterm infants, but a high level of evidence does not support this practice. The routine assessment of gastric residual volumes likely disrupts the natural production of hydrochloric acid in the stomach. Without an acidic gastric environment, preterm infants are at increased risk of bacterial colonization/overgrowth[17,18] and feeding intolerance due to the inactivation of the enzyme pepsin that digests protein-containing milk.[19] Limited clinical evidence consistently shows that optimizing gastric acidity reduces the risk of gastrointestinal complications. Not checking gastric residual volumes,[20,21] re-feeding gastric residual volumes,[13] and adding hydrochloric acid to infant formula[17] have been associated with a lower risk of feeding intolerance and NEC in randomized clinical trials. Observational studies also reported that avoiding antacid therapy is associated with a lower risk of NEC.[22]

In settings where the routine assessment of gastric residual volumes is no longer practiced, abdominal distension and emesis are the most common indications to withhold enteral feeding, particularly in preterm infants managed with noninvasive ventilation soon after birth. Although aerophagia and gaseous bowel distension occur in up to 83% of extremely preterm infants managed with noninvasive ventilation,[23] there is no evidence from randomized trials that noninvasive ventilation increases the risk of SIP or NEC.[24]

Routine abdominal radiographs have limited value in assessing feeding intolerance and NEC.[23] Several methods, including electrogastrography, abdominal tissue oxygenation using near-infrared spectroscopy, and bowel sound/acoustics, are being evaluated as diagnostic tools to assess feeding intolerance and identify infants at higher risk of intestinal disease.[24,25] Until the validity of these methods is sufficient to establish a risk stratification system, standardizing the clinical assessment of feeding intolerance with checklists that include questions about nutrition, motility, ischemia, and sepsis should be considered (**Box 1**)

CLINICAL EVIDENCE FOR FEEDING PROTOCOLS

This section summarizes evidence from randomized clinical trials in a questions and answers format and addresses specific clinical questions frequently discussed during bedside rounds.

Box 1	
Clinical assessment of feeding intolerance	
Nutrition	Has the patient received any formula feeds?
	Is the infant receiving more than trophic feeds (>25 mL/kg/d)?
Motility	Are the bowel sounds hypoactive or absent?
	Are there visible bowel loops?
	Is there abdominal distension with discoloration?
	Has the infant had an increase in abdominal girth?
	Has the infant had constipation?
	Has the infant had a bloody stool?
Ischemia	Is the infant's urine output low?
	Is the infant receiving support with vasopressors?
	Is the infant's lactate high?
	Is the infant showing signs of hypotension?
Sepsis	Is the infant experiencing abnormal heart rate characteristics?
	Has the infant had a relative increase in oxygen requirement?
	Is the infant having more apneas and bradycardia?

Should We Advocate for Enteral Fasting to Reduce the Risk of Necrotizing Enterocolitis?

Enteral fasting was previously considered a protective strategy to mitigate the risk of NEC in critically ill infants[25] because enteral feeding can alter splanchnic perfusion, increase the risk of ischemic injury,[26] cause osmotic injury to the mucosa, and promote bacterial overgrowth if enteral feeding results in the presence of undigested substrate in the intestinal lumen.[27,28] Subsequently, animal and clinical studies revealed a positive linear correlation between small feeding volumes of 12 to 50 mL/kg and gastrointestinal hormones that promote mucosal maturation.[29,30]

Multiple randomized clinical trials have since confirmed that early initiation of trophic feeding (ie, within the first 96 hours after birth) is a safe alternative to enteral fasting for critically ill preterm infants. In 2013, data from 9 randomized clinical trials of early initiation of trophic feeding with volumes up to 24 mL/kg/d in 754 very low birthweight infants were included in a meta-analysis.[31–40] NEC as an outcome was examined in the 9 trials included. Compared to enteral fasting, trophic feeding did not increase the risk of NEC (8% vs. 8%; risk ratio [RR]: 1.07; 95% confidence interval [CI]: 0.67–1.70; N = 748). Eight trials examined the time to establish full enteral feeding. In 3 trials, trophic feeding reduced the time to establish full enteral feeding.[33,36,39] Two trials reported data on sepsis. One noted fewer episodes of culture-positive sepsis in the trophic feeding group.[36] Mortality did not differ between groups (RR: 0.77; 95% CI: 0.46–1.30). The time to regain birthweight was not shorter in any of the 9 trials included in the meta-analysis.

This meta-analysis detected considerable heterogeneity across trials and included only a few extremely preterm infants. Still, no additional trials on this topic are anticipated. Feeding protocols should not favor a delay in initiation of trophic feeding beyond the first 96 hours after birth, even in critically ill infants with a history of low Apgar scores, acidosis, respiratory distress syndrome, hemodynamic instability, and/or persistent patency of the ductus arteriosus (PDA). Prolonging enteral fasting results in villous atrophy and complicates subsequent feeding. An unmasked trial excluded from all meta-analyses on early enteral feeding compared the effects of late minimal enteral feeding and progressive feeding after prolonged enteral fasting in 144 preterm infants born between 1996 and 2000. Because enteral feeding in both groups started after approximately 10 days of enteral fasting, all infants included in this trial likely had villous atrophy at the time of initiation of enteral feeding. Minimal enteral feeding compared to progressive feeding after prolonged enteral fasting delayed the establishment of full enteral feeding by approximately 13 days, extended hospital stay (mean difference between groups: 11 days), and resulted in a trend for a lower risk of NEC (RR:0.14; CI: 0.02–1.07).[41] However, these findings require a cautious interpretation.[42] Only 30% of infants in the trial received a human milk diet, and nearly 50% did not benefit from exposure to antenatal steroids. The use of antenatal steroids[43] and exclusive human milk feeding with either maternal or donated milk[44]—both effective strategies that reduce the risk of NEC—have increased substantially over the past 2 decades. Furthermore, late initiation of enteral feeding is now strongly discouraged, and the presence of umbilical catheters or infusions of vasopressor agents are no longer contraindications to initiate enteral feeding.[45,46]

Should We Promote Enteral Fasting During Patency of the Ductus Arteriosus Treatment or Blood Transfusions?

The evidence favoring enteral fasting to prevent NEC during PDA treatment or blood transfusions is predominantly limited to single-center observational studies with inconsistent results. Although it remains uncertain if enteral fasting can modify the baseline risk of NEC among high-risk infants requiring PDA treatment or blood transfusions, there is evidence from randomized trials that enteral fasting during PDA treatment increases the time to establish full enteral feeding and does not decrease the risk of NEC.[47] The potential benefits of enteral fasting to mitigate the risk of NEC during blood transfusions are currently being investigated in a randomized clinical trial.[48] However, it remains uncertain if intermittent exposure to blood transfusions transiently increases the risk of NEC.[49] Hemoglobin values below 7 g/dL and severity of anemia before a blood transfusion may be associated with a higher risk of NEC rather than the number of blood transfusions.[8]

Does Extending Enteral Fasting After Nonsurgical or Surgical Necrotizing Enterocolitis Prevent Complications Associated with Necrotizing Enterocolitis?

Observational studies recently questioned the benefits of prolonged enteral fasting after nonsurgical[50] and surgical NEC.[51] Shortening the duration of enteral fasting by 4 days (from 9 to 5 days) was associated with a 35% decrease in the time to establish full enteral feeding and a reduced need for central venous access after the diagnosis of nonsurgical NEC.[50] However, post-NEC strictures were not significantly lower after shortening the duration of enteral fasting (4% vs. 13%).[50] Similarly, the early reintroduction of enteral feeding after surgical NEC (≤7 days) was associated with a reduced need for parenteral nutrition 28 days postsurgical intervention in unadjusted analyses. In addition, exposure to early enteral feeding after surgical NEC was not associated with a higher risk of mortality (5% vs. 2%).[51] Clinical trials comparing shorter (3–5 days) versus extended (7–10 days) periods of enteral fasting after NEC are warranted.

If trophic feeding prevents villous atrophy, should we extend the duration of trophic feeding to reduce the risk of feeding intolerance and NEC?

By initiating a 3- to 7-day course of trophic feeding within the first 96 hours after birth,[11] most clinicians assume that preventing villous atrophy with an extended duration of trophic feeding will reduce the risk of feeding intolerance and NEC in preterm infants.[41,52,53] However, data from a recently updated meta-analysis of 14 randomized trials challenge this assumption. In the meta-analysis, early progressive feeding was

Table 1
Randomized trials of early progression of enteral feeding[1]

Study	Year	Study Population	Average GA	Initiation/Progression of Feeding
Ostertag et al,[89]	1986	38 infants with BW < 1500 g	28 wk (range: 26–32)	Initiation and progression on day 1 vs. day 7
Khayata et al,[88]	1987	12 infants with BW < 1500 g		Initiation and progression on day 2 vs. day 5
Davey et al,[85]	1994	62 infants with BW < 2000 g in stable condition	28.5 ± 3 wk	Initiation and progression on day 2 vs. day 5
Karagianni et al,[87]	2010	125 infants with GA 27–34 wk and BW < 10th percentile	31 wk (IQR: 27–34)	Initiation and progression on day 2 vs. day 7
Perez et al,[90]	2011	239 stable infants with GA 27–32 wk and BW < 1500 g	30 ± 2 wk	Initiation and progression on day 2 vs. day 5
Leaf et al,[55]	2012	404 infants with GA <35 wk and BW < 10th percentile	31 ± 2 wk	Initiation and progression on day 2 vs. day 5
Abdelmaaboud et al,[81]	2012	125 infants with GA <37 weeks and BW < 10th percentile	34 ± 3 wk	Initiation and progression on day 3 vs. day 6
Armanian et al,[82]	2013	82 infants with BW < 1500 g	30.5 ± 2 wk	Progression on day 4 vs. day 10
Arnon et al,[83]	2013	60 infants with GA <37 weeks and BW < 10th percentile	32 wk (IQR: 29–34)	Early initiation (<24 h) vs. late initiation
Dinerstein et al,[86]	2013	62 infants with BW < 1500 g	32 wk (IQR: 29–34)	Progression on day 2 vs. day 5
Srinivasan et al,[91]	2017	32 infants with GA < 37 wk and SGA	32 wk (SD: 2)	Progression on day 2 vs. day 5
Salas et al,[56]	2018	60 infants with GA <28 wk	26 wk (IQR: 24–28)	Early initiation (<72 h), progression on day 2 vs. day 5
Tewari et al,[92]	2018	62 infants with GA 27–32 wk and SGA	30 wk (range: 27–32)	Progression on day 1–2 vs. day 5–6
Bozkurt et al,[84]	2020	219 infants with BW < 1251 g	27 wk (range: 29–34)	Progression on day 2 vs. day 6

[1] *Abbreviations:* BW, birthweight; GA, gestational age; IQR, interquartile range; SGA, small for gestational age.

defined as the introduction of small increments of feeding volumes within the first 96 hours after birth. The trials included in the meta-analysis are summarized in **Table 1**.

Compared with delayed progression of feeding (after the first 96 hours), early progressive feeding reduced the time to full enteral feeding by 3 days on average without increasing the risk of NEC (8% vs. 7%; RR: 1.17, 95% CI: 0.80–1.70).[3] Six trials included in the meta-analysis also determined the effects of early progressive feeding on feeding intolerance. Data from 581 infants revealed an increased risk of feeding intolerance with early progressive feeding (51% vs. 41%; RR: 1.22, 95% CI: 1.02–1.46). Seven trials reported sepsis data (n = 872). Early progressive feeding compared to delayed progressive feeding reduced the risk of severe infection (22% vs. 31%; RR: 0.70, 95% CI: 0.56–0.87; P = .001). With an absolute risk reduction of 9% in the sepsis outcome, the number needed to treat with early progressive feeding to prevent one case of severe infection is 11.[3] Because preventing severe infections is more critical than preventing feeding intolerance among preterm infants, the current evidence supports the early progression of enteral feeding volumes within the first 96 hours after birth and questions the benefits of extending the duration of trophic feeding.

Although several trials in the meta-analysis did not include infants at the highest risk of NEC, the largest randomized trial on early progressive feeding included only high-risk preterm infants with evidence of intrauterine growth restriction (n = 404), and another randomized trial included only high-risk preterm infants 28 weeks of gestation or less (n =60). They were not powered for significant outcomes, but the results were consistent with the direction of effect for the outcomes reported in the meta-analysis.[54–56] These randomized clinical trials in infants considered at the highest risk of NEC due to either ischemia or extreme prematurity reported a potential reduction of culture-proven sepsis after early progression of enteral feeding volumes. Among extremely preterm infants, the risk difference in culture-proven sepsis (10% vs. 27%; P = .18) and culture-proven sepsis or death (13% vs. 27%; P = .20) did not reach statistical significance but favored the early progressive feeding group. The outcome of NEC or death did not differ between groups (27% vs. 20%; P = .56).[56]

The meta-analysis concluded that the effects of early progression of feeding volumes on long-term growth or neurodevelopment are unknown.[3] However, early feeding is associated with a lower risk of nosocomial sepsis,[57] mortality, and neurodevelopmental impairment in early childhood.[58] Therefore, it is plausible that early progression of enteral feeding volumes—by reducing sepsis—might reduce mortality and neurodevelopmental impairment in later childhood. Additional evidence from randomized trials on this topic is needed.

Does Slow Progression of Enteral Feeding Prevent Necrotizing Enterocolitis?

In randomized trials, slower rates of feeding progression (10–24 mL/kg/d) have been compared with faster rates (25–40 mL/kg/d). A 2021 Cochrane meta-analysis reviewed the cause–effect relationship between feeding progression rates and NEC risk.[4] The meta-analysis included 4033 infants from 14 randomized trials. Five trials, including the largest randomized trial,[59] enrolled only infants with birthweight less than 1500 g. The remaining trials listed birthweights ranging from less than 1000 g to 1000 to 2000 g as inclusion criteria. One trial included infants with gestational ages between 30 and 34 weeks. Another trial compared 15 mL/kg/d rates versus 35 mL/kg/d rates only in formula-fed infants.[60] Five trials did not include infants receiving formula. The remaining trials included infants receiving some human milk.

No significant differences in the risk of NEC were found between infants fed at slower or faster rates (6% vs. 5%; RR: 1.06, 95% CI: 0.83–1.37). Subgroup analyses of extremely low-birthweight infants, small-for-gestational-age infants, and infants with intrauterine growth found similar results, suggesting the generalizability of the findings to these high-risk populations. The effects of faster feeding progression rates on mortality, growth, neurodevelopment, and other comorbidities were also analyzed. Thirteen trials with mortality data did not find a risk reduction in mortality rates with slower feeding progression rates. Ten trials revealed that infants in the slower feeding progression group took longer to regain birthweight, but the largest randomized trial reported no differences in growth at the time of hospital discharge.[59] The 2021 meta-analysis also found an increased risk of feeding intolerance in infants fed at slower rates, though the certainty of this evidence was graded as low. Four trials reported longer lengths of stay in the group with slower rates.

The Speed of Increasing milk Feeds Trial (SIFT) contributed approximately 70% of the patients in the meta-analysis and was the only one that reported neurodevelopmental outcomes.[59] SIFT was a large, multicenter trial that enrolled 2804 patients across the United Kingdom and the Republic of Ireland. Infants less than 32 weeks of gestation or who had a birthweight of less than 1500 g were eligible and were randomized to receive either slow (18 mL/kg/d) or faster (30 mL/kg/d) feeding progression rates. The primary outcome of the trial was survival without moderate or severe neurodevelopmental disability at 24 months corrected age. Data were available for the primary outcome in 88% of recruited infants. No significant differences in survival or severe or moderate disability were found, but diagnosis of cerebral palsy was more frequent among infants in the faster feeding progression group (5.4% vs. 3.2%; $P = .015$). Infants in the faster feeding progression group reached full enteral feeding sooner and had fewer days of parenteral nutrition. Neither the analysis with all infants (n = 2793) nor the subgroup analysis with extremely preterm infants (n = 994) found an increased risk of NEC in the faster-feeding progression group.

Does, Early, Full Enteral Nutrition Increase the Risk of Necrotizing Enterocolitis?

As noted previously, randomized clinical trials demonstrated that early and faster progression of enteral feeding volumes does not increase the risk of adverse outcomes and may provide benefits in preterm infants.[3,59] With the availability of donated milk and the recognition that intravenous access increases the risk of sepsis, clinical trials have examined early full enteral feedings without requiring intravenous fluids or total parenteral nutrition. So far, 6 randomized clinical trials have been conducted in the past decade, including a combined total of 526 infants.[61]

In these trials, early full enteral feeding was typically defined as feeding volumes of 60 to 80 mL/kg/d beginning soon after birth. The control group received early progressive feeding with advances of 20 to 30 mL/kg/d until the establishment of full enteral feeding. All of these trials were conducted in resource-limited settings in India, and in 4 of the 6 trials, infants with insufficient maternal milk were supplemented with formula, whereas in 2 trials, donated milk was used to supplement maternal milk. None of the 6 trials included in the meta-analysis of randomized clinical trials masked group assignment.

Early full enteral feeding was associated with a higher weight z-score at discharge compared with early progressive feeding (risk difference [RD]: 0.24; 95% CI: 0.06–0.42). Infants in the early full enteral feeding group also regained birth weight faster (mean difference [MD]: −3 days; 95% CI: −4 to −2 days). In the largest randomized clinical trial of 180 very preterm infants, early full enteral feeding increased growth velocity somewhat (mean difference, 1.2 g/kg/d).[62] In the meta-analysis of randomized clinical trials, there was no difference in the rate of feeding intolerance (16% vs. 22%; RR: 0.74; 95% CI: 0.49–1.13; n = 393) or NEC between groups (3% vs. 3%; RR: 0.98; 95% CI: 0.38–2.54; n = 522).[61] There was also no difference in the rate of sepsis between groups (7% vs. 9%; RR: 0.72; 95% CI: 0.36–1.46; n = 359). Furthermore, there was no difference in hospital mortality between the groups (RR: 0.78; 95% CI: 0.36–1.70; n = 526). The practice of early full enteral feeding was associated with a decreased length of stay (mean difference, −3 days; 95% CI, −2 to −4 days).

These trials examined shorter-term hospital outcomes, but later growth and neuro-developmental outcomes were not reported. Overall, these trials included a few extremely preterm infants at the highest risk of adverse outcomes in high-income countries. Besides weight at discharge, anthropometric growth measures were not consistently reported in the included trials. Further trials that supplement maternal milk with donated milk in populations at high risk of NEC are recommended before adopting this practice in high-income countries. There are 2 such ongoing randomized clinical trials comparing early full enteral feeding to conventional feeding progression in the United States (E3NACT trial, NCT04337710) and the United Kingdom (FEED1 trial, ISRCTN89654042).

Does Limiting Enteral Intakes to Up 160 mL/kg/d Reduce the Risk of Necrotizing Enterocolitis?

Higher volume feedings are an emerging strategy to improve postnatal growth without increasing the risk of NEC. Minimum volumes of 120 mL/kg/d and maximum feeding volumes of 200 mL/kg/d have been proposed due to the risks of dehydration and over-hydration, respectively.[63,64] The typical volumes that reduce postnatal growth faltering differ between international guidelines and geographic locations. In North America, feeding volumes of approximately 140 to 160 mL/kg/d of fortified human milk or pre-term formula are typical.[65] Units in Europe, Australia, and New Zealand are more likely to use 161 to 180 mL/kg/d volumes. Few units in high-income countries with access to safe fortification use volumes above 180 mL/kg/d. However, feeding volumes up to 300 mL/kg/d are used internationally and have been reported to improve postnatal growth without evidence of fluid overload.[66]

Fluid overload has been associated with multiple adverse outcomes in preterm infants. In a meta-analysis of randomized clinical trials, restrictive fluid volume reduced the risk of patent ductus arteriosus, necrotizing enterocolitis, and intracranial hemorrhage compared with more liberal use of fluid.[67] Observational studies also report an association between excessive early fluid administration and adverse pulmonary outcomes, including BPD.[68] The proposed mechanism includes maintaining patency of the PDA and pulmonary edema from fluid overload. However, many of the studies of fluid volume reflected the use of early parenteral fluid administration rather than enteral feeding volumes. A randomized clinical trial among 60 preterm infants with bronchopulmonary dysplasia did not demonstrate a benefit of restricting fluids, although the trial was not powered for major neonatal morbidities.[69]

Several randomized clinical trials have compared higher with usual volume feedings in preterm infants.[66,70–72] The usual volume in high-income countries was approximately 140 to 160 mL/kg/d, with a higher volume defined as 180 to 200 mL/kg/d. In contrast, one trial conducted without human milk fortification defined the usual volume as 200 mL/kg/d and the higher volume as 300 mL/kg/d.[66] In a meta-analysis of randomized clinical trials, the authors defined usual volume fortified feedings as ≤180 mL/kg/d and higher volume fortified feedings as greater than 180 mL/kg day and included 2 studies.[73] The trial comparing 200 versus 300 mL/kg/d was included in a separate analysis of higher volume unfortified feedings that used a cut-off of ≤200 mL/kg/d in the lower group and greater than 200 mL/kg/d for the higher group.

Higher volume feedings increased growth velocity in preterm infants compared with usual volume feedings (MD: 2.6 g/kg/d; 95% CI: 1.4–3.8; n = 271). Other growth measures, including length and head circumference, did not differ statistically between groups, although in the largest study (n = 224) of feeding volumes included in the meta-analysis, linear growth, head circumference, and mid-arm circumference were significantly higher at discharge.[70,73] Improvements in postnatal growth failure at discharge did not reach significance (RR: 0.71; 95% CI: 0.50–1.02; n = 271).[73] In a secondary analysis of 86 of the 224 participants in the aforementioned higher volume feeding trial, there was no significant difference in the proportion of fat-free mass or percentage of body fat at discharge, suggesting that the increase in growth with higher volume feedings was not simply due to gains in fat.[74]

Trials of higher volume feedings have not reported increased risks of adverse outcomes. Fluid retention and edema rates did not differ between groups in one trial.[71] The largest trial on higher volume feedings found no difference in rates of PDA, BPD, the duration of respiratory support, or length of stay.[70] One trial reported a decreased length of stay with higher volume feedings in small for gestational age moderate-late preterm infants.[72] Other trials reported no difference in rates of tachypnea or PDA.[66] No difference in rates of NEC or feeding intolerance has been attributed to higher volume feedings after the establishment of full enteral feedings.[73] Limitations of these trials included the lack of masking and different growth measures used. Significantly, none of the studies were powered for major prematurity outcomes, and most included a few extremely preterm infants at the highest risk. Only one study reported neurodevelopmental outcomes, with no difference observed at 12 months of corrected age.[71]

FUTURE DIRECTIONS

There are multiple evidence-based potentially better nutritional practices that may reduce the time to full enteral feeding, reduce the need for parenteral nutrition, reduce the duration of central venous access, lower the risk of sepsis, and even reduce the length of hospital stay. Lack of masking introduces the possibility of bias and differential misclassification that might be expected to favor the traditional delayed and slower introduction of feedings. However, evidence from randomized clinical trials does not suggest that early progressive feeding, faster feeding rates, early full enteral feeding, or higher-volume feeding increase the risk of NEC. The baseline risk of NEC of approximately 3% to 8% in both groups of the clinical trials discussed above suggests a relatively high residual prevalence of NEC unexplained by feeding interventions and a need to investigate the pathogenesis of NEC further.

Although prolonged enteral fasting and the subsequent development of villous atrophy may have exacerbated the risk of NEC attributed to enteral feeding in earlier feeding trials, the increasing practice of exclusive human milk feeding in the latest trials is likely mitigating this risk. Only human milk feeding compared to formula feeding significantly reduces the risk of NEC. A recently updated meta-analysis found a nearly 50% relative risk reduction of NEC with human milk feeding (from 6.8% to 3.6%).[44] There are potential benefits of early and fast progression of enteral feeding, assuming adequate availability of exclusive human milk.[75] Early establishment of full enteral feeding using maternal or donated milk could lower the risk of feeding intolerance, NEC, and sepsis. High-risk preterm infants could benefit from an early progression of enteral feeding volumes by 20 to 25 mL/kg/d, ideally within the first 72 hours after birth. Moderate-risk preterm infants could be started on 30 to 40 mL/kg of enteral feeding within the first 24 hours after birth and have their feeding volumes increased daily by 30 to 40 mL/kg/d. Low-risk preterm infants could benefit from starting full enteral feeding volumes of 60 to 80 mL/kg/d within 24 hours after birth, avoiding the need for parenteral nutrition. This risk stratification strategy could decrease the wide variation in feeding practices.

Multicenter trials of early progressive feeding, full early enteral feeding, and higher volume feeding, including infants at the highest risk of adverse outcomes, are warranted. Without these adequately powered multicenter trials assessing longer-term outcomes of feeding practices, clinicians will continue to develop feeding protocols based on observational studies that are more susceptible to bias than randomized trials.[76] The need and timing of human milk fortification,[77] ideally based on postnatal age rather than volume, will also need further investigation if the goal of early full enteral feeding is achieved with new feeding protocols. Higher enteral protein intake might be required to minimize the risk of cerebral palsy reported in infants exposed to faster feeding rates.[59] Because human milk feeding,[44] probiotic administration,[78] and arginine supplementation[79,80] are the only feeding interventions that have shown superiority for the risk reduction of NEC, future trials should consider noninferiority designs to detect significant differences in the outcome of NEC.

SUMMARY

Preterm infants frequently experience malnutrition in the days and weeks after birth which may be preventable. Increasing energy and protein intake could attenuate critical illness, improve growth, and decrease the risk of short-term and long-term morbidity. The central aim of standardized feeding protocols should be the prevention of cumulative nutritional deficits in critically ill infants. Achieving this aim requires a shift in the current standards of care delivered to these infants. Thousands of preterm infants have been randomized to identify potentially better feeding practices that improve growth without increasing the risk of NEC. Although further randomized controlled trials are anticipated to optimize feeding strategies in the most vulnerable extremely preterm populations, there is sufficient data to standardize nutritional practices and improve growth for most very preterm infants.

Best practices

- High-risk preterm infants could benefit from an early progression of enteral feeding volumes by 20 to 25 mL/kg/d, ideally within the first 72 hours after birth.

- Moderate-risk preterm infants could be started on 30 to 40 mL/kg of enteral feeding within the first 24 hours after birth and have their feeding volumes increased daily by 30 to 40 mL/kg/d.

- Low-risk preterm infants could benefit from starting full enteral feeding volumes of 60 to 80 mL/kg/d within 24 hours after birth, avoiding the need for parenteral nutrition.

DISCLOSURE

The authors have no conflicts of interest relevant to this article to disclose. A.A. Salas received honoraria from the Lockwood Group for participation in Mead Johnson advisory board meetings and filed a patent for an instrumented feeding bottle. He is currently supported by the National Institute of Child Health and Human Development, United States (K23HD102554). C.P. Travers is currently supported by the National Heart, Lung, and Blood Institute, United States (K23HL157618).

REFERENCES

1. Ehrenkranz RA, Das A, Wrage LA, et al. Early nutrition mediates the influence of severity of illness on extremely LBW infants. Pediatr Res 2011;69(6):522–9.

2. Embleton NE, Pang N, Cooke RJ. Postnatal malnutrition and growth retardation: an inevitable consequence of current recommendations in preterm infants? Pediatrics 2001;107(2):270–3.

3. Young L, Oddie SJ, McGuire W. Delayed introduction of progressive enteral feeds to prevent necrotising enterocolitis in very low birth weight infants. Cochrane Database Syst Rev 2022;1:CD001970.

4. Oddie SJ, Young L, McGuire W. Slow advancement of enteral feed volumes to prevent necrotising enterocolitis in very low birth weight infants. Cochrane Database Syst Rev 2021;8:CD001241.

5. Rothman KJ. Epidemiology : an introduction. New York: Oxford University Press; 2002. p. 223, viii.

6. Kamoji VM, Dorling JS, Manktelow B, et al. Antenatal umbilical Doppler abnormalities: an independent risk factor for early onset neonatal necrotizing enterocolitis in premature infants. Acta Paediatr 2008;97(3):327–31.

7. Askie LM, Darlow BA, Finer N, et al. Association between oxygen saturation targeting and death or disability in extremely preterm infants in the neonatal oxygenation prospective meta-analysis collaboration. JAMA 2018;319(21):2190–201.

8. Patel RM, Knezevic A, Shenvi N, et al. Association of red blood cell transfusion, anemia, and necrotizing enterocolitis in very low-birth-weight infants. JAMA 2016; 315(9):889–97.

9. Dierikx TH, Deianova N, Groen J, et al. Association between duration of early empiric antibiotics and necrotizing enterocolitis and late-onset sepsis in preterm infants: a multicenter cohort study. Eur J Pediatr 2022;181(10):3715–24.

10. Swanson JR, Hair A, Clark RH, et al. Spontaneous intestinal perforation (SIP) will soon become the most common form of surgical bowel disease in the extremely low birth weight (ELBW) infant. J Perinatol 2022;42(4):423–9.

11. Salas AA, Kabani N, Travers CP, et al. Short versus extended duration of trophic feeding to reduce time to achieve full enteral feeding in extremely preterm infants: an observational study. Neonatology 2017;112(3):211–6.

12. Klingenberg C, Embleton ND, Jacobs SE, et al. Enteral feeding practices in very preterm infants: an international survey. Arch Dis Child Fetal Neonatal Ed 2012; 97(1):F56–61.

13. Salas AA, Cuna A, Bhat R, et al. A randomised trial of re-feeding gastric residuals in preterm infants. Arch Dis Child Fetal Neonatal Ed 2015;100(3):F224–8.

14. Hans DM, Pylipow M, Long JD, et al. Nutritional practices in the neonatal intensive care unit: analysis of a 2006 neonatal nutrition survey. Pediatrics 2009;123(1):51–7.

15. Mank E, Saenz de Pipaon M, Lapillonne A, et al. Efficacy and safety of enteral recombinant human insulin in preterm infants: a randomized clinical trial. JAMA Pediatr 2022;176(5):452–60.

16. Commare CE, Tappenden KA. Development of the infant intestine: implications for nutrition support. Nutr Clin Pract 2007;22(2):159–73.

17. Carrion V, Egan EA. Prevention of neonatal necrotizing enterocolitis. J Pediatr Gastroenterol Nutr 1990;11(3):317–23.

18. Munkstrup C, Krogfelt KA, Greisen G, et al. Feeding tube practices and the colonisation of the preterm stomach in the first week of life. Dan Med J 2022;69(8).

19. Neu J. Gastrointestinal maturation and implications for infant feeding. Early Hum Dev 2007;83(12):767–75.

20. Parker LA, Weaver M, Murgas Torrazza RJ, et al. Effect of gastric residual evaluation on enteral intake in extremely preterm infants: a randomized clinical trial. JAMA Pediatr 2019;173(6):534–43.

21. Torrazza RM, Parker LA, Li Y, et al. The value of routine evaluation of gastric residuals in very low birth weight infants. J Perinatol 2015;35(1):57–60.
22. Guillet R, Stoll BJ, Cotten CM, et al. Association of H2-blocker therapy and higher incidence of necrotizing enterocolitis in very low birth weight infants. Pediatrics 2006;117(2):e137–42.
23. Jaile JC, Levin T, Wung JT, et al. Benign gaseous distension of the bowel in premature infants treated with nasal continuous airway pressure: a study of contributing factors. AJR Am J Roentgenol 1992;158(1):125–7.
24. Salas AA, Carlo WA, Do BT, et al. Growth rates of infants randomized to continuous positive airway pressure or intubation after extremely preterm birth. J Pediatr 2021;237:148–153 e3.
25. McKeown RE, Marsh TD, Amarnath U, et al. Role of delayed feeding and of feeding increments in necrotizing enterocolitis. J Pediatr 1992;121(5 Pt 1):764–70.
26. Maheshwari A, Corbin LL, Schelonka RL. Neonatal necrotizing enterocolitis. Res Rep Neonatol 2011;1:39–53.
27. Bhatia AM, Feddersen RM, Musemeche CA. The role of luminal nutrients in intestinal injury from mesenteric reperfusion and platelet-activating factor in the developing rat. J Surg Res 1996;63(1):152–6.
28. Hsueh W, Caplan MS, Qu XW, et al. Neonatal necrotizing enterocolitis: clinical considerations and pathogenetic concepts. Pediatr Dev Pathol 2003;6(1):6–23.
29. Lucas A, Bloom SR, Aynsley-Green A. Gut hormones and 'minimal enteral feeding'. Acta Paediatr Scand 1986;75(5):719–23.
30. Slagle TA, Gross SJ. Effect of early low-volume enteral substrate on subsequent feeding tolerance in very low birth weight infants. J Pediatr 1988;113(3):526–31.
31. Morgan J, Bombell S, McGuire W. Early trophic feeding versus enteral fasting for very preterm or very low birth weight infants. Cochrane Database Syst Rev 2013;(3):CD000504.
32. Becerra M, Ambiado S, Kuntsman G, et al. Feeding VLBW infants: effect of early enteral stimulation (EES). Pediatr Res 1996;39:304A.
33. Dunn L, Hulman S, Weiner J, et al. Beneficial effects of early hypocaloric enteral feeding on neonatal gastrointestinal function: preliminary report of a randomized trial. J Pediatr 1988;112(4):622–9.
34. Meetze W, Valentine C, McGuigan J, et al. Gastrointestinal priming prior to full enteral nutrition in very low birth weight infants. J Pediatr Gastroenterol Nutr 1992;15:163–70.
35. Mosqueda E, Sapiegiene L, Glynn L, et al. The early use of minimal enteral nutrition in extremely low birth weight newborns. J Perinatol 2008;28(4):264–9.
36. McClure RJ, Newell SJ. Randomised controlled study of clinical outcome following trophic feeding. Arch Dis Child Fetal Neonatal Ed 2000;82(1):F29–33.
37. Schanler RJ, Shulman RJ, Lau C, et al. Feeding strategies for premature infants: randomized trial of gastrointestinal priming and tube-feeding method. Pediatrics 1999;103(2):434–9.
38. Saenz de Pipaon M, VanBeek RH, Quero J, et al. Effect of minimal enteral feeding on splanchnic uptake of leucine in the postabsorptive state in preterm infants. Pediatr Res 2003;53(2):281–7.
39. Troche B, Harvey-Wilkes K, Engle WD, et al. Early minimal feedings promote growth in critically ill premature infants. Biol Neonate 1995;67(3):172–81.
40. van Elburg RM, van den Berg A, Bunkers CM, et al. Minimal enteral feeding, fetal blood flow pulsatility, and postnatal intestinal permeability in preterm infants with intrauterine growth retardation. Arch Dis Child Fetal Neonatal Ed 2004;89(4):F293–6.

41. Berseth CL, Bisquera JA, Paje VU. Prolonging small feeding volumes early in life decreases the incidence of necrotizing enterocolitis in very low birth weight infants. Pediatrics 2003;111(3):529–34.
42. Engle WD, Lair CS. Early feeding of premature infants questioned. Pediatrics 2004;113(4):931–2.
43. Stoll BJ, Hansen NI, Bell EF, et al. Trends in care practices, morbidity, and mortality of extremely preterm neonates, 1993-2012. JAMA 2015;314(10):1039–51.
44. Quigley M, Embleton ND, McGuire W. Formula versus donor breast milk for feeding preterm or low birth weight infants. Cochrane Database Syst Rev 2019; 7:CD002971.
45. Tiffany KF, Burke BL, Collins-Odoms C, et al. Current practice regarding the enteral feeding of high-risk newborns with umbilical catheters in situ. Pediatrics 2003;112(1 Pt 1):20–3.
46. Havranek T, Johanboeke P, Madramootoo C, et al. Umbilical artery catheters do not affect intestinal blood flow responses to minimal enteral feedings. J Perinatol 2007;27(6):375–9.
47. Clyman R, Wickremasinghe A, Jhaveri N, et al. Enteral feeding during indomethacin and ibuprofen treatment of a patent ductus arteriosus. J Pediatr 2013;163(2): 406–11.
48. Gale C, Modi N, Jawad S, et al. The WHEAT pilot trial-WithHolding Enteral feeds Around packed red cell Transfusion to prevent necrotising enterocolitis in preterm neonates: a multicentre, electronic patient record (EPR), randomised controlled point-of-care pilot trial. BMJ Open 2019;9(9):e033543.
49. Kirpalani H, Bell EF, Hintz SR, et al. Higher or lower hemoglobin transfusion thresholds for preterm infants. N Engl J Med 2020;383(27):2639–51.
50. Patel EU, Head WT, Rohrer A, et al. A quality improvement initiative to standardize time to initiation of enteral feeds after non-surgical necrotizing enterocolitis using a consensus-based guideline. J Perinatol 2022;42(4):522–7.
51. Burdall O, Allin B, Ford K, et al. Association between timing of re-introduction of enteral feeding and short-term outcomes following laparotomy for necrotising enterocolitis. J Pediatr Surg 2022;57(7):1331–5.
52. Henderson G, Craig S, Brocklehurst P, et al. Enteral feeding regimens and necrotising enterocolitis in preterm infants: a multicentre case-control study. Arch Dis Child Fetal Neonatal Ed 2009;94(2):F120–3.
53. Jasani B, Patole S. Standardized feeding regimen for reducing necrotizing enterocolitis in preterm infants: an updated systematic review. J Perinatol 2017; 37(7):827–33.
54. Kempley S, Gupta N, Linsell L, et al. Feeding infants below 29 weeks' gestation with abnormal antenatal Doppler: analysis from a randomised trial. Arch Dis Child Fetal Neonatal Ed 2014;99(1):F6–11.
55. Leaf A, Dorling J, Kempley S, et al. Early or delayed enteral feeding for preterm growth-restricted infants: a randomized trial. Pediatrics 2012;129(5):e1260–8.
56. Salas AA, Li P, Parks K, et al. Early progressive feeding in extremely preterm infants: a randomized trial. Am J Clin Nutr 2018;107(3):365–70.
57. Flidel-Rimon O, Friedman S, Lev E, et al. Early enteral feeding and nosocomial sepsis in very low birthweight infants. Arch Dis Child Fetal Neonatal Ed 2004; 89(4):F289–92.
58. Stoll BJ, Hansen NI, Adams-Chapman I, et al. Neurodevelopmental and growth impairment among extremely low-birth-weight infants with neonatal infection. JAMA 2004;292(19):2357–65.

59. Dorling J, Abbott J, Berrington J, et al. Controlled trial of two incremental milk-feeding rates in preterm infants. N Engl J Med 2019;381(15):1434–43.

60. Rayyis SF, Ambalavanan N, Wright L, et al. Randomized trial of "slow" versus "fast" feed advancements on the incidence of necrotizing enterocolitis in very low birth weight infants. J Pediatr 1999;134(3):293–7.

61. Walsh V, Brown JVE, Copperthwaite BR, et al. Early full enteral feeding for preterm or low birth weight infants. Cochrane Database Syst Rev 2020;12:CD013542.

62. Nangia S, Vadivel V, Thukral A, et al. Early total enteral feeding versus conventional enteral feeding in stable very-low-birth-weight infants: a randomised controlled trial. Neonatology 2019;115(3):256–62.

63. Agostoni C, Buonocore G, Carnielli VP, et al. Enteral nutrient supply for preterm infants: commentary from the European society of paediatric gastroenterology, hepatology and nutrition committee on nutrition. J Pediatr Gastroenterol Nutr 2010;50(1):85–91.

64. Fusch C, Jochum F. Water, sodium, potassium and chloride. World Rev Nutr Diet 2014;110:99–120.

65. Klingenberg C, Muraas FK, Isaksen CE, et al. Growth and neurodevelopment in very preterm infants receiving a high enteral volume-feeding regimen - a population-based cohort study. J Matern Fetal Neonatal Med 2019;32(10):1664–72.

66. Thomas N, Cherian A, Santhanam S, et al. A randomized control trial comparing two enteral feeding volumes in very low birth weight babies. J Trop Pediatr 2012;58(1):55–8.

67. Bell EF, Warburton D, Stonestreet BS, et al. Effect of fluid administration on the development of symptomatic patent ductus arteriosus and congestive heart failure in premature infants. N Engl J Med 1980;302(11):598–604.

68. Oh W, Poindexter BB, Perritt R, et al. Association between fluid intake and weight loss during the first ten days of life and risk of bronchopulmonary dysplasia in extremely low birth weight infants. J Pediatr 2005;147(6):786–90.

69. Fewtrell MS, Adams C, Wilson DC, et al. Randomized trial of high nutrient density formula versus standard formula in chronic lung disease. Acta Paediatr 1997;86(6):577–82.

70. Travers CP, Wang T, Salas AA, et al. Higher- or usual-volume feedings in infants born very preterm: a randomized clinical trial. J Pediatr 2020;224:66–71 e1.

71. Kuschel CA, Evans N, Askie L, et al. A randomized trial of enteral feeding volumes in infants born before 30 weeks' gestation. J Paediatr Child Health 2000;36(6):581–6.

72. Zecca E, Costa S, Barone G, et al. Proactive enteral nutrition in moderately preterm small for gestational age infants: a randomized clinical trial. J Pediatr 2014;165(6):1135–1139 e1.

73. Abiramalatha T, Thomas N, Thanigainathan S. High versus standard volume enteral feeds to promote growth in preterm or low birth weight infants. Cochrane Database Syst Rev 2021;3:CD012413.

74. Salas AA, Travers CP, Jerome ML, et al. Percent body fat content measured by plethysmography in infants randomized to high- or usual-volume feeding after very preterm birth. J Pediatr 2021;230:251–254 e3.

75. Raban S, Santhakumaran S, Keraan Q, et al. A randomised controlled trial of high vs low volume initiation and rapid vs slow advancement of milk feeds in infants with birthweights </= 1000 g in a resource-limited setting. Paediatr Int Child Health 2016;36(4):288–95.

76. Tyson JE, Kennedy KA, Lucke JF, et al. Dilemmas initiating enteral feedings in high risk infants: how can they be resolved? Semin Perinatol 2007;31(2):61–73.
77. Thanigainathan S, Abiramalatha T. Early fortification of human milk versus late fortification to promote growth in preterm infants. Cochrane Database Syst Rev 2020;7:CD013392.
78. Sharif S, Meader N, Oddie SJ, et al. Probiotics to prevent necrotising enterocolitis in very preterm or very low birth weight infants. Cochrane Database Syst Rev 2020;10:CD005496.
79. Polycarpou E, Zachaki S, Tsolia M, et al. Enteral L-arginine supplementation for prevention of necrotizing enterocolitis in very low birth weight neonates: a double-blind randomized pilot study of efficacy and safety. JPEN J Parenter Enteral Nutr 2013;37(5):617–22.
80. Amin HJ, Zamora SA, McMillan DD, et al. Arginine supplementation prevents necrotizing enterocolitis in the premature infant. J Pediatr 2002;140(4):425–31.
81. Abdelmaaboud M, Mohammed A. A randomized controlled trial on early versus late minimal enteral feeding in preterm growth-restricted neonates with abnormal antenatal Doppler studies. J Neonatal Perinatal Med 2012;5(2):1–8.
82. Armanian AM, Mirbod SM, Kazemipour S, Hassanzade A. Comparison of prolonged low volume milk and routine volume milk on incidence of necrotizing enterocolitis in very low birth weight neonates. Pak J Med Sci, 2013;29(1 Suppl):312-316.
83. Arnon S, Sulam D, Konikoff F, et al. Very early feeding in stable small for gestational age preterm infants: a randomized clinical trial. J Pediatr 2013;89(4):388–93.
84. Bozkurt O, Alyamac Dizdar E, Bidev D, et al. Prolonged minimal enteral nutrition versus early feeding advancements in preterm infants with birth weight ≤1250 g: a prospective randomized trial. J Matern Fetal Neonatal Med 2020;25:1–7.
85. Davey AM, Wagner CL, Cox C, Kendig JW. Feeding premature infants while low umbilical artery catheters are in place: a prospective, randomized trial. J Pediatr 1994;124(5 Pt 1):795–9.
86. Dinerstein A, Nieto RM, Solana CL, et al. Early minimal enteral feeding with human milk in very low birth weight infants (VLBW): when to start? Pediatric Academic Societies Annual Meeting 2013;1514:579.
87. Karagianni P, Briana DD, Mitsiakos G, et al. Early versus delayed minimal enteral feeding and risk for necrotizing enterocolitis in preterm growth-restricted infants with abnormal antenatal Doppler results. Am J Perinatol 2010;27(5):367–73.
88. Khayata S, Gutcher G, Bamberger J, Heimler R. Early versus late feeding of low birth weight (LBW) infants: effect on growth and hyperbilirubinemia. Pediatr Res 1987;21:431A.
89. Ostertag SG, LaGamma EF, Reisen CE, Ferrentino FL. Early enteral feeding does not affect the incidence of necrotizing enterocolitis. Pediatrics 1986;77(3):275–80.
90. Pérez LA, Pradilla GL, Díaz G, Bayter SM. Necrotising enterocolitis among preterm newborns with early feeding. Biomédica 2011;31(4):485–91.
91. Srinivasan A, Nanavati RN, Kabra NS. Comparison of feeding regimens in preterm neonates with abnormal antenatal Doppler: a randomised controlled trial. Glob J Res Anal 2017;6(4):44–7.
92. Tewari VV, Dubey SK, Kumar R, et al. Early versus late enteral feeding in preterm intrauterine growth restricted neonates with antenatal doppler abnormalities: an open-label randomized trial. J Trop Pediatr 2018;64(1):4–14.

Human Milk Fortification for Very Preterm Infants
Toward Optimal Nutrient Delivery, Neonatal Intensive Care Unit Growth, and Long-Term Outcomes

Saharnaz Talebiyan, MD[a], Mandy Brown Belfort, MD, MPH[a,b,*]

KEYWORDS

- Neonatal • Enteral nutrition • Fortification • Macronutrients • Preterm infant
- Growth

KEY POINTS

- Human milk is the recommended diet for virtually all newborns, including those born very preterm at less than 32 weeks of gestation and/or very low birth weight (VLBW) at less than 1500 g.
- Human milk must be fortified during the neonatal intensive care unit (NICU) hospitalization to meet infant nutrient requirements.
- Existing approaches to human milk fortification include standard and adjustable approaches, whereas individually targeted fortification is a novel approach that uses human milk analysis at the point-of-care to identify and eliminate gaps in protein and energy delivery.
- Emerging data from randomized controlled trials suggest that some approaches to individually targeted fortification may be effective in closing nutrient intake gaps and improving growth in the NICU.

Funding Source: Dr M.B. Belfort is supported by the National Institutes of Health, United State (R01HD097327).
Financial Disclosure: The authors have no financial relationships relevant to this article to disclose.
Conflict of Interest: The authors have no conflicts of interest to disclose.
[a] Department of Pediatric Newborn Medicine, Brigham and Women's Hospital, 221 Longwood Avenue BL-341, Boston, MA 02115, USA; [b] Harvard Medical School, Boston, MA, USA
* Corresponding author. Department of Pediatric Newborn Medicine, Brigham and Women's Hospital, 221 Longwood Avenue BL-341, Boston, MA 02115.
E-mail address: mbelfort@bwh.harvard.edu

INTRODUCTION

The past decade has seen an increasing emphasis on breastfeeding and human milk, including in high-income countries, due to myriad health benefits for infants and mothers.[1] One specific setting in which human milk is strongly recommended is the neonatal intensive care unit (NICU), where human milk serves as the primary diet for very preterm (<32 weeks' gestation) and very low birth weight (VLBW, <1500 g) infants, due to short-term and long-term health and developmental benefits that are unique to this population.[2] In this context, human milk, as compared with infant formula, is well-tolerated,[3] reduces the risk of necrotizing enterocolitis,[4,5] and is associated with improved neurodevelopmental outcomes in infancy and childhood.[6,7]

The third trimester of pregnancy is a critical period for brain growth and development in the fetus. Due to an abrupt interruption of gestation at the time of very preterm birth and the need for intensive care technologies to support physiologic functions, very preterm infants experience this critical period in NICU environment. There, extrauterine sources of nutrition must support the rapid growth and development of the brain, processes that would normally occur in utero.[8] Nutrition may also play a role in recovery from perinatal brain injury to which this population is vulnerable.[9] During this period of neonatal hospitalization, human milk must be fortified to meet recommended macronutrient and micronutrient intakes,[10] which are estimated from fetal nutrient accretion rates and are substantially higher than those of full-term infants.

Within clinical practice, a major challenge to meeting nutrient intake requirements is the variability in maternal milk composition, both between individual mothers and within the same mother over time. This variability is driven by many factors, including gestational age at delivery, lactation duration, maternal diet, genetic factors,[11-13] and milk handling.[14,15] Additionally, pasteurized donor milk, which is the preferred alternative to preterm formula when maternal milk is in short supply or unavailable, is often lower in protein, fat, and energy than maternal milk.[16] Variable macronutrient content is clinically important. For example, infants fed with milk that is lower in protein demonstrate slower linear growth despite routine fortification,[17] suggesting that infants whose mother's milk is low in protein content could benefit from additional protein intake via fortification.

Common approaches to human milk fortification for very preterm infants in the NICU are standard fortification, in which a fixed dose of commercial multicomponent human milk fortifier is added to milk, and adjustable fortification, in which more protein and/or fat are added above the multicomponent fortifier based on low blood urea nitrogen (BUN) levels and/or growth faltering. Although effective in supporting growth[18,19] and highly feasible in clinical practice, these approaches may leave nutrient intake gaps for infants who receive milk with a nutrient content that is consistently below the reference.

In this article, we will (1) review standard and adjustable fortification strategies and (2) describe the rationale and synthesize emerging evidence, including several randomized, controlled trials (RCTs), for a new, individually targeted approach to human milk fortification in the NICU. Individually targeted approaches designed to reduce macronutrient intake gaps have the potential to improve growth and other nutrition-related outcomes, including neurodevelopment, in the nutritionally vulnerable very preterm and VLBW infant population. Although ensuring adequate intakes of both macronutrients and micronutrients is important, here we focus only on macronutrients because they are the target of existing and feasible individualized fortification strategies.

STANDARD AND ADJUSTABLE FORTIFICATION

International consensus-based guidelines recommend fortifying human milk with protein, fat, and/or carbohydrates, in addition to micronutrients, to support postnatal growth in very preterm and VLBW infants.[2,10,20,21] Two common approaches in clinical practice include standard fortification and adjustable fortification as reviewed recently[22] and briefly described here.

Standard fortification is practiced in neonatal units worldwide and involves adding a fixed dose of a commercial multicomponent fortifier to a specific volume of maternal or donor human milk, as per instructions on the product label. In lower-resource settings, infant formula powder may be used to fortify milk.[23] Existing commercial human milk fortifiers differ from each other in several ways, including their form (powder vs liquid), content and composition of protein (partially or extensively hydrolyzed), and balance of energy sources (fat vs carbohydrates).[24] Standard fortification is effective in promoting increased physical growth during the neonatal hospitalization. A Cochrane meta-analysis[25] of data from 14 clinical trials found that standard fortification, as compared with no fortification, increased weight gain by 1.8 g/kg/d (95% confidence interval [CI], 1.3, 1.2). The effect of fortification on weight gain was greater (2.2 g/kg/d, 95% CI, 1.5, 2.8) for trials including only very preterm or VLBW infants. Standard fortification is also effective in improving linear growth (meta-analysis estimate, 0.11 more cm/wk, 95% CI 0.08, 0.15) and head growth (0.06 more cm/wk, 95% CI 0.03, 0.08) as compared with no fortification. Fixed-dose standard fortification is straightforward to implement, even in settings without specialized expertise in neonatal dietetics, access to modular fortifiers, and/or staff available to prepare customized diets. However, standard fortification approaches fall short of optimal protein and/or energy intake for some individual infants with low intrinsic milk nutrient content and/or high nutrient requirements due to clinical illness or other factors. Overall, standard fortification approaches are effective in promoting average growth within a population, as compared with no fortification, and are straightforward to implement with commercially available products but may leave nutrient intake gaps for some individuals.

An alternative approach is *adjustable fortification*. This method builds on standard fortification by allowing for individualized adjustment of protein and/or energy intakes. As originally described,[18,26] adjustable fortification involves tracking serial BUN levels to indicate an infant's metabolic response to protein intake and guide adjustments in protein provision to ensure adequate intake while minimizing toxicity. Despite a lack of data on the optimal target level for BUN, this approach is effective in increasing weight gain and head growth, as compared with standard fortification while avoiding toxicity associated with excess protein intake.[27–29] In addition to short-term growth benefits, 2 small studies found higher neurodevelopmental scores in infants who received adjustable as compared with standard protein fortification.[30,31] An updated adjustable fortification protocol specifies target BUN levels of 10 to 16 mg/100 mL; levels below this range should prompt increased protein provision, whereas levels above this range indicate potential protein excess.[32,33]

The concept of adjustable fortification can be extended to include adjustment of protein intake for slow weight gain in combination with low BUN,[34] the inclusion of other biochemical markers such as prealbumin,[30] and the adjustment of protein and/or energy intakes for slow weight gain even without specific biochemical criteria. As compared with standard fortification, implementation of adjustable fortification requires additional blood sampling to trend biochemical markers, more specialized clinical expertise, and access to more nutritional products such as modular protein and energy fortifiers. Overall, evidence regarding the effectiveness of adjustable fortification in promoting early growth and potentially neurodevelopment suggests that investments to support adjustable fortification are worthwhile.

A limitation of both standard and adjustable fortification strategies involves the intrinsic variability in human milk composition, particularly protein and fat. Failing to address this variability leaves potential nutrient intake gaps for infants whose human milk is consistently low in protein and/or energy, and/or imbalanced in protein and energy content.[35-37] This concept is addressed in a new approach, individually targeted human milk fortification.

INDIVIDUALLY TARGETED FORTIFICATION
Overview

Human milk analysis techniques have evolved considerably over time (**Box 1**) but, until recently, their application in clinical settings was limited due to the need for substantial laboratory infrastructure. The "creamatocrit" was the first bedside technique for human milk analysis. This approach accurately estimates the caloric density of milk[38] but does not provide information about protein content. More recently, point-of-care analysis of all 3 human milk macronutrients (fat, protein, and carbohydrates) has become available, opening the door to clinical approaches that measure human milk composition in near real-time[39] and target protein, fat, and/or carbohydrates content to ensure that recommended daily intakes are reached. Fortification can also be targeted to achieve desired nutrient ratios. The effectiveness of individually targeted fortification, as compared with standard and/or adjustable fortification, can be evaluated in terms of nutrient delivery, short-term clinical outcomes such as postnatal growth, and longer term outcomes such as neurodevelopment.

To date, 10 published RCTs have evaluated the effectiveness of targeted human milk fortification (**Table 1**). These studies differ from each other in several ways. For example, some studies targeted fortification of only protein or only fat, whereas others targeted all 3 macronutrients. Some studies compared targeted fortification to standard, fixed-dose fortification, whereas others compared targeted to

---

Box 1
Historical perspective

Published reports of human milk composition and analysis date back to the nineteenth century. In 1847, Donne[57] described human milk as an emulsion with main components of "caseum" (protein), sugar (carbohydrate), and fat globules. He further proposed that milk volume and milk composition were both important criteria by which to judge the quality of milk produced by a wet nurse. Around the same time, Griffiths[58] identified changes in milk composition over time during lactation and proposed that the composition of the maternal diet also influenced the composition of milk. More recently, in 1978, Lucas and colleagues applied the technique of Fleet and Linzell[59] to estimated goat's milk fat with a hematocrit centrifuge and a standard glass capillary tube to determine human milk fat content and named it "Creamatocrit."[38] Within the dairy industry, by the late twentieth century, infrared milk analyzers were used widely to ensure high-quality cow's milk production.[60] Human milk scientists looking for an accurate method to analyze human milk in the clinical setting sought to apply these dairy industry approaches. For example, in 1988, Michaelsen and colleagues[61] showed that industrial infrared analyzers could accurately analyze human milk macronutrients in a single operation, although lactose was inaccurately measured due to interference from human milk oligosaccharides, which are not present in cow's milk. In 2018, the Food and Drug Administration approved for clinical use the first point-of-care human milk analyzer, a midinfrared spectroscopy device (MIRIS, Uppsala, Sweden).[62]

Table 1
Randomized trials of individually targeted human milk fortification: key aspects of study design

1st Author, Year, Country	Population Sample Size	Blinding	Milk Type	Frequency of Milk Analysis	Analyzer	Intervention Target(s)	Intervention Duration	Primary Growth Outcome(s)
Hair et al,[45] 2014, USA	BW 750–1250g n = 78	No	MM DM	Daily	Spectrastar NIR	Fat	Unspecified	Weight, length, HC velocity
McLeod et al,[47] 2016, Australia	GA ≤30 wk n = 40	Yes	MM DM	Weekly	Miris MIR	Protein, fat, carbohydrate	3 wk (Minimum)	Weight, length, and HC Weight gain velocity Body fat percent[a]
Maas et al,[46] 2017, Germany	GA <32 wk BW < 1500g n = 60	Partial	MM Formula	2x/week	Miris MIR	Protein, fat	Unspecified	Weight gain velocity
Agakidou et al,[40] 2019, Greece	BW < 1500 g GA = 25–32 wk n = 48	No	MM	Weekly	Milkoscan MIR	Protein	Unspecified	IGF-I and ghrelin plasma levels Weight, length, HC, BMI
Kadioglul et al,[43] 2019, Turkey	GA ≤32 wk BW ≤ 1500 g n = 60	Yes	MM	2x/week	Miris MIR	Protein	4 wk	Weight, length, HC gain
Bulut et al,[44] 2020, Turkey	GA ≤32 wk n = 32	No	MM	Daily	Miris MIR	Protein	4 wk	Weight, length, HC gain
Brion et al,[48] 2020, USA	GA<29 or <35 wk and SGA n = 120	Yes	MM DM	Daily	Spectrastar NIR	Protein, fat, carbohydrate	Unspecified	Weight gain, linear growth velocity

(continued on next page)

Table 1
(continued)

1st Author, Year, Country	Population Sample Size	Blinding	Milk Type	Frequency of Milk Analysis	Analyzer	Intervention Target(s)	Intervention Duration	Primary Growth Outcome(s)
Parat et al,[41] 2020, USA	BW < 1500 g n = 36	No	MM DM	Weekly	Calais MIR	Protein	Unspecified	Fat-free mass, body fat percent[a]
Quan et al,[42] 2020, China	BW = 800–1800g GA <34 wk n = 51	Yes	MM	2x/week	Miris MIR	Protein	10 d (Minimum)	Weight gain velocity
Rochow et al,[49] 2021, Canada	GA <30 wk n = 103	Yes	MM DM	3x/week	Spectrastar NIR	Protein, fat, carbohydrate	21 d (14 d minimum)	Weight gain velocity

Abbreviations: BW, birth weight; DM, donor milk; GA, gestational age; HC, head circumference; MIR, mid-infrared; MM, mother milk; NIR, near-infrared; wk, week
[a] Body composition measured with air displacement plethysmography.[56]

adjustable approaches. In terms of outcomes, all studies examined nutrient delivery and short-term weight gain, whereas some also focused on other aspects of growth, such as body length and/or body composition, biochemical markers, and/or growth-related hormones. Here, we review, contrast, and synthesize the existing published literature on individually targeted human milk fortification in the NICU setting.

Protein-Targeted Fortification

Five RCTs have evaluated the effectiveness of individually targeting protein fortification without targeting fat or other nutrients. Of these studies, 3 studies[40–42] compared protein-targeted fortification with standard, fixed-dose fortification using commercial human milk fortifier (HMF), 1 study[43] compared protein-targeted fortification with adjustable fortification, and 1 study[44] compared protein-targeted fortification with both standard and adjustable fortification (**Table 2**). It is useful to examine how average daily protein intakes differed both within and between studies due to study-specific differences in how milk was analyzed and fortified in control and intervention groups. In comparing protein-targeted fortification with standard fortification, Parat and colleagues[41] reported delivering, on average 4.1 g/kg/d of protein in the intervention group, which was substantially higher than the standard fortification group (3.1 g/kg/d). Similarly, Kadioglu and colleagues[43] reported an average of 4.5 g/kg/d in the intervention group as compared with 3.6 g/kg/d in the standard group. In contrast, Quan and colleagues[42] reported similar average protein intakes between groups (2.8 g/kg/d targeted vs 2.7 g/kg/d standard); notably, absolute enteral intakes in both groups fell short of current recommendations, possibly due to the more prolonged use of parenteral nutrition in that study. Agakidou and colleagues[40] also reported similar protein intakes between groups (4.0 g/kg/d targeted vs 4.2 g/kg/d standard); note that the intervention group received slightly *less* protein than the standard fortification group. Of 2 studies that compared protein delivery in targeted as compared with adjustable approaches, Bulut and colleagues[44] reported higher protein intake in the targeted group (4.5 vs 4.0 g/kg/d), and Kadioglu and colleagues[43] reported an average protein intake of 4.3 g/kg/d in the adjustable fortification group, which was intermediate between standard and targeted groups. Considered together, these studies indicate that individually targeting protein fortification sometimes, but not always, leads to higher average protein intakes as compared with standard or adjustable fortification. Additionally, even with targeted fortification, recommended average intakes may not be achieved.

Given observed differences in protein delivery, it is not surprising that weight gain also differed between groups in some but not all studies. Of the 3 studies that reported higher average protein intake in the targeted fortification group,[41,43,44] all reported improved growth outcomes: Parat and colleagues[41] found higher body length, flank skin fold thickness, and fat-free mass in the intervention group; Kadioglu and colleagues[43] found faster weight gain, linear growth, and head growth; and Bulut and colleagues[44] found faster weight gain and head growth. In contrast, both studies that reported similar average protein intake between groups also reported no difference in growth outcomes.[40,42] An exception is that Quan and colleagues[42] reported more rapid weight gain in the third week of the study within the targeted group, possibly a chance finding given the large number of outcomes assessed. Considered together, these studies illustrate that when targeted fortification shifts the average protein intake higher than standard fortification, average growth outcomes are also improved; in contrast, when targeted fortification fails to deliver higher average protein, growth outcomes are no different.

Table 2
Randomized trials of individually targeted human milk fortification: summary of main results

Intervention Target(s)	First Author	Control Approach	Results: Nutrient (g/kg/d) or Energy (Kcal/kg/d) Intakes Reported as Mean ± SD or Median (IQR)		Results: Growth Outcomes
			Control	Intervention	
Protein	Agakidou et al,[40] 2019	SF with multicomponent bovine HMF	Protein, 4.2 ± 0.4 Energy, 130 ± 9	Protein, 4.0 ± 0.3 Energy, 124 ± 9	No difference
	Parat et al,[41] 2020	SF with multicomponent bovine HMF	Protein, 3.1 ± 0.3 Energy, 117 ± 8	Protein, 4.1 ± 0.3 Energy, 107 ± 9	↑Flank skin-fold thickness, ↑fat-free mass nearly significant
	Quan et al,[42] 2020	SF with multicomponent bovine HMF	Protein, 2.7 ± 0.7 Energy,[a] 2336 (1706; 3122)	Protein, 2.8 ± 0.8 Energy,[a] 2249 (1659; 3660)	No difference
	Bulut et al,[44] 2020	AF with multicomponent bovine HMF + additional protein based on BUN	Protein, 4.0 ± 0.3 Energy, 144 ± 10	Protein, 4.5 ± 0.04 Energy, 145 ± 5.4	↑Weight, ↑HC
	Kadioglu et al,[43] 2019	SF with multicomponent bovine HMF / AF with multicomponent bovine HMF + additional protein based on BUN	Median protein, 3.6 Energy, 128 Median protein, 4.3 Energy, 131	Median protein, 4.5 Energy, 133	↑Weight, length, HC
Fat (human milk cream)	Hair et al,[45] 2014	SF with multicomponent human HMF	Not reported	Not reported	↑Weight and length gain velocity
Protein, fat	Maas et al,[46] 2016	SF with multicomponent bovine HMF + protein supplement	Protein, 3.5 ± 0.35 Energy, 129 ± 11	Protein, 4.1 ± 0.39 Energy, 130 ± 9	No difference
Protein, fat, carbohydrate	McLeod et al,[47] 2016	SF with multicomponent bovine HMF for non–fluid-restricted infants + additional protein and energy for fluid-restricted infants	Protein, 3.4 ± 0.5 Fat, 6.8 ± 1 Carbs, 13.5 ± 0.9 Energy, 129 ± 11	Protein, 3.3 ± 0.4 Fat, 6.8 ± 0.9 Carbs, 12.9 ± 1.1 Energy, 125 ± 11	No difference in growth or body composition outcomes

Brion et al,[48] 2020	AF with multicomponent bovine HMF + additional protein and energy based on weight gain, linear growth, BUN	Protein, 3.5 (0.6; 5.5) Energy, 115 (23, 173)	Protein, 3.3 (0.4; 5.1) Energy, 103 (14; 162)	No difference
Rochow et al,[49] 2021	SF with multicomponent bovine HMF	Protein, 3.6 ± 0.4 Fat, 7.1 ± 0.9 Carbs, 10.8 ± 0.8 Energy, 121 ± 10	Protein, 4.5 ± 0.3 Fat, 7.6 ± 0.9 Carbs, 13.6 ± 0.8 Energy, 140 ± 10	↑WGV ↑Body fat mass

Abbreviations: AF, adjustable fortification; HC, head circumference; HM, human milk; HMF, human milk fortifier; MM, mother milk; SF, standard fortification; TF, targeted fortification; WGV, weight gain velocity.

[a] Reported as total energy intake (Kcal/kg) from parenteral and enteral sources over entire study period.

Fat-Targeted Fortification

Only one study examined the effect of targeting energy intake through fat fortification. The intervention of Hair and colleagues[45] involved adding a human milk cream supplement targeting 20 kcal/ounce in the native milk, alongside standard fortification with multicomponent human HMF. That study did not report mean fat or energy intakes. Although 85% of participants in the intervention group received the cream supplement, how much additional fat or energy and on how many days was also not reported. The intervention group showed greater weight gain (14.0 vs 12.4 g/kg/d) and linear growth (1.0 vs 0.8 cm/wk), suggesting that the additional energy drove healthy tissue accretion rather than simply excess adiposity.

Protein and Fat-Targeted Fortification

Only one published study has examined targeting both protein and fat. Maas and colleagues[46] compared 3 groups: (1) a standard fortification, lower protein group receiving approximately 3.5 g/kg/d; (2) a fixed-dose higher protein group receiving 4.5 g/kg/d; and (3) an individually targeted higher protein group in which protein was targeted to 4.5 g/kg/d for infants weighing less than 1500 g and 4.0 g/kg/d for infants weighing 1500 g or more. Additionally, fat was individually targeted to meet a minimum of 4.8 g/kg/d. Primary analyses focused on differences between the lower protein group and the combined higher protein groups. In exploratory analyses comparing the fixed-dose higher protein group with the individually targeted higher protein group, protein intake was higher in the fixed-dose group (4.5 vs 4.2 g/kg/d), more variable (SD 0.3 vs 0.2), and less closely matched with the body weight-specific targets. Energy intakes (137 vs 140 kcal/kg/d) and weight gain (16.0 g/kg/d vs 16.1 g/kg/d) were similar between these higher protein groups. Overall, this study found that the protein delivery was not higher but was more closely matched to the specified targets with individually targeted fortification; average growth outcomes were not improved.

Protein, Fat, and Carbohydrates Targeted Fortification

Three published RCTs[47–49] have individually targeted all 3 macronutrients (protein, fat, and carbohydrates). Of these, only one reported substantial increases in nutrient delivery and weight gain. Rochow and colleagues[49] compared standard, fixed-dose fortification with individually targeted fortification to 3.0 g/dL protein, 4.4 g/dL fat, and 8.3 g/dL carbohydrates, intended to meet ESPGHAN[20] recommendations for intakes when fed at 150 mL/kg/d. Macronutrient intakes were higher in the intervention group (protein: 4.5 vs 3.6 g/kg/d, fat: 7.6 vs 7.1 g/kg/d, and carbohydrates: 13.6 vs 10.8 g/kg/d). Weight gain velocity (21.2 vs 19.3 g/kg/d), final weight at 36 weeks (2510 vs 2290g), and fat mass (608 vs 486 g) were also all higher in the intervention group. Differences between intervention and control groups were strongest in magnitude among infants with lower as compared with higher protein content in native milk, as discussed below. Additionally, infants with lower native milk protein content who received the intervention had higher fat-free mass (1946 vs 1744 g) at 36 weeks as compared with control infants. Overall, in this study, individually targeted fortification increased nutrient delivery and weight gain; the intervention was more effective for infants with low native milk protein content and led to higher fat-free mass at 36 weeks only in that group.

Two studies found no benefit of individually targeting all 3 macronutrients. McLeod and colleagues[47] provided variable amounts of multicomponent HMF, protein powder, and a carbohydrate-based energy supplement based on milk analysis and fluid allowance (restricted vs nonrestricted). The control group received a standard fixed dose of HMF, with additional protein and energy provided if fluid intake was restricted. Intakes of all macronutrients were similar between groups. Notably, average protein intake was 3.3 g/kg/d in the intervention group and 3.4 g/kg/d in the control group, both below recommended levels. Growth outcomes were not different between groups. Brion and colleagues[48] compared "optimized" (adjustable fortification based on infant's growth rate and serum biochemical markers) and "experimental" (individualized based on serial daily milk nutrient analysis results, then "optimized") groups. Results neither indicated statistical differences in average enteral protein or energy intakes between the "optimized" control group and the interventional group (protein: 3.5 vs 3.3 g/kg/d, energy: 115 vs 103 kcal/kg/d, respectively) nor observed differences in weight gain or other growth parameter. Of note, human milk comprised only 23% to 27% of enteral feedings in this study, with the remainder provided as formula.

DISCUSSION

Human milk must be fortified to meet nutrient requirements for growing very preterm and VLBW infants but the optimal approach to fortification is unknown. In this review, we have presented the rationale for individually targeted fortification of human milk in the NICU setting and summarized the published randomized trials that have investigated this approach to date. Considered together, published studies clearly demonstrate that individually targeted fortification is not a single approach. Rather, the term indicates a general approach to fortification that involves the application of real-time or nearly real-time human milk analysis to tailor protein and/or energy fortification for individual infants by accounting for the composition of their mother's milk and/or donor milk rather than relying on published reference values.

The details of how milk composition was analyzed and how the information was used varied markedly across studies. Studies also varied widely in the alternative approach to which individually targeted fortification was compared, and in other site-specific aspects of nutritional management in both intervention and control groups. Given these differences, it is not surprising that across studies, results differed markedly in terms of absolute nutrient delivery in intervention and control groups, as well as in whether between-group differences were seen in nutrient delivery and/or growth outcomes. Here, we distill factors that influenced study results, highlight clinical implications, and propose future research directions.

A key premise for individualized fortification is that intrinsic variation in human milk composition leads to cumulative between-infant differences in macronutrient intakes over time, most importantly below-target intakes occurring in those infants whose individual mother's milk is consistently low in nutrients. Another premise is that an upper limit exists to how much milk can be fortified routinely (eg, without knowledge of actual milk composition) to avoid toxicity associated with excess nutrient delivery above the acceptable range for those infants whose individual mother's milk is relatively high in nutrients. Standard fixed-dose fortification is intended to increase average nutrient delivery at a population level while remaining within the acceptable range for all infants, whereas individually targeted fortification is intended to benefit infants "at the margins," specifically infants whose individual mother's milk is lower than the reference values who can safely receive more fortification than the average infant.

Only one study explicitly addressed the fundamental concept that, by design, individually targeted fortification will mainly benefit infants with low nutrient milk. Rochow and colleagues[49] reported nutrient delivery and growth outcomes stratified by native milk protein content (low, mean 1 g/dL; high, mean 1.3–1.4 g/dL). In the low native milk protein group, the targeted fortification group received 1.2 g/kg/d more protein than the standard group, whereas in the high native milk protein group, the targeted group received only 0.8 g/kg/d more protein than the standard group. Growth outcomes aligned with the observed differences in protein delivery. In the high native milk protein group, body weight was 108 g higher in the targeted versus standard fortification group, whereas in the low native milk protein group, body weight was only 340 g higher. Importantly, only the low native milk protein group experienced an increase in fat-free mass with the intervention. This study emphasizes that individually targeted fortification mainly benefits infants whose nutrient intake is low due to low nutrient content in maternal milk. Future studies should report results stratified by intrinsic milk composition to reveal the full extent to which individually targeted fortification leads to higher nutrient intakes and/or growth outcomes in those infants it is designed to benefit.

It is notable that some studies[41,43–45,49] reported that targeted fortification resulted in substantially higher average protein and/or energy delivery than control fortification, whereas other studies reported similar or even lower average delivery in individually targeted as compared with control groups.[40,42,46–48] In theory, 3 key and related aspects of study design determine the extent to which average nutrient delivery will differ between individually targeted and control approaches: (1) the assumed (eg, reference) values for milk composition used under the control approach and how these values differ from actual measured milk composition; (2) the average actual nutrient delivery provided under the control approach and how this differs from the intended nutrient delivery; and (3) the choice of targets for milk composition and/or nutrient delivery under the individually targeted approach. A few examples illustrate these points.

Regarding assumed versus actual composition, McLeod and colleagues[47] assumed a reference value of 1.4 g/dL for protein, whereas the actual measured average protein content was 1.6 g/dL. As a result, the control group, whose milk was fortified based on the lower assumed reference value received *more* protein on average than the intervention group. Not surprisingly, there was no benefit of the individually targeted approach in terms of growth or body composition outcomes. Maas and colleagues[46] used a fixed-dose of protein fortifier to target 4.5 g/kg/d in a standard high protein control group using a reference value of 1.3 g/dL of milk protein. Individually targeting protein based on measured milk protein values of 1.6 g/dL at week 2 and 1.1 g/dL at week 4 resulted in less delivered protein (4.3 g/kg/d). Considered together, these examples illustrate that when reference values are lower than measured values, targeted fortification can result in lower nutrient delivery than standard, fixed-dose fortification.

In terms of nutrient delivery under the control approach and choice of targets, Parat and colleagues[41] reported delivering only 3.1 g/kg/d of protein with standard fixed-dose fortification using commercial multicomponent human milk fortifier, although notably protein delivery in this control group was calculated with an assumed reference value because milk was not directly analyzed. The intervention targeted 4 g/kg/d using a liquid protein fortifier, and this target was achieved on average, implying that many infants in the intervention group received additional protein over and above the standard fixed-dose fortifier. Under those conditions, simply adding a fixed dose of liquid protein fortifier as part of standard fortification might have been an effective and more straightforward way to meet the target protein delivery in many infants.

Individually targeting fortification requires a substantial investment of resources, including the purchase and maintenance of specialized equipment and staff training, and effort to sample and analyze milk and prepare specialized diets. Targeting multiple macronutrients is more labor intensive than targeting just protein or fat. Additionally, the frequency with which milk is analyzed contributes to the labor intensity, a concept that

Rochow and colleagues[50] addressed in a study that concluded that analyzing milk 3 times per week was the optimal frequency with respect to variability in milk composition. Costs of individually targeted fortification have not yet been explicitly measured or reported, nor has any study compared clinical outcomes across individually targeted approaches that are more versus less labor intensive. Additionally, the extent to which patient families prefer and/or value different strategies is a knowledge gap. Future work to quantify costs, benefits, and overall value of various individually targeted, standard, and adjustable approaches to fortification will be helpful to decision-makers.

A major rationale for optimizing nutritional support in the NICU is to support brain development during a critical period. More rapid weight gain, linear growth, and head growth in the NICU predict better neurodevelopmental outcomes,[51] and higher fat-free mass correlates with larger total and regional brain volumes and predicts neurodevelopment.[52–54] Therefore, growth and body composition represent reasonable short-term outcomes for studies of human milk fortification, although they are not perfect proxies. It is notable that to date, no study of individually targeted fortification has measured or compared long-term neurodevelopmental outcomes. Our in-progress RCT will help to address this gap by assessing brain development with MRI and neurodevelopmental outcomes through 2 years of corrected age in infants receiving individually targeted as compared with adjustable fortification.[55]

SUMMARY

Studies published in the past decade reveal mounting interest in the application of point-of-care human milk analysis to clinical fortification strategies in the NICU setting. Individualized human milk fortification holds promise as an approach to ensure target nutrient delivery for individual infants whose mother's milk is low in nutrients while avoiding toxicity for infants whose mother's milk is high in nutrients. We have identified many design elements that differ across studies and contribute to differences in results. Unfortunately, many studies do not explicitly state each of these inputs to their design. Standards for reporting of design and results would allow for greater insights into which approaches are most effective in closing nutrient intake gaps, and especially which approaches add value over standard and/or adjustable approaches that do not involve labor-intensive human milk analysis. Future studies should continue to focus on short-term growth outcomes, including fat-free mass as an indicator of healthy growth that correlates with brain development, while also evaluating long-term outcomes of neurodevelopment. Given the many remaining knowledge gaps, more research is needed before human milk analysis should be recommended for routine clinical care in the NICU.

Best practices box

- Human milk is the optimal diet for virtually all very preterm infants. Donor milk should be used if maternal milk is in short supply or unavailable. Milk should be fortified with a commercial multicomponent human milk fortifier, and additional protein and/or energy provided for growth faltering.

REFERENCES

1. Victora CG, Bahl R, Barros AJD, et al. Breastfeeding in the 21st century: epidemiology, mechanisms, and lifelong effect. The Lancet (British edition) 2016; 387(10017):475–90.

2. Parker MG, Stellwagen LM, Noble L, et al. Promoting human milk and breastfeeding for the very low birth weight infant. Pediatrics 2021;148(5). https://doi.org/10.1542/peds.2021-054272.

3. Sisk PM, Lovelady CA, Gruber KJ, et al. Human milk consumption and full enteral feeding among infants who weigh <=1250 grams. Pediatrics 2008;121(6):e1528–33.

4. Meinzen-Derr J, Poindexter B, Wrage L, et al. Role of human milk in extremely low birth weight infants' risk of necrotizing enterocolitis or death. J Perinatol 2009;29(1):57–62.

5. Quigley M, Embleton ND, McGuire W, et al. Formula versus donor breast milk for feeding preterm or low birth weight infants. Cochrane Libr 2019;2019(8):CD002971.

6. Belfort MB, Anderson PJ, Nowak VA, et al. Breast milk feeding, brain development, and neurocognitive outcomes: a 7-year longitudinal study in infants born at less than 30 Weeks' gestation. J Pediatr 2016;177:133–9.e1.

7. Lechner BE, Vohr BR. Neurodevelopmental outcomes of preterm infants fed human milk A systematic review. Clin Perinatol 2017;44(1):69–83.

8. Ramel SE, Georgieff MK, Uauy R, et al. Preterm nutrition and the brain. Nutritional Care of Preterm Infants 2014;110:190–200.

9. Volpe JJ. Dysmaturation of premature brain: importance, cellular mechanisms, and potential interventions. Pediatr Neurol 2019;95:42–66.

10. Kleinman RE, Greer FR. Pediatric nutrition. 8th edition. IL, USA: American Academy of Pediatrics; 2019.

11. Lee S, Kelleher SL. Biological underpinnings of breastfeeding challenges: the role of genetics, diet, and environment on lactation physiology. Am J Physiol Endocrinol Metab 2016;311(2):E405–22.

12. Keikha M, Bahreynian M, Saleki M, et al. Macro- and micronutrients of human milk composition: are they related to maternal diet? A comprehensive systematic review. Breastfeed Med 2017;12(9):517–27.

13. Golan Y, Assaraf YG. Genetic and physiological factors affecting human milk production and composition. Nutrients 2020;12(5):1500.

14. Gidrewicz DA, Fenton TR. A systematic review and meta-analysis of the nutrient content of preterm and term breast milk. BMC Pediatr 2014;14(1):216.

15. Paulsson M, Jacobsson L, Ahlsson F. Factors influencing breast milk fat loss during administration in the neonatal intensive care unit. Nutrients 2021;13(6):1939.

16. Perrin MT, Belfort MB, Hagadorn JI, et al. The nutritional composition and energy content of donor human milk: a systematic review. Adv Nutr 2020;11(4):960–70.

17. Belfort M, Cherkerzian S, Bell K, et al. Macronutrient intake from human milk, infant growth, and body composition at term equivalent age: a longitudinal study of hospitalized very preterm infants. Nutrients 2020;12(8):2249.

18. Arslanoglu S, Moro GE, Ziegler EE. Adjustable fortification of human milk fed to preterm infants: does it make a difference? J Perinatol 2006;26(10):614–21.

19. Brown JVE, Embleton ND, Harding JE, et al. Multi-nutrient fortification of human milk for preterm infants. Cochrane Libr 2016;2016(5):CD000343.

20. Agostoni C, Buonocore G, Carnielli VP, et al. Enteral nutrient supply for preterm infants: commentary from the European society of paediatric Gastroenterology, Hepatology and nutrition committee on nutrition. J Pediatr Gastroenterol Nutr 2010;50(1):85–91.

21. Koletzko B. 2nd edition. Nutritional care of preterm infants: scientific basis and practical guidelines, vol. 122. Karger; 2021.

22. Ong ML, Belfort MB. Preterm infant nutrition and growth with a human milk diet. Semin Perinatol 2021;45(2):151383.

23. Chinnappan A, Sharma A, Agarwal R, et al. Fortification of breast milk with preterm formula powder vs human milk fortifier in preterm neonates: a randomized noninferiority trial. JAMA Pediatr 2021;175(8):790–6.

24. Fusch S, Fusch G, Yousuf E, et al. Individualized target fortification of breast milk: optimizing macronutrient content using different fortifiers and approaches. Front Nutr 2021;8:652641.

25. McGuire W, Brown JVE, Lin L, et al. Multi-nutrient fortification of human milk for preterm infants. Cochrane Libr 2020;2020(7). https://doi.org/10.1002/14651858. CD000343.pub4.

26. Moro GE, Minoli I, Ostrom M, et al. Fortification of human milk: evaluation of a novel fortification scheme and of a new fortifier. J Pediatr Gastroenterol Nutr 1995;20(2):162–72.

27. Alan S, Atasay B, Cakir U, et al. An intention to achieve better postnatal in-hospital-growth for preterm infants: adjustable protein fortification of human milk. Early Hum Dev 2013;89(12):1017–23.

28. Morris SM Jr. Regulation of enzymes of urea and arginine synthesis. Annu Rev Nutr 1992;12(1):81–101.

29. Boehm G, Gedlu E, Müller MD, et al. Postnatal development of urea- and ammonia-excretion in urine of very-low-birth-weight infants small for gestational age. Acta Paediatr Hung 1991;31(1):31–45.

30. Ergenekon E, Soysal S, Hirfanoglu I, et al. Short- and long-term effects of individualized enteral protein supplementation in preterm newborns. Turk J Pediatr 2013;55(4):365–70.

31. Biasini A, Monti F, Chiara Laguardia M, et al. High protein intake in human/maternal milk fortification for ≤1250 gr infants: intrahospital growth and neurodevelopmental outcome at two years. Acta Biomed 2017;88(4):470–6.

32. Arslanoglu S, Bertino E, Coscia A, et al. Update of adjustable fortification regimen for preterm infants: a new protocol. J Biol Regul Homeost Agents 2012;26(3 Suppl):65–7.

33. Arslanoglu S. IV. Individualized fortification of human milk: adjustable fortification. J Pediatr Gastroenterol Nutr 2015;61(Suppl 1):S4–5.

34. Picaud JC, Houeto N, Buffin R, et al. Additional protein fortification is necessary in extremely low-birth-weight infants fed human milk. J Pediatr Gastroenterol Nutr 2016;63(1):103–5.

35. Fusch G, Mitra S, Rochow N, et al. Target fortification of breast milk: levels of fat, protein or lactose are not related. Acta Paediatr 2015;104(1):38–42.

36. Sauer CW, Boutin MA, Kim JH. Wide variability in caloric density of expressed human milk can lead to major underestimation or overestimation of nutrient content. J Hum Lact 2017;33(2):341–50.

37. Kashyap S, Ohira-Kist K, Abildskov K, et al. Effects of quality of energy intake on growth and metabolic response of enterally fed low-birth-weight infants. Pediatr Res 2001;50(3):390–7.

38. Lucas A, Gibbs JA, Lyster RL, et al. Creamatocrit: simple clinical technique for estimating fat concentration and energy value of human milk. Br Med J 1978; 1(6119):1018–20.

39. Kwan C, Fusch G, Rochow N, et al. Milk analysis using milk analyzers in a standardized setting (MAMAS) study: a multicentre quality initiative. Clin Nutr 2020; 39(7):2121–8.

40. Agakidou E, Karagiozoglou-Lampoudi T, Parlapani E, et al. Modifications of own mothers' milk fortification protocol affect early plasma IGF-I and Ghrelin levels in preterm infants. A randomized clinical trial. Nutrients 2019;11(12):3056.

41. Parat S, Raza P, Kamleh M, et al. Targeted breast milk fortification for very low birth weight (VLBW) infants: nutritional intake, growth outcome and body composition. Nutrients 2020;12(4):1156.

42. Quan M, Wang D, Gou L, et al. Individualized human milk fortification to improve the growth of hospitalized preterm infants. Nutr Clin Pract 2020;35(4):680–8.

43. Kadıoğlu Şimşek G, Alyamaç Dizdar E, Arayıcı S, et al. Comparison of the effect of three different fortification methods on growth of very low birth weight infants. Breastfeed Med 2019;14(1):63–8.

44. Bulut O, Coban A, Uzunhan O, et al. Effects of targeted versus adjustable protein fortification of breast milk on early growth in very low-birth-weight preterm infants: a randomized clinical trial. Nutr Clin Pract 2020;35(2):335–43.

45. Hair AB, Blanco CL, Moreira AG, et al. Randomized trial of human milk cream as a supplement to standard fortification of an exclusive human milk-based diet in infants 750-1250 g birth weight. J Pediatr 2014;165(5):915–20.

46. Maas C, Mathes M, Bleeker C, et al. Effect of increased enteral protein intake on growth in human milk–fed preterm infants: a randomized clinical trial. JAMA Pediatr 2016;171(1):16–22.

47. McLeod G, Sherriff J, Hartmann PE, et al. Comparing different methods of human breast milk fortification using measured v. assumed macronutrient composition to target reference growth: a randomised controlled trial. Br J Nutr 2016;115(3):431–9.

48. Brion LP, Rosenfeld CR, Heyne R, et al. Optimizing individual nutrition in preterm very low birth weight infants: double-blinded randomized controlled trial. J Perinatol 2020;40(4):655–65.

49. Rochow N, Fusch G, Ali A, et al. Individualized target fortification of breast milk with protein, carbohydrates, and fat for preterm infants: a double-blind randomized controlled trial. Clin Nutr 2021;40(1):54–63.

50. Rochow N, Fusch G, Zapanta B, et al. Target fortification of breast milk: how often should milk analysis Be done? Nutrients 2015;7(4):2297–310.

51. Belfort MB, Rifas-Shiman SL, Sullivan T, et al. Infant growth before and after term: effects on neurodevelopment in preterm infants. Pediatrics 2011;128(4):E899–906.

52. Bell KA, Matthews LG, Cherkerzian S, et al. Associations of growth and body composition with brain size in preterm infants. J Pediatr 2019;214:20–6.e2.

53. Pfister KM, Zhang L, Miller NC, et al. Early body composition changes are associated with neurodevelopmental and metabolic outcomes at 4 years of age in very preterm infants. Pediatr Res 2018;84(5):713–8.

54. Bua J, Risso FM, Bin M, et al. Association between body composition at term equivalent age and Bayley scores at 2 years in preterm infants. J Perinatol 2021;41(8):1852–8.

55. Belfort MB, Woodward LJ, Cherkerzian S, et al. Targeting human milk fortification to improve very preterm infant growth and brain development: study protocol for Nourish, a single-center randomized, controlled clinical trial. BMC Pediatr 2021;21(1):167.

56. COSMED - PEA POD: Gold standard for non-invasive Infant Body Composition. Available at: https://www.cosmed.com/en/products/body-composition/pea-pod. Accessed March 4, 2022.

57. WET NURSES–COMPOSITION OF MILK. The Boston Medical and Surgical Journal (1828-1851). 1847;37(7):0_1-.
58. Chem Gaz P 192. Analysis of Human Milk. The Medico-Chirurgical Review, and Journal of Medical Science. 1849;(VI):526-.
59. Fleet IR, Linzell JL. Rapid method of estimating fat in very small quantities of milk. In: Journal of Physiology-London. Vol 175. CAMBRIDGE UNIV PRESS 40 WEST 20TH STREET, NEW YORK, NY 10011-4211; 1964:P15.
60. Lucey JA, Otter D, Horne DS, et al. 100-Year Review: progress on the chemistry of milk and its components. J Dairy Sci 2017;100(12):9916–32.
61. Michaelsen KF, Pedersen SB, Skafte L, et al. Infrared analysis for determining macronutrients in human milk. J Pediatr Gastroenterol Nutr 1988;7(2):229–35.
62. Miris Test for Nutrient Levels in Breast Milk Receives FDA Authorization | Aacc.org. Available at: https://www.aacc.org/cln/articles/2019/march/miris-test-for-nutrient-levels-in-breast-milk-receives-fda-authorization. Accessed April 7, 2022.

Human Milk Fortification Strategies in the Neonatal Intensive Care Unit

Ting Ting Fu, MD[a,b,]*, Brenda B. Poindexter, MD, MS[c]

KEYWORDS

- Human milk • Fortification • Nutrition • Macronutrients • Preterm infant • Growth

KEY POINTS

- There is insufficient evidence to support the choice of human milk-based human milk fortifiers over bovine milk-based human milk fortifiers.
- Increased amounts of fortifier or modular agents beyond standard fortification can improve growth, especially with the use of pasteurized donor breast milk, the use of human milk-based human milk fortifier, and in clinical cases of growth faltering. This can be provided either in a fixed or individualized approach.
- Additional studies regarding a newer generation of fortifier products and fortification strategies are needed.

INTRODUCTION

Human milk is the ideal nutrition for infants and provides macronutrients, micronutrients, and physiologic factors to support growth and development.[1] For the preterm population, especially higher risk infants born very low birth weight (VLBW, born weighing <1500 g), breast milk alone is often not adequate to meet their metabolic demands and recommended nutritional goals, and higher intakes of protein, calcium, and phosphorus in particular are crucial to support organ development and bone deposition in preterm infants.[2,3] Although there is no definitive association between human milk fortification and long-term neurodevelopmental outcomes, greater gains in growth during the neonatal intensive care unit (NICU) hospitalization are related to better developmental outcomes.[4–7] Thus, human milk fortification has become the standard of care in the NICU to support short-term growth.[2,3,8] However, there

[a] Division of Neonatology, Perinatal Institute, Cincinnati Children's Hospital Medical Center, 3333 Burnet Avenue, Cincinnati, OH 45229, USA; [b] Department of Pediatrics, University of Cincinnati College of Medicine, Cincinnati, OH, USA; [c] Division of Neonatology, Department of Pediatrics, Children's Healthcare of Atlanta and Emory University School of Medicine, 2015 Uppergate Drive Northeast, Atlanta, GA 30322, USA
* Corresponding author.
E-mail address: tingting.fu@cchmc.org

Clin Perinatol 50 (2023) 643–652
https://doi.org/10.1016/j.clp.2023.04.006
0095-5108/23/© 2023 Elsevier Inc. All rights reserved.

is no consensus on how or when to fortify human milk, and different strategies and products are used. In this review, the authors examine the various approaches to common challenges relating to human milk fortification.

FORTIFIER PRODUCTS

Human milk fortifier (HMF) agents are available in two primary categories: multicomponent and single component. As the name suggests, multicomponent fortifiers provide a range of nutrients, including protein, fat, carbohydrates, vitamins, and minerals. Single-component agents are typically used in conjunction with multicomponent fortifiers to enhance further the delivery of individual nutrients. Fortifiers may also be classified based on its milk source (bovine milk or human milk) and formulation (powder or liquid).

Although standard doses of multicomponent HMF may increase the caloric density similarly, different manufacturers achieve this through varying distributions of macronutrients. For example, HMF agents may provide 0.8 to 1.8 g protein/100 mL human milk, and some HMFs contain a higher proportion of carbohydrates, whereas others provide more fat.[9] Furthermore, there is variation in protein type (whey vs casein) and whether the protein is intact or hydrolyzed, either partially or extensively.[10,11] However, further studies are needed to determine whether any specific HMF nutrient profile or source may be more beneficial.

Human Milk-Based Human Milk Fortifiers

With the increasing prevalence of donor breast milk (DBM) as the preferred alternative to preterm formula when maternal breast milk (MBM) is not available, the use of human milk-based HMF (HM-HMF) to promote an exclusive human milk diet (EHMD) has been evaluated.[12–14] HM-HMF is an expensive liquid product that is offered in a range of caloric preparations, but it displaces a high proportion of MBM, especially at higher caloric densities. As of 2018, HM-HMF was available in 22% of neonatal facilities in the United States reporting the use of any HMF.[12]

The proposed benefit of HM-HMF and an EHMD is extrapolated from the studies demonstrating the association between preterm formula and an increased incidence of necrotizing enterocolitis (NEC).[15,16] The first randomized controlled trials examining an EHMD compared with MBM fortified with bovine milk-based HMF (BM-HMF) but supplemented with preterm formula, not DBM fortified with BM-HMF.[17,18] Consequently, a true head-to-head comparison of the impact of bovine versus human milk-based HMF added to a base diet of human milk (either donor or maternal) is not possible in these trials. A secondary analysis focusing on infants who received an EHMD and those who received exclusively MBM fortified with BM-HMF (no formula exposure at all) reported a higher incidence of NEC in the BM-HMF group, though it is unclear how generalizable the results are, given that the incidence (15.6%) was remarkably higher than national average at baseline.[19,20] A separate randomized controlled trial (OptiMOM) directly comparing the use of HM-HMF and BM-HMF found no difference in feeding tolerance (primary outcome), incidence of NEC, mortality, or infection.[21] Moreover, HM-HMF has not been shown to have any impact on the preterm infant microbiome compared with BM-HMF with microbial diversity influenced primarily by exposure to MBM.[22–24] At present, there is not sufficient conclusive evidence for the benefit of human milk-based fortifier versus bovine fortifier in preterm infants exclusively receiving human milk.

Poor growth has also been a concern with the use of HM-HMF. In the initial trial comparing an EHMD with preterm formula as sole diet, the EHMD group had worse linear growth.[17] However, adequate growth can be achieved in VLBW infants when feeding higher caloric density human milk prepared with HM-HMF.[25] Similarly, the OptiMOM trial also reported no difference in growth z-score trajectories between HM-HMF and BM-HMF with the HM-HMF group receiving a higher caloric density (26 kcal/oz) at minimum.[21] A human milk-based cream product can also provide caloric enrichment, though its use may exacerbate negative linear growth trajectories when compared with the use of higher caloric densities with HM-HMF.[26,27]

Thus, at present, there is insufficient evidence to recommend the choice of HM-HMF over BM-HMF. Additional studies are warranted to assess the benefits of HM-HMF versus newer liquid BM-HMF formulations with partially or extensively hydrolyzed protein.

STRATEGIES FOR FORTIFICATION

Standard fortification, the most common approach to human milk fortification, occurs by adding a fixed amount of multicomponent HMF. The standard degree of fortification is generally regarded as 24 kcal/oz or 80 kcal/dL to support short-term growth.[8] One problem with this approach is that it assumes all human milk provides a similar distribution of nutrients, but many infant and maternal factors contribute to individual milk composition, leading to variability.[28–30] Furthermore, the two most common HMF products in the American market presumes a protein concentration of 1.6 to 1.7 g/dL in preterm human milk, but this assumption may not be accurate after the early weeks of lactation.[10,11,30,31]

In practice, clinicians may provide additional fortification to increase nutrient delivery, either in a fixed or an individualized approach. The fixed approach can be accomplished with an increased amount of HMF (greater than manufacturers' instructions) or with a specified amount of modular agents, such as a liquid protein fortifier (LPF). The use of higher concentrations of HMF has been described particularly with DBM feedings and with fortification using HM-HMF and associated with appropriate growth.[21,25,32] Salas and colleagues reported increased fat-free mass, weight, and length with protein-enrichment using LPF compared with standard fortification alone.[33]

Individualized approaches include adjustable and targeted. Adjustable fortification provides additional protein enrichment based on blood urea nitrogen levels as a proxy for protein intake and has been related to higher weight and head circumference velocities.[34] Targeted fortification involves regular macronutrient analysis of human milk (weekly or more frequent) and adding modular products to achieve targeted nutrient goals. In the largest randomized control trial to date and the only to target all three macronutrients, the infants in the targeted fortification group had greater weight gain.[35] Two small trials have compared adjustable and protein-targeted fortification with inconsistent results.[36,37] However, both methods require careful measurements of modular agents. Moreover, human milk analysis may be prohibitive due to both cost, availability, and the time and labor needed to provide frequent, accurate, and reliable analyses.[38,39]

Regardless of method of fortification strategy, one concern that sometimes arise is exceeding an enteral feeding osmolality of 450 mOsm/kg. This threshold was delineated by the American Academy of Pediatrics in 1976 and based on the association of hyperosmolar formula feedings with delayed gastric emptying and NEC.[40] The theoretic risk with hyperosmolar feedings has not been demonstrated with human milk or modern fortifiers.[41] Standard fortification to 24 kcal/oz with one HMF in the American market already yields an osmolality greater than 450 mOsm/kg, presumably due to its hydrolyzed protein and carbohydrate content.[42] Additional research may assuage further concerns, though practically, it is likely that many of these existing studies of fortified human milk also exceed the theoretical risk threshold without alarming reports of gastrointestinal adverse effects.

TIMING OF FORTIFICATION

The optimal timing to initiate human milk fortification is unclear. As such, there is wide practice variation. In addition to the osmolality apprehension described above, one other area of theoretical concern is the potential risk for NEC and feeding intolerance with early timing of fortification, despite lack of evidence of this association.[43–45] Furthermore, there are no studies to support the practice of slower incremental fortification by 1 to 2 kcal/oz versus fortifying directly to 24 kcal/oz.

Complicating the issue is that the trials examining timing of fortification are heterogenous with their definitions of early and late. A Cochrane review from 2020 evaluated two small randomized control trials with early fortification occurring at enteral feeding volume of 20 to 40 mL/kg/d versus 100 mL/kg/d and found there was insufficient evidence to support either early or late initiation; of note, one trial used HM-HMF, and the other used BM-HMF.[44] However, a larger retrospective study reported that early fortification before 60 mL/kg/d could be safe with improved growth outcomes.[46] Interestingly, two other studies have compared early fortification at the time of enteral feeding initiation versus late timing and found no difference in clinical outcomes, including incidences of NEC and feeding intolerance.[47,48] Similarly, early protein enrichment at the time of enteral feeding initiation can be tolerated in stable infants.[49]

Although the evidence does not strongly identify a particular timepoint for initiation of fortification, one point of consideration is the specific relationship of enteral protein intake with brain development. Early enteral protein intake in very preterm infants has been positively associated with global and regional brain volumes and fractional anisotropy on brain imaging at term-equivalent age.[50,51] Emerging evidence may also suggest an association between early enteral protein intake and the ratio of enteral to parenteral intake with neurodevelopmental outcomes at 2 years of age.[52,53] Not only would earlier fortification support short-term constitutional growth, but the increased early provision of enteral protein may have long-term impact.

Last, duration of human milk fortification remains controversial, though continuing an enriched diet after NICU discharge may still confer benefit.[54] A companion article in this volume ("Nutrition Management of High-Risk Neonates After Discharge") provides additional insight.

SPECIAL CONSIDERATIONS FOR DONOR BREAST MILK

The availability of pasteurized DBM as an alternative feeding source to supplement MBM has increased in recent years.[12,13] The use of DBM in the VLBW population is recommended primarily due to a decreased risk of NEC associated with DBM.[55,56] However, compared with preterm MBM, the nutritional profile of DBM is more similar to mature milk of mothers of term infants, the most common donors, and typically contains less protein and total energy.[57] Furthermore, milk processing subjects donated milk to increased freeze-thaw cycles and additional handling that results in fat loss, and heat pasteurization and retort processing reduce the bioactivity and concentration of nonnutritive factors that may influence digestion, growth, and metabolic regulation.[58–62] Thus, infants receiving predominantly DBM may require higher caloric densities to attain clinically appropriate growth.[25,49] Protein enrichment may also be considered to increase the baseline content of DBM before multicomponent fortification.[49]

Similarly, some milk banks have incorporated human milk analysis in their workflow to target caloric and protein intake, though this step is not required by the Human Milk Banking Association of North America.[63] Some examples of this include strategic pooling of milk from multiple donors to target a particular nutrient goal or the addition of skimmed fat from a different sample specifically to increase total caloric content.[32] Thus, nationally, not all DBM is equivalent, and this may limit the generalizability of studies evaluating DBM and growth. Providers may wish to inquire whether any targeted methods are used by their milk bank source. However, milk analysis of pooled DBM is typically conducted before dispensing into individual bottles, which may lead to inaccurate nutrient labeling. In a study that analyzed "high calorie DBM" sourced from five milk banks, there were significant differences between measured and reported calorie and protein content.[64]

Furthermore, targeting macronutrient intake alone may not attenuate the physiologic differences between DBM and MBM. Infants who receive primarily unpasteurized MBM compared with primarily pasteurized DBM demonstrate increased weight gain.[49,65] In a different observational study, preterm infants fed target-fortified MBM had higher weight and length velocities compared with infants fed target-fortified DBM; when MBM intake was further classified into pasteurized and unpasteurized, the greatest weight gain was seen with unpasteurized MBM.[66] These findings reinforce that other human milk components, such as bioactive factors that currently cannot be supplemented with HMF, may play a role in regulating growth as well. Hence, supporting lactation and promoting the provision of MBM are critical efforts that directly impact the growth of these high-risk infants, beyond the general benefits of human milk exposure alone. The availability of DBM as an intervention to bridge maternal supply and encourage milk expression may have some positive influence, though studies have been conflicting.[67-71]

HOW TO APPROACH SUBOPTIMAL GROWTH

Numerous observational studies have reported lower growth rates in preterm infants fed human milk than those fed preterm formula. These differences in growth are typically thought to be magnified when comparing donor human milk to preterm formula. Indeed, a recent systematic review compared outcomes of preterm infants fed formula versus donor human milk when sufficient MBM is not available. With 12 trials and 1879 infants, higher rates of in-hospital weight gain, linear growth, and head growth were found in formula-fed infants, but no effect on long-term growth or neurodevelopment.[15] However, a recent multicenter cohort study of VLBW infants from Massachusetts evaluated the association of human milk feeding and growth and found that fortified human milk was not associated with suboptimal growth compared with preterm formula.[72] Thus, growth faltering no longer needs to be accepted as an inevitable consequence of a human milk diet in preterm infants.

Perhaps the most important strategy to prevent growth faltering is simply recognizing the change in macronutrient composition of human milk over time and differences in macronutrient composition between donor human milk and preterm maternal milk. Understanding and anticipating the impact of these differences is the key in developing fortification strategies to optimize growth. In the first few weeks of lactation, the protein content of preterm human milk is highest in the first weeks of lactation and gradually decreases over time, reaching the protein content of term milk.[9] Given these differences in macronutrient composition, earlier fortification of donor milk seems prudent. Furthermore, additional protein supplementation may be needed for infants receiving donor human milk for the majority of their enteral intake.

Fu and colleagues have demonstrated the feasibility of this approach.[49] It is also important to recognize the vulnerable transition period when enteral nutrition is increasing and parenteral nutrition is being weaned. Without human milk fortification, significant deficits in protein intake can accrue as parenteral intake is reduced.[73]

SUMMARY

In conclusion, human milk fortification is beneficial to support the short-term growth of preterm infants during the postnatal hospital course. Either HM-HMFs or BM-HMFs may be used, though long-term advantages are unclear. Questions remain regarding the optimal methods and products to use, and additional research is warranted to address these uncertainties. Most importantly, individual infant growth and nutritional assessments are needed to provide tailored support, and lactation support and maternal milk provision must be emphasized.

Best practices

- Human milk is the preferred nutrition source for preterm infants and should be fortified with a multicomponent fortifier to support short-term growth during the NICU course.
- Additional fortification or modular agents may be necessary to attain optimal growth in high-risk infants.

DISCLOSURE

The authors have no conflicts of interest to disclose.

FUNDING

Ting Ting Fu is supported by a Procter Scholar Award from the Cincinnati Children's Research Foundation.

REFERENCES

1. Ballard O, Morrow AL. Human milk composition: nutrients and bioactive factors. Pediatr Clin North Am. Feb 2013;60(1):49–74.
2. Agostoni C, Buonocore G, Carnielli VP, et al. Enteral nutrient supply for preterm infants: commentary from the European society of paediatric gastroenterology, hepatology and nutrition committee on nutrition. J Pediatr Gastroenterol Nutr 2010;50(1):85–91.
3. American Academy of Pediatrics. Committee on nutrition, kleinman RE, greer FR. *Pediatric nutrition*. 8th edition. xii: American Academy of Pediatrics; 2020. p. 1731.
4. Ehrenkranz RA, Dusick AM, Vohr BR, et al. Growth in the neonatal intensive care unit influences neurodevelopmental and growth outcomes of extremely low birth weight infants. Pediatrics 2006;117(4):1253–61.
5. Ramel SE, Demerath EW, Gray HL, et al. The relationship of poor linear growth velocity with neonatal illness and two-year neurodevelopment in preterm infants. Neonatology 2012;102(1):19–24.
6. Belfort MB, Rifas-Shiman SL, Sullivan T, et al. Infant growth before and after term: effects on neurodevelopment in preterm infants. Pediatrics 2011;128(4): e899–906.

7. Guellec I, Lapillonne A, Marret S, et al. Effect of intra- and extrauterine growth on long-term neurologic outcomes of very preterm infants. J Pediatr 2016;175: 93–9.e1.

8. Brown JV, Lin L, Embleton ND, et al. Multi-nutrient fortification of human milk for preterm infants. Cochrane Database Syst Rev 2020;6:CD000343.

9. Picaud JC, Vincent M, Buffin R. Human milk fortification for preterm infants: a review. World Rev Nutr Diet 2021;122:225–47.

10. Abbott Nutrition. Similac® Human Milk Fortifier Hydrolyzed Protein Concentrated Liquid. Accessed October 18, 2022, https://www.abbottnutrition.com/our-products/similac-human-milk-fortifier-hydrolyzed-protein-concentrated-liquid.

11. Mead Johnson & Company. Enfamil® Liquid Human Milk Fortifier Standard Protein. Accessed October 18, 2022, https://www.hcp.meadjohnson.com/s/product/a4R4J000000PpQmUAK/enfamil-liquid-human-milk-fortifier-standard-protein.

12. Perrin MT. Donor human milk and fortifier use in United States level 2, 3, and 4 neonatal care hospitals. J Pediatr Gastroenterol Nutr 2018;66(4):664–9.

13. Perrine CG, Scanlon KS. Prevalence of use of human milk in US advanced care neonatal units. Pediatrics 2013;131(6):1066–71.

14. Elliott MJ, Golombek SG. Evolution of preterm infant nutrition from breastfeeding to an exclusive human milk diet: a review. NeoReviews 2022;23(8):e558–71.

15. Quigley M, Embleton ND, McGuire W. Formula versus donor breast milk for feeding preterm or low birth weight infants. Cochrane Database Syst Rev 2019; 7:CD002971.

16. Lucas A, Cole TJ. Breast milk and neonatal necrotising enterocolitis. Lancet 1990; 336(8730–8731):1519–23.

17. Cristofalo EA, Schanler RJ, Blanco CL, et al. Randomized trial of exclusive human milk versus preterm formula diets in extremely premature infants. J Pediatr 2013; 163(6):1592–5.e1.

18. Sullivan S, Schanler RJ, Kim JH, et al. An exclusively human milk-based diet is associated with a lower rate of necrotizing enterocolitis than a diet of human milk and bovine milk-based products. J Pediatr 2010;156(4):562–567 e1.

19. Han SM, Hong CR, Knell J, et al. Trends in incidence and outcomes of necrotizing enterocolitis over the last 12 years: a multicenter cohort analysis. J Pediatr Surg. Jun 2020;55(6):998–1001.

20. Lucas A, Boscardin J, Abrams SA. Preterm infants fed cow's milk-derived fortifier had adverse outcomes despite a base diet of only mother's own milk. Breastfeed Med 2020;15(5):297–303.

21. O'Connor DL, Kiss A, Tomlinson C, et al. Nutrient enrichment of human milk with human and bovine milk-based fortifiers for infants born weighing <1250 g: a randomized clinical trial. Am J Clin Nutr 2018;108(1):108–16.

22. Kumbhare SV, Jones WD, Fast S, et al. Source of human milk (mother or donor) is more important than fortifier type (human or bovine) in shaping the preterm infant microbiome. Cell Rep Med 2022;24:100712.

23. Ford SL, Lohmann P, Preidis GA, et al. Improved feeding tolerance and growth are linked to increased gut microbial community diversity in very-low-birth-weight infants fed mother's own milk compared with donor breast milk. Am J Clin Nutr 2019;109(4):1088–97.

24. Embleton ND, Sproat T, Uthaya S, et al. Effect of an exclusive human milk diet on the gut microbiome in preterm infants: a randomized clinical trial. JAMA Netw Open 2023;6(3):e231165.

25. Hair AB, Hawthorne KM, Chetta KE, et al. Human milk feeding supports adequate growth in infants </= 1250 grams birth weight. BMC Res Notes 2013;6:459.

26. Hair AB, Blanco CL, Moreira AG, et al. Randomized trial of human milk cream as a supplement to standard fortification of an exclusive human milk-based diet in infants 750-1250 g birth weight. J Pediatr 2014;165(5):915–20.

27. Knake LA, King BC, Gollins LA, et al. Optimizing the use of human milk cream supplement in very preterm infants: growth and cost outcomes. Nutr Clin Pract 2020;35(4):689–96.

28. Underwood MA. Human milk for the premature infant. Pediatr Clin North Am 2013;60(1):189–207.

29. Tudehope DI. Human milk and the nutritional needs of preterm infants. J Pediatr 2013;162(3 Suppl):S17–25.

30. de Halleux V, Rigo J. Variability in human milk composition: benefit of individualized fortification in very-low-birth-weight infants. Am J Clin Nutr 2013;98(2): 529S–35S.

31. Gidrewicz DA, Fenton TR. A systematic review and meta-analysis of the nutrient content of preterm and term breast milk. BMC Pediatr 2014;14:216.

32. Fu TT, Schroder PE, Poindexter BB. Macronutrient analysis of target-pooled donor breast milk and corresponding growth in very low birth weight infants. Nutrients 2019;11(8):1884.

33. Salas AA, Jerome M, Finck A, et al. Body composition of extremely preterm infants fed protein-enriched, fortified milk: a randomized trial. Pediatr Res 2022; 91(5):1231–7.

34. Arslanoglu S, Moro GE, Ziegler EE. Adjustable fortification of human milk fed to preterm infants: does it make a difference? J Perinatol 2006;26(10):614–21.

35. Rochow N, Fusch G, Ali A, et al. Individualized target fortification of breast milk with protein, carbohydrates, and fat for preterm infants: a double-blind randomized controlled trial. Clin Nutr 2020. https://doi.org/10.1016/j.clnu.2020.04.031.

36. Bulut O, Coban A, Uzunhan O, et al. Effects of targeted versus adjustable protein fortification of breast milk on early growth in very-low-birth-weight preterm infants: a randomized clinical trial. Nutr Clin Pract 2020;35(2):335–43.

37. Kadioglu Simsek G, Alyamac Dizdar E, Arayici S, et al. Comparison of the effect of three different fortification methods on growth of very low birth weight infants. Breastfeed Med 2019;14(1):63–8.

38. Kwan C, Fusch G, Rochow N, et al. Milk analysis using milk analyzers in a standardized setting (MAMAS) study: a multicentre quality initiative. Clinical Nutrition 2019. https://doi.org/10.1016/j.clnu.2019.08.028.

39. Ramey SR, Merlino Barr S, Moore KA, et al. Exploring innovations in human milk analysis in the neonatal intensive care unit: a survey of the United States. Front Nutr 2021;8:692600.

40. American Academy of Pediatrics. Commentary on breast-feeding and infant formulas, including proposed standards for formulas. Pediatrics 1976;57(2):278–85.

41. Ellis ZM, Tan HSG, Embleton ND, et al. Milk feed osmolality and adverse events in newborn infants and animals: a systematic review. Arch Dis Child Fetal Neonatal Ed 2019;104(3):F333–40.

42. Donovan R, Kelly SG, Prazad P, et al. The effects of human milk fortification on nutrients and milk properties. J Perinatol 2017;37(1):42–8.

43. Senterre T. Practice of enteral nutrition in very low birth weight and extremely low birth weight infants. World Rev Nutr Diet 2014;110:201–14.

44. Thanigainathan S, Abiramalatha T. Early fortification of human milk versus late fortification to promote growth in preterm infants. Cochrane Database Syst Rev 2020;7(7):Cd013392.

45. Ziegler EE. Human milk and human milk fortifiers. World Rev Nutr Diet 2014;110: 215–27.

46. Huston R, Lee M, Rider E, et al. Early fortification of enteral feedings for infants <1250 grams birth weight receiving a human milk diet including human milk based fortifier. J Neonatal Perinat Med 2020;13(2):215–21.

47. Tillman S, Brandon DH, Silva SG. Evaluation of human milk fortification from the time of the first feeding: effects on infants of less than 31 weeks gestational age. J Perinatol 2012;32(7):525–31.

48. Alizadeh Taheri P, Sajjadian N, Asgharyan Fargi M, et al. Is early breast milk fortification more effective in preterm infants?: a clinical trial. J Perinat Med 2017; 45(8):953–7.

49. Fu TT, Kaplan HC, Fields T, et al, Folger AT, Gordon K, Poindexter BB. Protein enrichment of donor breast milk and impact on growth in very low birth weight infants. Nutrients 2021;13(8). https://doi.org/10.3390/nu13082869.

50. Coviello C, Keunen K, Kersbergen KJ, et al. Effects of early nutrition and growth on brain volumes, white matter microstructure, and neurodevelopmental outcome in preterm newborns. Pediatrics 2018;83(1–1):102–10.

51. Schneider J, Fischer Fumeaux CJ, Duerden EG, et al. Nutrient intake in the first two weeks of life and brain growth in preterm Neonates. Pediatrics 2018; 141(3). https://doi.org/10.1542/peds.2017-2169.

52. Cormack BE, Bloomfield FH, Dezoete A, et al. Does more protein in the first week of life change outcomes for very low birthweight babies? J Paediatr Child Health 2011;47(12):898–903.

53. Henkel RDFT, Barnes-Davis ME, Parikh NA. Effects of early enteral vs. Parenteral protein intake on growth and neurodevelopment in very low birth weight preterm infants. Chicago, IL: Midwest Society for Pediatric Research Annual Meeting; 2022.

54. Lucas A, Sherman J, Fewtrell M. Postdischarge nutrition in preterm infants. NeoReviews 2022;23(8):e541–57.

55. O'Connor DL, Gibbins S, Kiss A, et al. Effect of supplemental donor human milk compared with preterm formula on neurodevelopment of very low-birth-weight infants at 18 Months: a randomized clinical trial. JAMA 2016;316(18):1897–905.

56. Committee On N, Section On B, Committee On F, et al. Donor human milk for the high-risk infant: preparation, safety, and usage options in the United States. Pediatrics 2017;139(1):e20163440.

57. Perrin MT, Belfort MB, Hagadorn JI, et al. The nutritional composition and energy content of donor human milk: a systematic review. Adv Nutr 2020;11(4):960–70.

58. Chang FY, Fang LJ, Chang CS, et al. The effect of processing donor milk on its nutrient and energy content. Breastfeed Med 2020;15(9):576–82.

59. Colaizy TT. Effects of milk banking procedures on nutritional and bioactive components of donor human milk. Semin Perinatol 2021;45(2):151382.

60. Friend LL, Perrin MT. Fat and protein variability in donor human milk and associations with milk banking processes. Breastfeed Med 2020;15(6):370–6.

61. Vieira AA, Soares FVM, Pimenta HP, et al. Analysis of the influence of pasteurization, freezing/thawing, and offer processes on human milk's macronutrient concentrations. Early Hum Dev 2011;87(8):577–80.

62. Andersson Y, Savman K, Blackberg L, et al. Pasteurization of mother's own milk reduces fat absorption and growth in preterm infants. Acta Paediatr 2007;96(10): 1445–9.

63. Human Milk Banking Association of North America Guidelines Committee. HMBANA Standards for Donor Human Milk Banking: An Overview, https://www.

hmbana.org/file_download/inline/95a0362a-c9f4-4f15-b9ab-cf8cf7b7b866. Accessed 21 October, 2022.

64. Jo DB, Hagadorn JI, Smith KC, et al. Macronutrient analysis of donor human milk labelled as 24 kcal/oz. J Perinatol 2020;40(4):666–71.

65. Montjaux-Régis N, Cristini C, Arnaud C, et al. Improved growth of preterm infants receiving mother's own raw milk compared with pasteurized donor milk. Acta Paediatr 2011;100(12):1548–54.

66. de Halleux V, Pieltain C, Senterre T, et al. Growth benefits of own mother's milk in preterm infants fed daily individualized fortified human milk. Nutrients 2019;11(4). https://doi.org/10.3390/nu11040772.

67. Delfosse NM, Ward L, Lagomarcino AJ, et al. Donor human milk largely replaces formula-feeding of preterm infants in two urban hospitals. J Perinatol 2013;33(6): 446–51.

68. Kantorowska A, Wei JC, Cohen RS, et al. Impact of donor milk availability on breast milk use and necrotizing enterocolitis rates. Pediatrics 2016;137(3): e20153123.

69. Williams T, Nair H, Simpson J, et al. Use of donor human milk and maternal breastfeeding rates: a systematic review. J Hum Lact 2016;32(2):212–20.

70. Parker MG, Burnham L, Mao W, et al. Implementation of a donor milk program is associated with greater consumption of mothers' own milk among VLBW infants in a US, level 3 NICU. J Hum Lact 2016;32(2):221–8.

71. Fu TTAM, Schulz A, Ward LP, et al. Standardizing feeding strategies in moderately preterm infants. Chicago, IL: Midwest Society for Pediatric Research Annual Meeting; 2022.

72. Soldateli B, Parker M, Melvin P, et al. Human milk feeding and physical growth in very low-birth-weight infants: a multicenter study. J Perinatol 2020;40(8):1246–52.

73. Poindexter BB, Cormack BE, Bloomfield FH. Approaches to growth faltering. World Rev Nutr Diet 2021;122:312–24.

Nutrition Management of High-Risk Neonates After Discharge

Shruti Gupta, MD, Sarah N. Taylor, MD*

KEYWORDS

- Infant • Nutrition • Breastfeeding • Growth • Neurodevelopment
- Body composition

KEY POINTS

- Discharge nutrition plans for the high-risk infant need to address the family's feeding plan, the infant's metabolic demand, and the infant's oral ability.
- With the benefits of breastfeeding, if a family chooses to breastfeed, it must be prioritized in the transition from NICU to home.
- Research is needed to identify how long to continue enriched nutrition for the preterm infant.

INTRODUCTION

Nutrition management after neonatal intensive care unit (NICU) hospital discharge requires consideration of the infant's oral feeding ability, nutritional needs, and their family's expectations for breastfeeding and human milk intake. Many high-risk neonates are discharged home before oral feeding maturation is complete or with diseases, such as bronchopulmonary dysplasia, which limit their feeding ability and may increase nutritional needs. Preterm infant growth trajectory postterm age and its relationship with neurodevelopment is not as well-studied as the impact of preterm infant growth before term age but available evidence reflects the potential for posthospital discharge growth to relate positively with brain development especially in the first 3 to 4 months corrected age.

The basic tenants of infant nutrition at hospital discharge are to first ensure that the infant has adequate intake to maintain hydration. Second, the priority is to provide

Dr S. Gupta has no conflicts of interest to disclose. Dr S.N. Taylor has received a honorarium from Astarte Medical; serves as the site principal investigator for research at Yale School of Medicine sponsored by Ferring Pharmaceuticals, Pfizer, and Prolacta Bioscience; and receives collaborative funding via Beth Israel Deaconess Medical Center, United States from Mead Johnson Nutrition.
Department of Pediatrics, Yale School of Medicine, PO Box 208064, New Haven, CT 06520, USA
* Corresponding author.
E-mail address: sarah.n.taylor@yale.edu

Clin Perinatol 50 (2023) 653–667
https://doi.org/10.1016/j.clp.2023.04.011

adequate nutrition for growth and development. Third, posthospital nutrition should support the family's infant feeding plan especially if it includes a plan to breastfeed. During pregnancy, many families develop a strategy for how they plan to feed their infant. Decisions such as breast or bottle and, if breast, exclusive versus partial, and the duration of breastfeeding likely have been considered. When pregnancy is complicated by either a preterm birth or an NICU hospitalization, family feeding goals may change as the family adapts to this complication or the family may prefer to maintain their original infant feeding goal. Therefore, a goal of nutrition management of high-risk neonates should include attention to the family's ideal feeding intention, which often includes a plan to breastfeed. For most, the preterm infant will not reach their full breastfeeding potential until after hospital discharge. Hence, nutrition management is best if it bridges inpatient and outpatient care.

Oral Feeding Development

Preterm infant oral feeding development is more intricate than putting the infant to breast or providing a bottle at a specific gestational age. Oral feeding development is an individualized complex interplay of central neurologic maturation, respiratory status, and peripheral nervous system sucking and swallowing skills.[1] Developing bottle feeding skills may be further complicated by variations in nipple flow rates and variations in how family members and various hospital care providers feed the infant.[2]

Evidence-Based Methods to Support Preterm Infant Oral Feeding Skills

Evidence-based methods to improve preterm infant oral feeding development include nonnutritive experiences such as kangaroo care, nonnutritive sucking on a pacifier or an emptied breast, or oral motor stimulation.[3–5] With bottle feeding, tools to assist in oral feeding progress include cue-based or infant-driven feeding and metrics to assess oral feeding readiness and feeding quality.[6–8] Infant breastfeeding assessment scales, such as the Preterm Breastfeeding Assessment Tool and LATCH score[9] are not reliable in predicting volume of milk intake in preterm infant breastfeeding.[10] Instead, test weighing is a validated method to measure milk transfer with breastfeeding.[10–12] Nipple shields are a tool to assist with establishment of preterm infant milk transfer with breastfeeding.[13,14] Supplementing breastfeeds with a method other than bottle feeding, such as cup feeding or tube feeding, is related to a higher likelihood of breastfeeding at hospital discharge and at 3 months and 6 months postdischarge although the studies on this topic are limited.[15] Specific tools to consider to support high-risk infant oral feeding posthospital discharge are listed in **Table 1**.

High-Risk Infant Oral Feeding Safety

Recently in the NICU, greater attention has been given to oral feeding safety with recognition that swallowing maturation may lag oropharyngeal expression and suck maturation. High-risk infants are at risk for dysphagia with aspiration and/or the potential to develop oral aversion.[16,17] Infants in the NICU with neurologic injury, such as hypoxic ischemic encephalopathy, are at the highest risk for oral feeding difficulties.[18] Although general approaches to feeding skill development are adequate for most NICU infants, some high-risk infants exhibit persistent bradycardia, desaturations, coughing, gagging, arching, feed refusal, or poor nippling with feeds. These infants need a specialized, individualize examination of suck and swallowing ability and/or airway protection.[19]

Table 1
Tools to support high risk oral feeding after hospital discharge

Tools	Use	Considerations
Breast pumps	Breast pumps are critical in NICU to maintain milk supply while infant is unable to nurse. Even after discharge, most mothers need to pump for several feeds as infants transition to direct breastfeeding	A hospital-grade double electric pump is considered the ideal way to express milk for lactating mothers who are separated from their infants and require full replacement of breastfeeding by pumping[69] Home breast pump should be arranged before discharge. Some mothers experience PTSD[70] after NICU discharge and may not want to hear the noise of a pump. Changing to manual or silicone pump with proper teaching may reduce anxiety
Digital scales	Test weighs are performed by weighing the infant before and after a feed to determine how much breast milk infant consumed during a breastfeed[11,71]	Not all digital scales are accurate.[72] It can create undue anxiety if infant does not gain enough weight and parents may not learn infant's cues and signs of satiety. A clinical trial of test weighing at home did not show improved breastfeeding[54]
Nipple shields	A nipple shield is a thin piece of silicone that is placed on mother's areola and nipple. It is a short-term tool when baby is having trouble latching or due to maternal reasons such as nipple pain, flat nipples, and engorgement	Ongoing lactation support is essential to support use and weaning off nipple shield. Improper use of nipple shield could decrease breastfeeding duration[73]
Slow flow or specialty nipples	Infant's ability to self-regulate flow may be compromised so custom flow restrictions may be warranted to meet each infant's unique feeding needs[74]	High-risk infants using variable flow nipples should be followed up by feeding specialists such as speech pathologists[75]

Nutritional Needs

Preterm infants have greater nutritional needs than full-term infants during the preterm period. Whether they have ongoing higher nutritional needs after term equivalent age is unclear. Certainly, preterm infants, who amassed nutritional deficits before term age, may need ongoing correction of those deficits after hospital discharge. Additionally, preterm infants with cardiovascular or respiratory disease may have increased metabolic demand necessitating increased nutritional intake.

Micronutrient Needs

Iron, calcium, and phosphorus are specific micronutrients for which preterm infants may have inadequate stores at hospital discharge and, therefore, need supplementation. The American Academy of Pediatrics recommends 2 mg/kg/d iron supplementation be provided to preterm infant by 1 month of age and extended through 12 months as either medicinal iron or in iron-fortified foods.[20] For calcium and phosphorus, 120 to 200 mg/kg/d calcium and 70 to 120 mg/kg/d phosphorus are recommended for preterm infants to match the intrauterine accretion of these minerals and to avoid metabolic bone disease of prematurity. How long these supplements are needed is not well established.[21]

Macronutrient Needs

The impact of posthospital discharge intake of specific macronutrients on preterm infant outcomes has not been studied. Instead, existing studies are of multinutrient supplementation either as a postdischarge formula, preterm infant formula, or fortification of human milk and include how these feeding types influence growth, neurodevelopment, and bone mineralization.

Postdischarge Feeding Type and Preterm Infant Outcomes

Randomized, controlled trials of postdischarge formula (1.8–1.9 g protein, 72–27 kcal energy, 70–80 mg calcium per 100 mL) and preterm infant formula (2.2–2.3 g protein, 80–90 kcal energy, 100–108 calcium per 100 mL) compared with standard formula (1.4–1.5 g protein, 67 kcal energy, 35–54 mg per 100 mL) have compared these feeding types for 1 to 12 months postterm or posthospital discharge.[22,23] Additionally, 3 randomized, controlled trials have studied supplementation to mother's milk posthospital discharge.[24–27] The results of these 3 studies are shown in **Table 2**. Growth, brain development, and bone mineralization are the primary outcomes compared between feeding types.

Postdischarge Feeding Type and Growth

In meta-analysis of randomized, controlled trials, postdischarge formula was not associated with higher weight, length, or head circumference gains except for increased weight and length at 9 months that was not sustained at 12 months. Alternatively, preterm infant formula for 2 to 6 months posthospital discharge related to higher weight gain at 12 months and 18 months postterm, higher length gain at 18 months postterm, and higher head circumference at 9-month, 12-month, and 18-month postterm age.[22] In a small trial of mother's milk feedings, fortifying 50% of feeds with human milk fortifier for 12 weeks posthospital discharge was associated with increased weight and length at 12 months correct age and greater head circumference for infants born less than 1250 g.[24,25] In only one retrospective cohort study was preterm infant growth compared between infants discharged home on formula versus those discharged home on human milk and formula. Groups had similar

Table 2
Nutrient-enrichment versus no enrichment of breastmilk posthospital discharge

Study	Population	Intervention	Outcomes Reaching Statistically Significance
O'Connor et al,[24] 2008 Aimone et al,[25] 2009	39 ≥ 80% breastmilk and 750–1800 g at birth infants	Protein 0.8 g/kg Calories 10–15/kg Fortified with HMF 50% of feeds for 12 wk	Intervention infants at 12 mo: • Heavier by 1.2 kg • Longer • Greater bone mineral content Infants born <1250 g at 12 mo: • Greater head circumference Intervention infants at 18 mo: • No difference in Bayley II scale
Zachariassen et al,[27] 2011	320 infants born 24–32 wk PMA receiving breastmilk at discharge	Protein 1.37 g/d Calories 17/d For 4 mo	At 12 mo: • No difference in growth
De Cunha et al,[26] 2016	53 exclusively breastfed VLBW infants	Protein 0.5 g/d Calories 20/d For 4–6 mo	At 12 mo: • No difference in Bayley III scale • No difference in developmental delay

Data from Arslanoglu S, Boquien CY, King C, et al. Fortification of Human Milk for Preterm Infants: Update and Recommendations of the European Milk Bank Association (EMBA) Working Group on Human Milk Fortification. Front Pediatr. 2019;7:76.

catch-up growth in weight, length, and head circumference at 12 to 15 months corrected age.[28]

Postdischarge Feeding Type and Preterm Infant Neurodevelopment

No studies of postdischarge feeding type have exhibited improved neurodevelopmental scores with enriched feeds compared with standard feeds.[22,25,29–31]

Postdischarge Feeding Type and Bone Mineralization

In a small study of fortifying 50% of feeds with human milk fortifier for 12 weeks posthospital discharge, bone mineral content was greater at 12 months corrected age.[25] In studies of nutrient-enriched formula, bone outcomes have not differed by feeding type except for contrary findings in 2 studies of postdischarge formula with one showing greater bone mineral content at 9 months corrected age[32] and the other showing lower bone mass at the 12-month study end.[33]

Breastfeeding and Human Milk Posthospital Discharge in the High-Risk Infant Population

For the hospitalized very preterm infants, great emphasis is placed on establishing and sustaining maternal milk supply because intake of maternal milk relates to a decrease in the risk of necrotizing enterocolitis, sepsis, and retinopathy of prematurity.[34] Less emphasis is placed on establishing breastfeeding and maintaining breastfeeding posthospital discharge for the high-risk infant to meet the American Academy of Pediatrics' and the World Health Organization's recommendations to breastfeed for at least first 6 months after birth.[35,36] Breastfeeding relates to lower prevalence of acute and chronic pediatric disorders including ear, gastrointestinal, and respiratory infections; autoimmune diseases such as inflammatory bowel disease; allergic disease; childhood leukemia; and diabetes mellitus. For the mother, type 2 diabetes mellitus, at least 3 types of cancer, and hypertension risks are lower with breastfeeding.[35] Although these outcomes have not been studied specifically in the breastfed preterm or high-risk newborn population, mechanistically, these infants and their mothers should receive similar, if not greater, benefit.

Postdischarge Mother's Milk Intake and Very Preterm Infant Neurodevelopment

Although the evidence is limited because randomized, controlled trials cannot be performed, intake of breast milk through the first postnatal months relates to improved neurodevelopmental outcomes in very preterm infants. In a study of 280 very-low birthweight infants, breast milk feeding for greater than or equal to 8 months was associated with an adjusted mean verbal IQ 6 points higher at 7 years of age when compared with infants who received no breast milk.[37] In a recent study to investigate the long-term effect of probiotics to very-low birthweight infants during the neonatal period, in 2467 primary school-aged children, breastfeeding for greater than or equal to 3 months related to improved behavior with lower prevalence of conduct disorders and less inattention/hyperactivity.[38]

High-Risk Infant Postdischarge Growth and Neurodevelopment

Postdischarge growth trajectories also seem to relate positively to neurodevelopmental outcomes. Many preterm infants remain below their expected growth trajectories at hospital discharge. Numerous studies show how preterm infant growth before term equivalent age relates to neurodevelopmental outcomes.[39] Less is known about how preterm infant growth postterm age relates to infant outcomes. In a study of 945 preterm and low birthweight infants, more rapid linear growth from term age to

4 months was linked to better neurodevelopmental outcomes but also a higher likelihood of overweight or obesity at 8 and 18 years of age.[40] In a nationwide study in Taiwan, 1791 very low birthweight infants were assessed at 6, 12, and 24 months of corrected age. Postdischarge failure to thrive, defined as body weight below the third percentile of the standard growth curve for Taiwanese children, was associated with poor neurodevelopmental outcomes after controlling for other risk factors.[41]

Optimal Growth Patterns Posthospital Discharge

Overall, for preterm infants, especially those born extremely preterm, growth faltering occurs initially, followed by accelerated growth. Accelerated growth for preterm infants is often termed catch-up growth and is a positive increase in a growth z-score toward the infant's birth percentile or toward growth parameters within the normal range for the infant's chronologic age. Sixteen studies of extremely preterm infant growth were included in a 2020 systematic review and overall showed growth faltering until term corrected age and sometimes up to a year of age. In this systematic review, growth faltering was followed by catch-up growth, which sometimes continued until adulthood although overall these extremely low birthweight infants remained small. The best pattern for catch-up growth has yet to be determined.[42] Although some studies have shown both better neurodevelopmental scores and higher likelihood of obesity or overweight with higher growth trajectory,[40] in one study, extremely low birthweight infants with catch-up growth exhibited no difference in neurodevelopment and a lower percentage body fat at 11 years of age when compared with those without catch-up growth.[43] This inability to define optimal catch-up growth significantly hinders development of general guidelines for optimal preterm infant discharge nutrition.

Postdischarge Expectations for the High-Risk Infant

Until optimal catch-up growth is defined, postdischarge nutrition should be provided to ensure preterm infant growth along a steady trajectory. Unfortunately, even when attention is given to nutrition and growth at hospital discharge, growth faltering occurs. In one study of infants discharged from an NICU with a standard guideline to provide discharge nutrition to achieve at least 25 g/d weight gain, in the first weeks post-NICU discharge, 37% exhibited moderate growth failure, defined as 20 to 29 g/d, and 14% exhibited severe growth failure, defined as less than 20 g/d, and 1% exhibited weight loss even when most were receiving nutritionally dense feeds.[44] Hence, postdischarge growth trajectories are difficult to predict before hospital discharge. Consequently, frequent, expert postdischarge monitoring is recommended. Additionally, if the family plans to breastfeed, it is often not established before discharge, so ongoing expert guidance is needed.

Methods to Sustain Parent Milk Supply

Support of a family's plan to breastfeed starts at infant birth even when the infant will have a long hospitalization because the breast milk supply must be established in the first weeks. The practices associated with sustaining milk until at least 40 weeks' gestation include milk expression by 6 hours postbirth, kangaroo care, and expressing milk at least 5 times per day. The practices associated with maintaining an adequate supply until at least hospital discharge include use of a double, electric pump, producing 500 mL/d by day 10, and an NICU environment that is adequately staffed with nurses who have a high level of lactation education and who are supportive of breastfeeding.[45–50] Maintaining milk supply after the infant is discharged from the hospital is less studied but seems to be difficult for families of high-risk infants.

Sustained Breastfeeding for the High-Risk Infant

If the family feeding plan includes breastfeeding, breastfeeding should be initiated in the hospital stay. Initiating breastfeeding before bottle feeding is associated with an increased likelihood of sustained breastfeeding.[47,51] Proper breastfeeding support of high-risk infants includes both specialized lactation consultants and an educated, supportive nursing staff.[52] Other factors related to breastfeeding outcomes include a shorter length of hospitalization, use of test weighing procedures to estimate the volume of intake in a breastfeed, and kangaroo care or skin-to-skin time.[3,53–55] In one study of very preterm infants, the average daily minutes of kangaroo care in the hospital positively related to the duration of breastfeeding up to 6 months corrected age.[55] In a randomized trial comparing unlimited kangaroo care with standard kangaroo care practices in moderately and late preterm infants, the group who received unlimited kangaroo care experienced a longer duration of breastfeeding (5 vs 2 months) and a longer duration of exclusive breastfeeding.[3] Nipple shields are a tool to increase milk transfer in preterm infants,[13] although their study is limited. Most NICUs have low direct breastfeeding rates.[56] Even in hospitals with programs to prioritize breastfeeding, infants are discharged home before breastfeeding is completely established. A detailed, proactive discharge plan may alleviate postdischarge stress and lead to a family achieving their breastfeeding goal. Barriers to sustaining breastfeeding for the high-risk infant after hospital discharge are detailed in **Table 3**.

Fortification of Human Milk

Fortification of human milk is challenging as no human milk fortifier is specifically formulated for the postdischarge or postterm age time. One human milk fortifier was studied posthospital discharge[24] but it is expensive and is not sold in stores. Hence, although not studied, the most common approach to supplement breast milk feeds posthospital discharge is to enrich milk with postdischarge formula powder or to use postdischarge formulas for a portion of the feedings.[57] Because these forms of supplementation have not been studied, no guidelines are available as to how long to supplement. Practices vary with some based on continuing until a specific corrected gestational age such as 46 or 52 weeks; corrected age and others continuing until the infant exhibits a specified amount of catch-up growth.[58] Plans for supplementation additionally should account for maternal lactation goals and milk supply. Supplementation may give the impression that formula is more nutritious than breast milk. With the stressed environment at home soon after discharge and anxiety of whether the infant is growing well, the perception of formula as nutritionally superior may promote cessation of lactation.[59]

Strategies to Optimize Discharge Feeding Plan

- Integrate family feeding plans to the strategy including how much parental leave is remaining and who will be the primary caregivers postdischarge.[60] This would help determine whether exclusive direct breastfeeding is feasible and a goal for the mother.
- Allow parents to room in with their baby before discharge to mimic home environment as much as possible. Although rooming-in, the parents or caregivers provide all physical care and supervision for their infant, including home equipment for feeding and breast pumping.[61,62]
- Ensure all aspects of the discharge feeding plan are communicated with the family well in advance so they can obtain supplies before discharge. The recent formula shortages[63] caused undue anxiety to NICU families.

Table 3
Barriers to sustaining breastfeeding for the high-risk infant

Barriers/Reasons	Assessment	Tools
Not receiving enough milk by direct breastfeeding[77]	a. Assess latch b. Evidence of swallowing c. Optimize any breastfeeding that is occurring by teaching breast massage and breast compressions[57]	Electronic Scales—prefeeding and postfeeding test weighs[71,72]
Infant not latching/fussy[78]	a. Assess latch[57] b. Teach strategies to latch before infant is crying c. May start with a bottle feed and then finish at the breast	Nipple Shields can be an essential tool but there must be a plan for monitoring and weaning[73]
Poor growth[79]	a. Assess for proportional growth on multiple data points b. Obtain detailed feeding history	Growth charts Fortification plans[76]
Low milk production[80]	a. Quantity at each pumping session b. Frequency of pumping c. Frequency of breastfeeding	Breast pumps[69] Pumping/feeding log
Maternal exhaustion[81]	a. Obtain detailed feeding history b. Assess support at home	Avoid triple feeding (breastfeed, pump, bottle feed at each feeding time) Social support
Maternal anxiety[70]	a. Explore reasons for anxiety b. Assess for depression c. Assess for posttraumatic stress disorder from NICU admission[70]	Assess depression[82] Psychosocial support[59]
Conflicting information[80]	a. Assess the concern b. Assess from where is the information is coming?	Family involvement Pediatrician Lactation specialist Peer support[83]

- Flexibility with options for modifications as needed is an important component of successful discharge plan. As was experienced with the recent formula shortages,[63] families need alternative options in case the recommended feeding type is not available or the family's feeding plan changes.
- Assess the infant's degree of risk for nutritional deficits such as very preterm birth, small for gestational age at birth, less than the 10th percentile for any growth parameters at hospital discharge, bronchopulmonary dysplasia, metabolic bone disease, diuretic therapy, or cardiovascular disease. If an infant has protein or mineral deficiency persisting at the time of hospital discharge, a discharge plan should include ongoing measures to assess and correct these deficiencies.[57]
- Some high-risk infants have adequate but tenuous feeding ability at hospital discharge. Risk factor include taking less than 150 mL/kg/d feed volume, requiring caloric density greater than 24 kcal/oz to maintain acceptable growth velocity, taking greater than 20 minutes for each bottle feed, and less than 30 g/d average weight gain on the discharge feeding plan. Infants with these risk factors require intensive postdischarge follow-up.
- Predischarge feeding assessment should include a comprehensive lactation consult if the infant is receiving any maternal milk at the time of discharge.[57,64] Even if a mother is pumping only, a discharge lactation plan including the availability and optimization breast pumping and safe milk storage practices for home.
- Once the above assessments are complete, the team should create discharge instructions that are clear, simple, concise, and devoid of medical jargon. When possible, these instructions should be translated in family's native language.[65] Medical team can help parents gain confidence by preparing this individualized education plan. This can also prevent the risk of readmission soon after discharge from the NICU.[66]

Postdischarge Assessment of High-Risk Infant Nutrition

- Posthospital discharge care providers should obtain a careful feeding history from the family and the details should include nutrition type, volume, frequency, and duration of the feed. If concern exists, observation of a feeding session provides excellent information. Although initial weight loss is concerning, it may be temporary, improve with maturation, and may not require a large change to the nutritional plan. Exploring the potential reasons for poor growth and schedule a follow up visit within a few days.
- If a mother is breastfeeding, ensure it is optimized for maximal transfer of milk. The main reason identified as to why mothers stop breastfeeding shortly after discharge is that they are concerned their baby might not be getting enough milk by direct feeding.[67] Ideally families should have a full lactation assessment with test weights done at the initial visit and then again at 40 weeks gestation. Once infant is term equivalent age and breastfeeding is established, tools like nipple shields should be weaned.
- Availability of lactation support or programs designed to specifically care for preterm infants can significantly increase success of breastfeeding postdischarge.
- Arranging for an NICU representative to call or meet via video visit shortly after discharge to ensure family is following all feeding directions and has understood discharge instructions correctly.[65,68] One NICU follow-up program found that 18.5% of families were mixing feeds erroneously despite having detailed instruction from an NICU registered dietitian before hospital discharge.[44]

SUMMARY

Nutritional management of the high-risk infant after hospital discharge is complicated by differences in preceding nutritional and growth deficits, oral feeding skills, and the family's feeding plan. Previously studies of preterm infant postdischarge nutrition do not provide a clear nutritional management choice likely due to these individual differences. Therefore, instead of a one-size-fits-all nutrition plan, nutrition management is individualized to achieve an acceptable growth pattern while supporting the family's plan feeding. More information is needed to define the optimal posthospital discharge growth pattern to ensure brain growth and maturation. However, the benefits of breastfeeding until 6 months of age necessitate development of nutritional management plans, which protect and promote breastfeeding.

CLINICS CARE POINTS

- High-risk infants, especially those who are preterm or who have neurologic injury, are at risk of incomplete oral feeding skill maturation at hospital discharge.
- High-risk infants, especially those preterm or with cardiovascular or respiratory disease, are at greatest risk for growth faltering posthospital discharge.
- For formula-fed preterm infants, preterm infant formula for 1 to 6 months postterm equivalent age has the greatest positive impact on growth trajectory.
- High-risk infants likely receive the same, if not greater, benefit with breastfeeding, and therefore, breastfeeding for at least 6 months should promoted and protected.
- Greater research is needed to identify the rate of a catch-up growth related to optimal neurodevelopment and body composition outcomes.

REFERENCES

1. Lau C, Geddes D, Mizuno K, et al. The development of oral feeding skills in infants. Int J Pediatr 2012;2012:572341.
2. Pados BF. Milk flow rates from bottle nipples: what we know and why it matters. Nurs Womens Health 2021;25(3):229–35.
3. Hake-Brooks SJ, Anderson GC. Kangaroo care and breastfeeding of mother-preterm infant dyads 0-18 months: a randomized, controlled trial. Neonatal network 2008;27(3):151–9.
4. Foster JP, Psaila K, Patterson T. Non-nutritive sucking for increasing physiologic stability and nutrition in preterm infants. Cochrane Database Syst Rev 2016; 10(10):CD001071.
5. Chen D, Yang Z, Chen C, et al. Effect of oral motor intervention on oral feeding in preterm infants: a systematic review and meta-analysis. Am J Speech Lang Pathol 2021;30(5):2318–28.
6. Crowe L, Chang A, Wallace K. Instruments for assessing readiness to commence suck feeds in preterm infants: effects on time to establish full oral feeding and duration of hospitalisation. Cochrane Database Syst Rev 2016;2016(8): CD005586.
7. Lau C. To individualize the management care of high-risk infants with oral feeding challenges: what do we know? What can we do? Front Pediatr 2020;8:296.
8. Thoyre SM, Shaker CS, Pridham KF. The early feeding skills assessment for preterm infants. Neonatal Netw 2005;24(3):7–16.

9. Altuntas N, Kocak M, Akkurt S, et al. LATCH scores and milk intake in preterm and term infants: a prospective comparative study. Breastfeed Med 2015; 10(2):96–101.

10. Perrella SL, Nancarrow K, Rea A, et al. Estimates of preterm infants' breastfeeding transfer volumes are not reliably accurate. Adv Neonatal Care 2020;20(5): E93–9.

11. Haase B, Barreira J, Murphy PK, et al. The development of an accurate test weighing technique for preterm and high-risk hospitalized infants. Breastfeed Med 2009;4(3):151–6.

12. Funkquist EL, Tuvemo T, Jonsson B, et al. Influence of test weighing before/after nursing on breastfeeding in preterm infants. Adv Neonatal Care 2010;10(1):33–9.

13. Perrella SL, Nancarrow K, Rea A, et al. Longitudinal follow-up of preterm breastfeeding to 12 Weeks corrected gestational age. Adv Neonatal Care 2022;22(6): 571–7.

14. Meier PP, Brown LP, Hurst NM, et al. Nipple shields for preterm infants: effect on milk transfer and duration of breastfeeding. J Hum Lactation 2000;16(2):106–14 [quiz: 129–31].

15. Allen E, Rumbold AR, Keir A, et al. Avoidance of bottles during the establishment of breastfeeds in preterm infants. Cochrane Database Syst Rev 2021;10(10): CD005252.

16. Horton J, Atwood C, Gnagi S, et al. Temporal trends of pediatric dysphagia in hospitalized patients. Dysphagia 2018;33(5):655–61.

17. Stoll BJ, Hansen NI, Bell EF, et al. Trends in care practices, morbidity, and mortality of extremely preterm neonates, 1993-2012. JAMA 2015;314(10):1039–51.

18. Jensen PS, Gulati IK, Shubert TR, et al. Pharyngeal stimulus-induced reflexes are impaired in infants with perinatal asphyxia: does maturation modify? Neuro Gastroenterol Motil 2017;29(7). https://doi.org/10.1111/nmo.13039.

19. Jadcherla SR, Peng J, Moore R, et al. Impact of personalized feeding program in 100 NICU infants: pathophysiology-based approach for better outcomes. J Pediatr Gastroenterol Nutr 2012;54(1):62–70.

20. Baker RD, Greer FR. Diagnosis and prevention of iron deficiency and iron-deficiency anemia in infants and young children (0-3 years of age). Pediatrics 2010;126(5):1040–50.

21. Taylor SN. Calcium, magnesium, phosphorus, and vitamin D. World Rev Nutr Diet 2021;122:122–39.

22. Young L, Embleton ND, McGuire W. Nutrient-enriched formula versus standard formula for preterm infants following hospital discharge. Cochrane Database Syst Rev 2016;12(12):CD004696.

23. Teller IC, Embleton ND, Griffin IJ, et al. Post-discharge formula feeding in preterm infants: a systematic review mapping evidence about the role of macronutrient enrichment. Clin Nutr 2016;35(4):791–801.

24. O'Connor DL, Khan S, Weishuhn K, et al. Growth and nutrient intakes of human milk-fed preterm infants provided with extra energy and nutrients after hospital discharge. Pediatrics 2008;121(4):766–76.

25. Aimone A, Rovet J, Ward W, et al. Growth and body composition of human milk-fed premature infants provided with extra energy and nutrients early after hospital discharge: 1-year follow-up. J Pediatr Gastroenterol Nutr 2009;49(4):456–66.

26. da Cunha RD, Lamy Filho F, Rafael EV, et al. Breast milk supplementation and preterm infant development after hospital discharge: a randomized clinical trial. J Pediatr 2016;92(2):136–42.

27. Zachariassen G, Faerk J, Grytter C, et al. Nutrient enrichment of mother's milk and growth of very preterm infants after hospital discharge. Pediatrics 2011;127(4): e995–1003.
28. Fernandes AI, Gollins LA, Hagan JL, et al. Very preterm infants who receive transitional formulas as a complement to human milk can achieve catch-up growth. J Perinatol 2019;39(11):1492–7.
29. Cooke RJ, Embleton ND, Griffin IJ, et al. Feeding preterm infants after hospital discharge: growth and development at 18 months of age. Pediatr Res 2001; 49(5):719–22.
30. Jeon GW, Jung YJ, Koh SY, et al. Preterm infants fed nutrient-enriched formula until 6 months show improved growth and development. Pediatr Int 2011;53(5):683–8.
31. Agosti M, Vegni C, Calciolari G, et al. Post-discharge nutrition of the very low-birthweight infant: interim results of the multicentric GAMMA study. Acta Paediatr Suppl 2003;91(441):39–43.
32. Lucas A, Bishop NJ, King FJ, et al. Randomised trial of nutrition for preterm infants after discharge. Arch Dis Child 1992;67(3):324–7.
33. Koo WW, Hockman EM. Posthospital discharge feeding for preterm infants: effects of standard compared with enriched milk formula on growth, bone mass, and body composition. Am J Clin Nutr 2006;84(6):1357–64.
34. Miller J, Tonkin E, Damarell RA, et al. A systematic review and meta-analysis of human milk feeding and morbidity in very low birth weight infants. Nutrients 2018;10(6):707.
35. Meek JY, Noble L. Policy statement: breastfeeding and the use of human milk. Pediatrics 2022;150(1). e2022057988.
36. Maternal, newborn, child and adolescent health; guidelines on optimal feeidng of low birth-weight infants in low- and middle-income countries. 2011; Available at: https://www.who.int/publications/i/item/9789241548366, 2022. Accessed October 12, 2022.
37. Horwood LJ, Darlow BA, Mogridge N. Breast milk feeding and cognitive ability at 7-8 years. Arch Dis Child Fetal Neonatal Edition 2001;84(1):F23–7.
38. Härtel C, Spiegler J, Fortmann I, et al. Breastfeeding for 3 Months or longer but not probiotics is associated with reduced risk for inattention/hyperactivity and conduct problems in very-low-birth-weight children at early primary school age. Nutrients 2020;12(11):3278.
39. Taylor SN, Buck CO. Monitoring of growth and body composition: new methodologies. World Rev Nutr Diet 2021;122:32–45.
40. Belfort MB, Gillman MW, Buka SL, et al. Preterm infant linear growth and adiposity gain: trade-offs for later weight status and intelligence quotient. J Pediatr 2013; 163(6):1564–1569 e1562.
41. Hsu CT, Chen CH, Lin MC, et al. Post-discharge body weight and neurodevelopmental outcomes among very low birth weight infants in Taiwan: a nationwide cohort study. PLoS One 2018;13(2):e0192574.
42. Van de Pol C, Allegaert K. Growth patterns and body composition in former extremely low birth weight (ELBW) neonates until adulthood: a systematic review. Eur J Pediatr 2020;179(5):757–71.
43. Raaijmakers A, Jacobs L, Rayyan M, et al. Catch-up growth in the first two years of life in Extremely Low Birth Weight (ELBW) infants is associated with lower body fat in young adolescence. PLoS One 2017;12(3):e0173349.
44. Zhang X, Donnelly B, Thomas J, et al. Growth in the high-risk newborn infant post-discharge: results from a neonatal intensive care unit nutrition follow-up clinic. Nutr Clin Pract 2020;35(4):738–44.

45. Furman L, Minich N, Hack M. Correlates of lactation in mothers of very low birth weight infants. Pediatrics 2002;109(4):e57.

46. Hallowell SG, Rogowski JA, Spatz DL, et al. Factors associated with infant feeding of human milk at discharge from neonatal intensive care: cross-sectional analysis of nurse survey and infant outcomes data. Int J Nurs Stud 2016;53:190–203.

47. Casavant SG, McGrath JM, Burke G, et al. Caregiving factors affecting breast-feeding duration within a neonatal intensive care unit. Adv Neonatal Care 2015; 15(6):421–8.

48. Fewtrell MS, Kennedy K, Ahluwalia JS, et al. Predictors of expressed breast milk volume in mothers expressing milk for their preterm infant. Arch Dis Child Fetal Neonatal Ed 2016;101(6):F502–6.

49. Parker LA, Krueger C, Sullivan S, et al. Demographic, social, and personal factors associated with lactation cessation by 6 Weeks in mothers of very low birth weight infants. J Hum Lactation 2021;37(3):511–20.

50. Lai CT, Rea A, Mitoulas LR, et al. Short-term rate of milk synthesis and expression interval of preterm mothers. Arch Dis Child Fetal Neonatal Ed 2020;105(3):266–9.

51. Pineda R. Direct breast-feeding in the neonatal intensive care unit: is it important? J Perinatol 2011;31(8):540–5.

52. Flacking R, Tandberg BS, Niela-Vilén H, et al. Positive breastfeeding experiences and facilitators in mothers of preterm and low birthweight infants: a meta-ethnographic review. Int Breastfeed J 2021;16(1):88.

53. Smith MM, Durkin M, Hinton VJ, et al. Initiation of breastfeeding among mothers of very low birth weight infants. Pediatrics 2003;111(6 Pt 1):1337–42.

54. Hurst NM, Meier PP, Engstrom JL, et al. Mothers performing in-home measurement of milk intake during breastfeeding of their preterm infants: maternal reactions and feeding outcomes. J Hum Lactation 2004;20(2):178–87.

55. Flacking R, Ewald U, Wallin L. Positive effect of kangaroo mother care on long-term breastfeeding in very preterm infants. J Obstet Gynecol Neonatal Nurs 2011;40(2):190–7.

56. Gertz B, DeFranco E. Predictors of breastfeeding non-initiation in the NICU. Matern Child Nutr 2019;15(3):e12797.

57. Noble LM, Okogbule-Wonodi AC, Young MA. ABM clinical protocol #12: transitioning the breastfeeding preterm infant from the neonatal intensive care unit to home, revised 2018. Breastfeed Med 2018;13(4):230–6.

58. McCormick K, King C, Clarke S, et al. The role of breast milk fortifier in the post-discharge nutrition of preterm infants. Br J Hosp Med 2021;82(3):42–8.

59. Gianni ML, Bezze EN, Sannino P, et al. Maternal views on facilitators of and barriers to breastfeeding preterm infants. BMC Pediatr 2018;18(1):283.

60. Purdy IB, Craig JW, Zeanah P. NICU discharge planning and beyond: recommendations for parent psychosocial support. J Perinatol 2015;35(Suppl 1):S24–8.

61. Bowles JD, Jnah AJ, Newberry DM, et al. Infants with technology dependence: facilitating the road to home. Adv Neonatal Care 2016;16(6):424–9.

62. Aydon L, Hauck Y, Murdoch J, et al. Transition from hospital to home: parents' perception of their preparation and readiness for discharge with their preterm infant. J Clin Nurs 2018;27(1–2):269–77.

63. Doherty T, Coutsoudis A, McCoy D, et al. Is the US infant formula shortage an avoidable crisis? Lancet 2022;400(10346):83–4.

64. Maastrup R, Hansen BM, Kronborg H, et al. Factors associated with exclusive breastfeeding of preterm infants. Results from a prospective national cohort study. PLoS One 2014;9(2):e89077.

65. Smith VC, Love K, Goyer E. NICU discharge preparation and transition planning: guidelines and recommendations. J Perinatol 2022;42(Suppl 1):7–21.
66. Smith VC, Hwang SS, Dukhovny D, et al. Neonatal intensive care unit discharge preparation, family readiness and infant outcomes: connecting the dots. J Perinatol 2013;33(6):415–21.
67. Goldstein RF, Malcolm WF. Care of the neonatal intensive care unit graduate after discharge. Pediatr Clin North Am 2019;66(2):489–508.
68. Kripalani S, Jackson AT, Schnipper JL, et al. Promoting effective transitions of care at hospital discharge: a review of key issues for hospitalists. J Hosp Med 2007;2(5):314–23.
69. Bartick M, Hernandez-Aguilar MT, Wight N, et al. ABM clinical protocol #35: supporting breastfeeding during maternal or child hospitalization. Breastfeed Med 2021;16(9):664–74.
70. Schecter R, Pham T, Hua A, et al. Prevalence and longevity of PTSD symptoms among parents of NICU infants analyzed across gestational age categories. Clin Pediatr (Phila) 2020;59(2):163–9.
71. Rankin MW, Jimenez EY, Caraco M, et al. Validation of test weighing protocol to estimate enteral feeding volumes in preterm infants. J Pediatr 2016;178:108–12.
72. Savenije OE, Brand PL. Accuracy and precision of test weighing to assess milk intake in newborn infants. Arch Dis Child Fetal Neonatal Ed 2006;91(5):F330–2.
73. Maastrup R, Walloee S, Kronborg H. Nipple shield use in preterm infants: prevalence, motives for use and association with exclusive breastfeeding-Results from a national cohort study. PLoS One 2019;14(9):e0222811.
74. McGrattan KE, McFarland DH, Dean JC, et al. Effect of single-use, laser-cut, slow-flow nipples on respiration and milk ingestion in preterm infants. Am J Speech Lang Pathol 2017;26(3):832–9.
75. Orton JL, Olsen JE, Ong K, et al. NICU graduates: the role of the allied health team in follow-up. Pediatr Ann 2018;47(4):e165–71.
76. Arslanoglu S, Boquien CY, King C, et al. Fortification of human milk for preterm infants: update and recommendations of the European Milk Bank Association (EMBA) working group on human milk fortification. Front Pediatr 2019;7:76.
77. Meier PP, Furman LM, Degenhardt M. Increased lactation risk for late preterm infants and mothers: evidence and management strategies to protect breastfeeding. J Midwifery Wom Health 2007;52(6):579–87.
78. Pinchevski-Kadir S, Shust-Barequet S, Zajicek M, et al. Direct feeding at the breast is associated with breast milk feeding duration among preterm infants. Nutrients 2017;9(11):1202.
79. Koletzko B, Li Z. Feeding after discharge. World Rev Nutr Diet 2021;122:325–39.
80. Dosani A, Hemraj J, Premji SS, et al. Breastfeeding the late preterm infant: experiences of mothers and perceptions of public health nurses. Int Breastfeed J 2016;12:23.
81. Elder M, Murphy L, Notestine S, et al. Realigning expectations with reality: a case study on maternal mental health during a difficult breastfeeding journey. J Hum Lact 2022;38(1):190–6.
82. Yawn BP, Pace W, Wollan PC, et al. Concordance of edinburgh postnatal depression scale (EPDS) and patient health questionnaire (PHQ-9) to assess increased risk of depression among postpartum women. J Am Board Fam Med 2009;22(5):483–91.
83. Dennis CL, Hodnett E, Gallop R, et al. The effect of peer support on breastfeeding duration among primiparous women: a randomized controlled trial. CMAJ (Can Med Assoc J) 2002;166(1):21–8.

Red Blood Cell Transfusion, Anemia, Feeding, and the Risk of Necrotizing Enterocolitis

Anand Salem, DO, Ravi M. Patel, MD, MSc*

KEYWORDS

- Red blood cell • Gut injury • Neonate • Infant • Preterm

KEY POINTS

- Both severe anemia and red blood cell (RBC) transfusion may induce intestinal injury and inflammation.
- Evidence to support the withholding of feeding during RBC transfusion is uncertain.
- Ongoing large trials may provide more certainty regarding approaches to feeding during transfusion.

INTRODUCTION

Necrotizing enterocolitis (NEC) is a leading cause of morbidity and mortality in preterm infants and can lead to prolonged hospital stays and increased health care costs.[1–4] NEC has a multifactorial pathophysiology that includes a combination of intestinal barrier immaturity, abnormal inflammatory and microvascular regulation, microbial dysbiosis, and genetic predisposition.[5,6] Clinically, NEC typically presents in a preterm infant with feeding intolerance, abdominal distension, and sometimes bloody stools after the first week of age. Radiographic findings may include pneumatosis intestinalis and portal venous gas, although cases of NEC may present without either[7] and a variety of diagnostic approaches have been proposed.[8] Many potential risk factors for NEC have been reported in the literature,[9] although there is uncertainty with regards to the causality of several factors, including severe anemia, red blood cell (RBC) transfusion, and approaches to feeding during RBC transfusion.[10] In this narrative review, we highlight studies evaluating the effects of severe anemia, RBC transfusion, and feeding during transfusion on the risk of NEC.

Department of Pediatrics, Emory University and Children's Healthcare of Atlanta, 2015 Uppergate Drive Northeast, Atlanta, GA 30322, USA
* Corresponding author.
E-mail address: rmpatel@emory.edu

Clin Perinatol 50 (2023) 669–681
https://doi.org/10.1016/j.clp.2023.04.014
0095-5108/23/© 2023 Elsevier Inc. All rights reserved.

ETIOLOGY OF NECROTIZING ENTEROCOLITIS

Although there is often uncertainty regarding the etiology of NEC in a specific infant, data from mechanistic and clinical studies suggest a multifactorial etiology. Intestinal inflammation, tissue hypoxia, microbial dysbiosis, and toll-like receptor 4 (TLR-4) activation have all been implicated in the pathogenesis of NEC.[11–14] In preclinical models, platelet activating factors (PAFs) and lipopolysaccharide (LPS) have been linked to intestinal bowel injury and necrosis,[12,13] while LPS appears to drive inflammation through TLR-4 and NF-KB activation. In murine models, administration of an LPS-antagonist reduces production of the pro-inflammatory cytokine, TNF-alpha, by macrophages, highlighting the roles of LPS and macrophage activation in NEC. Additionally, Jilling and colleagues 2006[13] reported in a neonatal murine model that TLR-4 expression localized to the apical membrane of intestinal epithelium was increased in formula-fed and asphyxiated rats, which could model similar exposures, such as formula feeding and hypoxia, that preterm infants are exposed to during their stay in the intensive care unit.

THE ROLE OF OXYGENATION IN NECROTIZING ENTEROCOLITIS

Mechanistic insights from preclinical studies suggesting that tissue hypoxia is an important risk factor for NEC have been supported by data from clinical trials. Specifically, arterial oxygenation saturation targets have been studied in several clinical trials and shown to impact the risk of NEC. The NeoProM meta-analysis[14] assessed 5 randomized trials with a total of 4965 participants. The study found no significant difference between a lower SpO_2 target range (85%–89%) compared with a higher SpO_2 target range (91%–95%) on the primary composite outcome of death or major disability at a corrected age of 18 to 24 months, corresponding to a risk difference of 1.7% (95% CI −1.3% to 4.6%) and a relative risk of 1.04 (95% CI 0.98–1.09). However, among secondary outcomes, infants in the lower saturation target group had an increased risk of death and a higher risk of severe NEC (9.2% vs 6.9%, with a corresponding risk difference of 2.3% and a relative risk of 1.33 (95% CI 1.10–1.61)). In addition to arterial oxygen saturation, regional tissue oxygenation saturation may be a useful measure to assess oxygen delivery to the intestinal or mesenteric tissue bed. Near-infrared spectroscopy (NIRS) has been used to quantify oxygenation trends in mesenteric vasculature with regards to RBC transfusion and feeding. Marin and colleagues[15] found that when evaluating enteral feedings and RBC transfusions on mesenteric tissue oxygenation with NIRS, infants who developed NEC following transfusion showed greater variability than those without NEC. Additionally, the cerebral-splanchnic oxygenation ratio (CSOR) may be a measure to evaluate relative tissue oxygenation with lower values (eg, <0.75) in some studies associated with gut injury,[16] but not others.[15] Relevant to tissue oxygenation and the adequacy of oxygen delivery is the tolerance of anemia, which might influence an infant's arterial oxygen content. In the next section, we discuss the data from clinical trials on RBC transfusion and anemia, because it relates to the primary outcomes from these trials, and NEC.

RED BLOOD CELL TRANSFUSION THRESHOLD TRIALS IN PRETERM INFANTS

Very preterm infants are susceptible to anemia due to iatrogenic causes such as frequent blood sampling, impaired RBC production, or bleeding. Because of this, very preterm infants are commonly transfused with RBCs, and more liberal versus conservative approaches have been studied in several trials. The Prematures in Need of Transfusion (PINT) trial[17] was conducted to determine if a restrictive hemoglobin transfusion threshold, compared with a liberal one, would impact the primary composite outcome of either death before discharge or survival with severe morbidity. There was no statistically significant difference in the primary composite outcome of death or neonatal morbidity, which some clinicians may have used to justify a lower transfusion threshold given the lack of benefit of a higher threshold. A post hoc analysis showed that mild-to-moderate cognitive delay was reduced in the higher hemoglobin threshold arm, suggesting an adverse effect of more tolerance of anemia.[18] Based on this finding, a larger trial was conducted to determine if a more liberal transfusion threshold could improve survival without neurodevelopmental impairment in preterm infants. The transfusion of prematures (TOP) trial was a multicenter randomized trial in 41 neonatal units within the *Eunice Kennedy Shriver* NICHD Neonatal Research Network that enrolled and randomized 1824 infants.[19] The trial found no significant difference in the risk of death or neurodevelopmental impairment at 22 to 26 months of corrected age. This finding was consistent with the ETTNO trial,[20] which also found no difference in death or disability at 24 months corrected age when comparing conservative versus liberal transfusion strategies. In all of the aforementioned trials, NEC was assessed as a secondary outcome, and there were no differences in the incidence of NEC when comparing higher versus lower transfusion threshold arms. Additionally, meta-analyses of these 3 trials, in addition to other smaller trials, have not found a difference in the risk of NEC when comparing higher versus lower RBC transfusion thresholds.[21]

Because the aforementioned trials did not show a significant difference in higher versus lower transfusion thresholds with regards to death, major morbidity (including NEC), and neurodevelopmental outcomes around 2 years of age, the results support the safety of tolerance of anemia using the lower transfusion thresholds studied in the trials. However, the safety of tolerating anemia below the levels studied in the trials is uncertain. Relevant to the potential concerns about the effects of severe anemia are data from preclinical studies that have shown anemia to cause gut inflammation and injury. Although these studies may not translate into commensurate effects of specific thresholds in human infants, they provide mechanistic insight into the potential effects of anemia in the gut. Murine phlebotomy-induced anemia models have been particularly useful in demonstrating the effects of anemia, specifically its severity, duration, and role in gut inflammation and barrier dysfunction.[22,23] Arthur and colleagues[22] showed that severe anemia induced significant increases in intestinal tissue hypoxia that extended into the crypts, which led to macrophage activation and interferon-gamma production by tissue macrophages. This macrophage-mediated inflammation led to barrier dysfunction, with increases in paracellular intestinal permeability and associated changes in tight junction proteins. The relevance of these findings to preterm infants is supported by a paired clinical study where cytokine samples collected from infants over a span of 4 years showed a significant negative correlation between hemoglobin and the pro-inflammatory cytokine interferon-gamma ($P<.0001$), supporting the role of anemia as a driver of systemic inflammation. MohanKumar et al.[23] demonstrated that severe anemia in a murine model was associated with decreased adherens junctions, increased intestinal permeability, and elevated plasma LPS, potentially from bacterial translocation. Taken together, these preclinical murine studies show that severe anemia may drive gut inflammation and impaired intestinal barrier function and could have a potential role in the pathogenesis of NEC.

Observational studies have supported the potential role of more severe anemia in the pathogenesis of gut inflammation and injury. Kalteren and colleagues[24] demonstrated that lower hemoglobin levels were associated with higher urinary intestinal fatty acid binding protein (I-FABP) levels prior to any RBC transfusion in preterm infants. In their study, they used I-FABP as a biomarker of intestinal injury and showed in multivariable analysis that decreasing hemoglobin levels were significantly associated with increased levels of urinary I-FABP. With regards to NEC, a multicenter observational cohort study by Patel and colleagues[25] showed that severe anemia in a given week (hemoglobin ≤8 g/dL) was associated with a higher rate of NEC (adjusted cause-specific hazard ratio 6.0; 95% CI 2.0–18.0) in a cohort of 598 low birth weight infants. In additional analysis, each 1 g/dL decrease in the nadir hemoglobin in a given week was associated with a higher rate of NEC (cause specific hazard ratio 1.65; 95% CI 1.23–2.12). Similar results were reported by Singh and colleagues[26] in a study of 333 preterm infants with matched controls, with each one % point decrease in the nadir hematocrit associated with a 10% increase in the odds of NEC. Taken together, these preclinical and observational studies highlight the potential importance of the degree of anemia on intestinal inflammation and gut injury. However, within the context of clinical trials to date, it is likely that levels of anemia tested in the lower thresholds of the trials are unlikely to lead to a higher rate of NEC, when compared with those levels in infants threatened with higher transfusion thresholds.

MECHANISTIC AND OBSERVATIONAL STUDIES OF TRANSFUSION-ASSOCIATED NECROTIZING ENTEROCOLITIS

Whereas there is no consensus definition of transfusion-associated NEC, most studies have characterized the entity as the development of NEC within 48 hours following an RBC transfusion. As most infants receiving RBC transfusions are anemic, it is difficult to differentiate the effect of the RBC transfusion from the effect of the degree of anemia that led to the RBC transfusion. The potential interaction between anemia and its treatment (RBC transfusion) was clearly shown in a murine model. MohanKumar et al.[27] demonstrated that RBC transfusions triggered gut injury in anemic mouse pups that received RBC transfusions, with experiments supporting the occurrence through a TLR-4-mediated mechanism that also depends on the duration of storage of the transfused RBCs. When RBCs were transfused in the absence of anemia, there was no evidence of gut injury. Additionally, mouse pups that received multiple RBC transfusions sustained more severe gut injuries. These data support the possibility that anemia may prime the gut for macrophage-mediated inflammation, with a subsequent RBC transfusion adding a second inflammatory insult, leading to increases in gut inflammation and injury. Observational studies indirectly support the role of antecedent anemia prior to RBC transfusion in the potential risk of NEC. Mally and colleagues[28] identified several risk factors among neonates that developed late NEC: a close temporal association with RBC transfusion (<48 hours), the degree of anemia (hematocrit ~ 25%), and the elective nature of RBC transfusion.

In considering the summary of observational studies, an initial meta-analysis in 2012 of 12 observational studies, largely case-control, by Mohamed and Shah[29] showed an association between exposure to RBC transfusion and a higher risk of NEC. However, since that meta-analysis, there have been additional studies with conflicting findings. Sharma and colleagues,[30] using a matched case-control study, did not identify a statistically significant temporal or dose-response relationship between RBC transfusions and NEC. Hay and colleagues[31] used the GRADE approach to evaluate the certainty of evidence as to whether the RBC transfusions were associated with an increased risk of NEC and found that the overall certainty of evidence was low, with inconsistency and significant heterogeneity across studies. This raises the possibility that a true association may not exist. Rai and colleagues[32] performed a separate systemic review and meta-analysis of observational studies comparing the risk of developing NEC in infants who were exposed to a recent RBC transfusion (within 48 hours) to those who were either unexposed or who were exposed greater than 48 hours prior to the diagnosis of NEC. The study found a statistically significant reduction in the unadjusted odds of NEC in infants who were recently transfused (OR 0.55; 95% CI 0.31–0.98) and a potentially significant protective effect with regards to NEC. A more recent meta-analysis by Garg and colleagues[33] of 17 observational studies found no significant association between RBC transfusions and the risk of NEC; findings tended to differ based on study design, with case-control studies suggesting an association with RBC transfusion and NEC, whereas cohort studies suggeste RBC transfusion to be protective against NEC. In aggregate, there appears to be conflicting evidence about the role of RBC transfusion in causing NEC in clinical studies. This may reflect the heterogeneity of the studies, the varying degrees of pretransfusion anemia, or other potential factors that might influence the risk, such as feeding approaches, which are discussed in the next section. Additionally, preclinical studies can provide biologic plausibility and mechanistic insight into how RBC transfusion may cause gut injury, although it is unclear if this phenomenon consistently translates to an increase in the risk of NEC in the clinical setting, as highlighted by the uncertainty from the meta-analyses by Hay and colleagues[31] and Garg and colleagues[33]

FEEDING DURING RED BLOOD CELL TRANSFUSION AND THE RISK OF NECROTIZING ENTEROCOLITIS

Based on the rationale that NEC risk may be increased following RBC transfusion, some observational studies have evaluated if withholding feeding around RBC transfusion may reduce NEC risk. We have highlighted some of these studies in **Table 1**, which examined the associations between varying feeding protocols during RBC transfusion and the incidence of NEC following transfusion. Of note, this is not a systematic review of all studies conducted to date but is intended to provide an overview of the various approaches used to withholding feeding and the results from these studies. Of the 10 studies examined,[34–43] only 1 study[42] reported a statistically significant decrease in the incidence of NEC after withholding feeds during transfusion. Other studies did report a decrease in NEC rates after the implementation of feeding protocols, but these were not statistically significant. However, some of these studies had small sample sizes or had other changes as part of the implementation of feeding protocols (eg, increases in breast milk provision) that may confound the effects of withholding feeding during RBC transfusion. Additionally, most studies were conducted at a single center, and only one was a randomized trial.[38] The study populations differed (eg, preterm infants <32 weeks' gestation, low birth weight infants <2500 g) and decisions of when to transfuse were variable among these studies.

In a systematic review and meta-analysis by Jasani and colleagues,[44] 7 studies[35–37,39–41,43] with 7492 infants that examined the association between withholding of feeding and NEC following RBC transfusion were pooled together. The study reported moderate GRADE certainty of evidence because of a "large sample size, narrow CIs, and mild statistical heterogeneity," with withholding of feeding during RBC transfusion associated with a lower risk of NEC: RR 0.47; 95 CI 0.28 to 0.80. In a separate article, Killion[45] conducted a review (not a meta-analysis) of 6 studies[34–38,46] that evaluated feeding practices during RBC transfusion in relation to the development of NEC following RBC transfusion and noted inconclusive evidence regarding the practice of withholding feedings around RBC transfusion and its effect on the risk of NEC. The authors noted the need for adequately powered randomized controlled trials (RCTs). We have highlighted such large ongoing RCTs in **Table 2**. The WHEAT trials

Table 1
Summary of completed studies on withholding feeding during transfusion

Study Name[ref]	Sample Size	Population	Intervention	Main Results
Clarke-Pounder et al,[34] 2015	145	Infants < 32 wk GA	Feeding withheld during the immediate time of transfusion and restarting feeds at the previous volume immediately posttransfusion.	No significant difference in incidence of NEC between the 2 groups.
Derienzo et al,[35] 2014	1380	VLBW infants (<1500 g)	Oral food and fluids withheld from infants for 4 h before, during, and after transfusion, at which time feeds are restarted at 50% of the original volume for 12 h and then advanced to the original volume.	Significant reduction in the incidence of NEC with a nonsignificant reduction in TANEC.
Doty et al,[36] 2016	108	VLBW infants (500–1500 g)	Feedings withheld at least 3 h before a transfusion and restarted following the transfusion as determined by the provider.	No significant difference in the incidence of NEC between the 2 groups.
Bajaj et al,[37] 2019	125	Infants with BW < 1250 g who survived beyond 1 wk of age	Feeding withheld for 12–24 h during and after the blood transfusion.	No significant decrease in rates of NEC or TANEC.
Sahin et al,[38] 2020	112	VLBW infants (≤1500 g) or infants with GA ≤ 32 wk	Feeding withheld during transfusion vs continued.	No significant difference in rates of NEC.
Rindone et al.[39] (Abstract)	1577	Infants with GA < 34 wk	Feeding withheld for >24 h after transfusion.	Nonsignificant reduction in TANEC rates after intervention implementation.

Mohamed et al.[40] (Abstract)	2422	VLBW infants (<1500 g)	Feeding withheld during RBC transfusion.	Nonsignificant reduction in TANEC cases postimplementation.
Meneses et al.[41] (Abstract)	1201	LBW infants	Feeding withheld 3 h before and 9 h after every RBC transfusion.	Nonsignificant reduction in TANEC cases.
El-Dib et al,[42] 2011	25	Preterm infants <32 wk GA and LBW <2500 g with case-control methodology (matched with controls with similar BW, GA, and gender)	Feeding withheld immediately before and during the period of transfusion, then resumed immediately after completion.	Withholding feeds during transfusion was associated with a significant reduction in the incidence of NEC ($P = .047$).
Perciaccante and Young[43] (Abstract)	595	VLBW infants	Feedings withheld 4 h before, during, and after the completion of the transfusion	Nonsignificant reduction in TANEC cases after implementation.

Abbreviations: BW, birth weight; GA, gestational age; LBW, low birth weight; NEC, necrotizing enterocolitis; NPO, nil per os; TANEC, transfusion-associated NEC; VLBW, very low birth weight.

Table 2
Summary of ongoing large randomized trials evaluating the withholding of feeding during transfusion

Trial Name	Location	Target Sample Size	Estimated Completion Year	Population	Intervention	Outcome
WHEAT	Australia, New Zealand	4437[a]	2025	Preterm infants <30 wk gestation	All enteral feeds will be discontinued for 4 h prior to the red cell transfusion, during the transfusion, and until 4 h posttransfusion.	NEC stage 2 or more
WHEAT	Canada and United Kingdom	4333[b]	2025	Same as above	Same as above	Same as above

[a] Enrollment as of March 2023 was 90 infants. Data from the Australian New Zealand Clinical Trials Registry. WithHolding or continuing Enteral feeds Around blood Transfusion (WHEAT) to prevent necrotising enterocolitis (NEC) in preterm infants. Available at: https://www.anzctr.org.au/Trial/Registration/TrialReview.aspx?id=377274. Accessed Apr 13 2023.
[b] Enrollment as of March 2023 was 63 infants. Data from neoEPOCH. WHEAT International Trial. Available at: http://neoepoch.com/wheat-trial. Accessed Apr 13 2023.

are two similar multicenter randomized trials, with one being conducted in Australia and New Zealand and the other in Canada and the UK, based on the design of a pilot trial in the UK.[47] The target sample sizes of these trials are among the largest that have enrolled preterm infants, and together they will exceed 8500 infants. However, based on the data available at the time of this review article, around 2% of the target sample size had been enrolled. Therefore, it will be some time before data could possibly become available (eg, 2025). Until more data are available, we have highlighted in **Box 1** some considerations regarding whether to withhold feedings or not during an RBC transfusion. Among these is the low absolute risk of NEC within 48 hours following RBC transfusion (estimated to be ~0.5%).[25,48]

EFFECT OF FEEDING PROTOCOLS ON THE RISK OF NECROTIZING ENTEROCOLITIS

As shown in **Table 1**, there is variability in feeding approaches to RBC transfusion, with some studies reporting on changes as part of broader standardized feeding protocols. Therefore, separating the effect specifically of withholding feeding during RBC transfusion from other changes in practice is challenging, as noted by DeRienzo et al.[35] Although formula feeding is a risk factor for NEC, the benefits of maternal breast milk feeding are well-established, and many centers now provide donor milk when maternal breast milk is unavailable or have worked to improve maternal breast milk provision. Both of these factors are likely to influence the risk of NEC as part of feeding strategies and could bias preimplementation and postimplementation studies of feeding protocols that change many feeding parameters. As noted in the study by DeRienzo et al.,[35] this may have explained the reduction in risk of NEC over time. Dako and colleagues[49] explored the implementation of an institution wide standardized, slow enteral feeding regimen on the risk on the NEC and transfusion-associated NEC in preterm infants.[50] They implemented a protocol in which infants had a prolonged NPO period in the first 1 to 2 weeks, depending on birth weight, followed by a period of trophic feedings of human milk for 1 week that was advanced slowly until 100 mL/kg/d, where a human milk fortifier was introduced. Full feeds were achieved by day 44 to 52, compared with a prior feeding protocol of day 14 to 18. This study showed a decrease in rates of NEC in relation to RBC transfusion as well as NEC rates overall. By contrast, the EPIPAGE 2 and EPIFLORE studies

---

Box 1
Considerations regarding feeding or withholding feeding during RBC transfusion

Favors Not Withholding Feeding
1. Low absolute risk of NEC within 48 hours after RBC transfusion (~0.5%).[25,48]
2. Lack of data from randomized trials to support the efficacy of withholding feeding on the risk of NEC.
3. Low overall incidence of NEC results in many infants with feedings withheld who are unlikely to develop NEC.
4. Uncertainty about the optimal duration of withholding feeding during and around transfusion.
5. May result in additional treatments (eg, intravenous fluids) that would otherwise not be needed.

Favors Withholding of Feeding
1. Observational studies support a potential reduction in the risk of NEC (**Table 1**).
2. Meta-analysis shows a large magnitude relative risk reduction (eg, ~50%).[44]
3. Approach is limited to a short period of higher NEC risk following RBC transfusion.
4. Feasible to apply in the clinical setting.

evaluated 3161 preterm infants and the associations between advancement of enteral feeding and risk of NEC and found that a slower rate of progression of enteral feeding was significantly associated with an increased incidence of NEC.[51]

Schindler and colleagues[46] examined 3 different enteral feeding regimens during a single red cell transfusion in preterm infants using NIRS and calculating the mean splanchnic–cerebral oxygenation ratio and a mean splanchnic fractional oxygen extraction before, during, and after RBC transfusion. The study found no differences in splanchnic oxygenation when enteral feeds were withheld or restricted in relation to an RBC transfusion. Taken together, it appears that outside of specifically evaluating the withholding of feeding during RBC transfusion, different approaches to early feeding (slow vs fast) or restricting feeding do not consistently influence the risk of NEC, despite evidence that the use of a standardized feeding regimen is associated with an important reduction in the risk of NEC.[52]

SUMMARY

Severe anemia and RBC transfusions are associated with gut inflammation and injury in preclinical models and observational studies. However, there is uncertainty about the role of these factors in the pathogenesis of NEC. Given the results of recent randomized trials of lower versus higher RBC transfusion thresholds, it appears that the lower thresholds studied in the trials are safe with regards to the risk of NEC. Observational studies have shown that withholding feeding during RBC transfusion may lower the risk of NEC, although confirmatory data from randomized trials are lacking. Ongoing large trials may provide more certainty regarding approaches to feeding during transfusion, although given the target sample sizes of these trials, the data are unlikely to be available in the near term.

DISCLOSURE

R.M. Patel serves as a consultant for Noveome, Inc and serves on the data-safety monitoring committee for Infant Bacterial Therapeutics/Premier research.

FUNDING

This review was supported by the NHLBI K23 HL128942 to Ravi Patel.

REFERENCES

1. Neu J, Walker WA. Necrotizing enterocolitis. N Engl J Med 2011;364(3):255–64.
2. Patel RM, Kandefer S, Walsh MC, et al. Causes and timing of death in extremely premature infants from 2000 through 2011. N Engl J Med 2015;372:331–40.
3. Alganabi M, Lee C, Bindi E, et al. Recent advances in understanding necrotizing enterocolitis. F1000Res 2019;8:F1000. Faculty Rev-107.
4. Cotten CM, Oh W, McDonald S, et al. Prolonged hospital stay for extremely premature infants: risk factors, center differences, and the impact of mortality on selecting a best-performing center. J Perinatol 2005;25(10):650–5.
5. Hackam D, Caplan M. Necrotizing enterocolitis: pathophysiology from a historical context. Semin Pediatr Surg 2018;27(1):11–8.
6. Lin PW, Stoll BJ. Necrotising enterocolitis. Lancet 2006;368(9543):1271–83.
7. Battesrby C, Longford N, Coseloe K, et al. Development of a gestational age-specific case definition for neonatal necrotizing enterocolitis. JAMA Pediatr 2017;171(3):256–63.

8. Patel RM, Ferguson J, McElroy SJ, et al. Defining necrotizing enterocolitis: current difficulties and future opportunities. Pediatr Res 2020;88:10–5.
9. Rose AT, Patel RM. A critical analysis of risk factors for necrotizing enterocolitis. Semin Fetal Neonatal Med 2018;23(6):374–9.
10. Rose AT, Saroha V, Patel RM. Transfusion-related gut injury and necrotizing enterocolitis. Clin Perinatol 2020;47(2):399–412.
11. Carlisle EM, Morowitz MJ. The intestinal microbiome and necrotizing enterocolitis. Curr Opin Pediatr 2013;25(3):382–7.
12. Caplan MS, Simon D, Jilling T. The role of PAF, TLR, and the inflammatory response in neonatal necrotizing enterocolitis. Semin Pediatr Surg 2015;14(3): 145–51.
13. Jilling T, Simon D, Lu J, et al. The roles of bacteria and TLR4 in rat and murine models of necrotizing enterocolitis. J Immunol 2006;177(5):3273–82.
14. Askie LM, Darlow BA, Finer N, et al. Association between oxygen saturation targeting and death or Di, sability in extremely preterm infants in the neonatal oxygenation Prospective meta-analysis Collaboration. JAMA 2018;319(21):2190–201.
15. Marin T, Moore J, Kosmetatos N, et al. Red blood cell transfusion-related necrotizing enterocolitis in very-low-birthweight infants: a near-infrared spectroscopy investigation. Transfusion 2013;53(11):2650–8.
16. Fortune PM, Wagstaff M, Petros AJ. Cerebro-splanchnic oxygenation ratio (CSOR) using near infrared spectroscopy may be able to predict splanchnic ischaemia in neonates. Intensive Care Med 2001;27(8):1401–7.
17. Kirpalani H, Whyte RK, Andersen C, et al. The Premature Infants in Need of Transfusion (PINT) study: a randomized, controlled trial of a restrictive (low) versus liberal (high) transfusion threshold for extremely low birth weight infants. J Pediatr 2006;149(3):301–7.
18. Whyte RK, Kirpalani H, Asztalos EV, et al. Neurodevelopmental outcome of extremely low birth weight infants randomly assigned to restrictive or liberal hemoglobin thresholds for blood transfusion. Pediatrics 2009;123(1):207–13.
19. Kirpalani H, Bell EF, Hintz SR, et al. Higher or lower hemoglobin transfusion thresholds for preterm infants. N Engl J Med 2020;383(27):2639–51.
20. Franz AR, Engel C, Bassler D, et al. Effects of liberal vs restrictive transfusion thresholds on survival and neurocognitive outcomes in extremely low-birth-weight infants: the ETTNO randomized clinical trial. JAMA 2020;324(6):560–70 [published correction appears in JAMA. 2022 Jul 12;328(2):217].
21. Wang P, Wang X, Deng H, et al. Restrictive versus liberal transfusion thresholds in very low birth weight infants: a systematic review with meta-analysis. PLoS One 2021;16(8):e0256810.
22. Arthur CM, Nalbant D, Feldman HA, et al. Anemia induces gut inflammation and injury in an animal model of preterm infants. Transfusion 2019;59(4):1233–45.
23. MohanKumar K, Namachivayam K, Sivakumar N, et al. Severe neonatal anemia increases intestinal permeability by disrupting epithelial adherens junctions. Am J Physiol Gastrointest Liver Physiol 2020;318(4):G705–16.
24. Kalteren WS, Bos AF, van Oeveren W, et al. Neonatal anemia relates to intestinal injury in preterm infants. Pediatr Res 2022;91(6):1452–8.
25. Patel RM, Knezevic A, Shenvi N, et al. Association of red blood cell transfusion, anemia, and necrotizing enterocolitis in very-low-birth-weight infants. JAMA 2016; 315(9):889–97.
26. Singh R, Visintainer PF, Frantz ID 3rd, et al. Association of necrotizing enterocolitis with anemia and packed red blood cell transfusions in preterm infants. J Perinatol 2011;31(3):176–82.

27. MohanKumar K, Namachivayam K, Song T, et al. A murine neonatal model of necrotizing enterocolitis caused by anemia and red blood cell transfusions. Nat Commun 2019;10(1):3494.

28. Mally P, Golombek SG, Mishra R, et al. Association of necrotizing enterocolitis with elective packed red blood cell transfusions in stable, growing, premature neonates. Am J Perinatol 2006;23(8):451–8.

29. Mohamed A, Shah PS. Transfusion associated necrotizing enterocolitis: a meta-analysis of observational data. Pediatrics 2012;129(3):529–40.

30. Sharma R, Kraemer DF, Torrazza RM, et al. Packed red blood cell transfusion is not associated with increased risk of necrotizing enterocolitis in premature infants. J Perinatol 2014;34(11):858–62.

31. Hay S, Zupancic JA, Flannery DD, et al. Should we believe in transfusion-associated enterocolitis? Applying a GRADE to the literature. Semin Perinatol 2017;41(1):80–91.

32. Rai SE, Sidhu AK, Krishnan RJ. Transfusion-associated necrotizing enterocolitis re-evaluated: a systematic review and meta-analysis. J Perinat Med 2018;46(6):665–76.

33. Garg P, Pinotti R, Lal CV, et al. Transfusion-associated necrotizing enterocolitis in preterm infants: an updated meta-analysis of observational data. J Perinat Med 2018;46(6):677–85.

34. Clarke-Pounder J, Howlett J, Burnsed J, et al. Withholding feeding during transfusion: Standardization of practice and nutritional outcomes in premature infants. J Neonatal Perinatal Med 2015;8(3):199–205.

35. Derienzo C, Smith PB, Tanaka D, et al. Feeding practices and other risk factors for developing transfusion-associated necrotizing enterocolitis. Early Hum Dev 2014;90(5):237–40.

36. Doty M, Wade C, Farr J, et al. Feeding during blood transfusions and the association with necrotizing enterocolitis. Am J Perinatol 2016;33(9):882–6.

37. Bajaj M, Lulic-Botica M, Hanson A, et al. Feeding during transfusion and the risk of necrotizing enterocolitis in preterm infants. J Perinatol 2019;39(4):540–6.

38. Sahin S, Gozde Kanmaz Kutman H, Bozkurt O, et al. Effect of withholding feeds on transfusion-related acute gut injury in preterm infants: a pilot randomized controlled trial. J Matern Fetal Neonatal Med 2020;33(24):4139–44.

39. Rindone S, Knee A, Rothstein R. Assessing the impact of holding feedings during PRBC transfusion on the incidence of transfusion related gut injury (TRAGI) in preterm infants. Internet. Pediatric Academic Societies Abstract Archive. cited 2022 Oct 25.

40. Mohamed A, Ayed M, Shah P. Withholding feeds during blood transfusion and risk of transfusion associated necrotizing enterocolitis (TANEC). Paediatr Child Health 2015;20:62 (abstr).

41. Meneses J, Figueredo J, Macedo A. Does witholding feedings during transfusions decrease the incidence of necrotizing enterocolitis in preterm infants? Internet. Pediatric Academic Societies Abstract Archive. Available at: http://www.abstracts2view.com/pasall. Accessed October 25, 2022.

42. El-Dib M, Narang S, Lee E, et al. Red blood cell transfusion, feeding and necrotizing enterocolitis in preterm infants. J Perinatol 2011;31(3):183–7. https://doi.org/10.1038/jp.2010.157.

43. Perciaccante JV, Young TE. Necrotizing enterocolitis associated with packed red blood cell transfusions in premature neonates Internet. Pediatric Academic Societies Abstract Archive. cited 2022 Oct 25.

44. Jasani B, Rao S, Patole S. Withholding feeds and transfusion-associated necrotizing enterocolitis in preterm infants: a systematic review. Adv Nutr 2017;8(5): 764–9.
45. Killion E. Feeding practices and effects on transfusion-associated necrotizing enterocolitis in premature neonates. Adv Neonatal Care 2021;21(5):356–64.
46. Schindler T, Yeo KT, Bolisetty S, et al. FEEding DURing red cell transfusion (FEE-DUR RCT): a multi-arm randomised controlled trial. BMC Pediatr 2020;20(1):346.
47. Gale C, Modi N, Jawad S, et al. The WHEAT pilot trial-WithHolding Enteral feeds Around packed red cell Transfusions to prevent necrotizing enterocolitis in preterm neonates: a multicenter, electronic patient record (EPR), randomized controlled point-of-care pilot trial. BMJ Open 2019;9(9):e033543.
48. Paul DA, Mackley A, Novitsky A, et al. Increased odds of necrotizing enterocolitis after transfusion of red blood cells in premature infants. Pediatrics 2011;127(4): 635–41.
49. Dako J, Buzzard J, Jain M, et al. Slow enteral feeding decreases risk of transfusion associated necrotizing enterocolitis. J Neonatal Perinatal Med 2018;11(3): 231–9.
50. Pietz J, Achanti B, Lilien L, et al. Prevention of necrotizing enterocolitis in preterm infants: a 20-year experience. Pediatrics 2007;119(1):e164–70.
51. Rozé JC, Ancel PY, Lepage P, et al. Nutritional strategies and gut microbiota composition as risk factors for necrotizing enterocolitis in very-preterm infants. Am J Clin Nutr 2017;106(3):821–30.
52. Jasani B, Patole S. Standardized feeding regimen for reducing necrotizing enterocolitis in preterm infants: an updated systematic review. J Perinatol 2017; 37(7):827–33.

Current Practices, Challenges, and Recommendations in Enteral Nutrition After Necrotizing Enterocolitis

Elena Itriago, MD[a], Kimberly Fernandez Trahan, MD[a],
Leonor Adriana Massieu, RD, LD, CNSC[a], Parvesh M. Garg, MD[b],
Muralidhar H. Premkumar, MD[a],*

KEYWORDS

- Necrotizing enterocolitis • Enteral nutrition • Parenteral nutrition • Intestinal failure
- Prematurity • Breast milk

KEY POINTS

- The evidence behind the current nutritional management of infants following necrotizing enterocolitis (NEC) is weak.
- The institutional policies and expert opinions form the basis for most post-NEC nutritional practices.
- Standardizing the post-NEC nutritional regimen will likely decrease practice variability and improve outcomes.

INTRODUCTION

Necrotizing enterocolitis (NEC) is an inflammatory bowel that occurs in about 7% of very low birthweight premature infants with a mortality rate ranging from 15% to 30%.[1] The pathophysiology of NEC is not entirely understood, yet multiple risk factors have been described. Prematurity is one of NEC's most recognized risk factors, and the risk is inversely associated with birthweight and gestational age.[1–3] A breast milk-based diet is associated with protection against NEC, whereas a formula-based diet is associated with a higher prevalence of NEC.[4] Intestinal dysbiosis is another risk

[a] Department of Pediatrics, Section of Neonatology, Baylor College of Medicine, Texas Children's Hospital, Houston, TX, USA; [b] Wake Forest School of Medicine, Brenner Children's Hospital, Atrium Health Wake Forest Baptist, Winston-Salem, NC, USA
* Corresponding author. Texas Children's Hospital, 6621 Fannin, Suite A5590, Houston, TX 77030.
E-mail address: premkuma@bcm.edu

Clin Perinatol 50 (2023) 683–698
https://doi.org/10.1016/j.clp.2023.04.009
0095-5108/23/© 2023 Elsevier Inc. All rights reserved.

perinatology.theclinics.com

factor in the development of NEC characterized by decreased diversity and increased colonization of pathogenic microbiota replacing the beneficial strains.[5]

Nutritional management plays a significant role in the prevention and treatment of NEC. However, much of the current literature and evidence-based nutritional guidelines in NEC focuses on prevention. Similar evidence-based, high-quality guidelines regarding nutritional management following NEC are lacking. Most nutritional strategies practiced in the recovery and rehabilitation period after NEC are based on institutional policies and expert opinion. This review describes the nutritional rehabilitation process following NEC and its challenges and provides practical recommendations.

CURRENT CLINICAL PRACTICES THAT AFFECT ENTERAL NUTRITION AFTER NECROTIZING ENTEROCOLITIS

Historically, medical and surgical NEC management has involved bowel rest, nasogastric decompression, parenteral nutrition, and the prolonged use of intravenous antibiotics.[6] Because of the lack of evidence to support those practices, variations in nutritional management after NEC is challenging (**Table 1**).

- Duration of bowel rest following NEC

NEC is a state of marked intestinal inflammation associated with ongoing cellular repair, compromised permeability, and dysmotility due to ileus. Hence, the infants are kept nil per os (NPO) for variable periods to allow the healing process to complete. Infants are placed on bowel rest for 7 to 14 days after the diagnosis of NEC.[6] These recommendations are arbitrary and not based on strong evidence. No randomized controlled trials comparing different periods of bowel rest to determine the optimal duration exist. Once feeds are initiated, they are advanced cautiously because of the concern that enteral nutrition (EN) could be associated with the development of recurrent NEC or result in an intestinal stricture.[7] One consequence of the lack of strong evidence in the literature is the practice variation among neonatologists, pediatric surgeons, and institutions. Zani and colleagues[8] evaluated the current practice of surgeons in managing medical and surgical NEC in 20 European countries through a survey. For medical NEC, 41% of providers kept the infants in bowel rest for 7 days and 49% for 10 days. For surgical NEC, 46% of the infants were held nil by mouth for 5 to 7 days, 42% for more than 7 days, and 12% for less than 5 days.

- Duration of antibiotics

Several studies have shown intestinal dysbiosis in infants with NEC, and over 40% of infants with NEC demonstrate positive blood cultures for bacterial growth.[5,9] These

Table 1	
Factors that promote tolerance to enteral nutrition after necrotizing enterocolitis	
Predictors and Variables that Affect Enteral Nutrition After NEC	
Medical and Surgical NEC	**Surgical NEC with Short Bowel Syndrome**
Earlier initiation of feeds	Postmenstrual age at onset of disease
Standardization of nutritional regimen	Residual bowel length
Antibiotic stewardship	Presence of ileocecal valve
Prevention of bloodstream infection	Presence of colon
	Presence of mucus fistula
	Intestinal rehabilitation program

associations between dysbiosis and NEC support antibiotic therapy as a standard component of the treatment of NEC. The duration of antibiotic therapy in NEC is based on the severity; neonates with medical NEC receive shorter courses, and those with surgical NEC receive more prolonged antibiotics. The adopted antibiotic durations are arbitrary and not based on high-quality evidence. Interestingly, feeding practices following NEC are closely linked to the period of antibiotic coverage. The practice of withholding feeds until the completion of the antibiotic course is common. The intent to withhold feeds until the completion of antibiotic therapy, perhaps, is to ensure that the bacteria-induced inflammation has entirely resolved. Withholding feeds until the completion of antibiotics makes logical sense, but has not been systematically studied. A study of 34 neonatal intensive care units under the Children's Hospital Neonatal consortium demonstrated a direct correlation between the duration of antibiotics and the time to full feeds and length of stay in medical and surgical NEC patients.[10] The centers with longer durations of antibiotics had much more extended periods of bowel rest.

- Lack of standardization of practices

Variation in practices is one common narrative in the practices mentioned above: the duration of NPO and the duration of antibiotics. Standardized feeding practices have shown improved outcomes in neonates with a reduction in the incidence of NEC.[11] In the previously mentioned post-NEC antibiotic study, centers with higher variability in the use of antibiotics had longer durations of antibiotics, took much longer to initiate feeds, and thus reached full feeds later.[10] This suggests that standardization of antibiotic regimens and feeding practices within and across various centers will likely facilitate shorter durations of antibiotic treatment and earlier initiations of enteral feeds after NEC.

CONSEQUENCES OF DELAYED ENTERAL FEEDS

Prolonged periods of bowel rest and slow feeding advancement have several negative consequences for infants with NEC, as enumerated in **Box 1**.

- Oral aversion

The benefits of oral feeding include sensory stimulation at multiple levels, such as the positive aspect of touch, taste, smell, and satiety. Patients with prolonged bowel

---

Box 1
Current practice, challenges, and consequences of post-necrotizing enterocolitis enteral nutrition advancement

Current Practice
  Prolonged period of nil by mouth
  Prolonged duration of antibiotics

Current Challenges
  Variation within individual practice
  Variation among individual and institutional practice
  Lack of evidence-based recommendations

Consequences
  Oral aversion
  Gastrointestinal mucosal atrophy
  Intestinal dysmotility
  Intestinal failure-associated liver disease (IFALD)
  Central line-associated bloodstream infection (CLABSI)

rest are at risk of developing oral aversion. The prolonged use of parenteral nutrition (PN) and tube feeding deprives infants of the positive experience of oral feeding, thus leading to oral aversion and delaying the establishment of normal suck and swallow patterns.[12] Patients with a prolonged nasogastric tube develop negative experiences secondary to tube insertion, airway, and gastrointestinal suctioning that could be associated with stressful and painful experiences. These negative experiences may trigger a response of feeding avoidance when oral feedings are delayed in premature infants and negatively affect parent–child bonding.

- Gastrointestinal effects

The prolonged deprivation of EN could cause several gastrointestinal effects, including mucosal villous atrophy, dysbiosis, small intestinal bacterial overgrowth, and intestinal dysmotility.[13,14] Starvation has been shown to induce mucosal atrophy in animal models as manifested by decreased villous height and shallow crypts due to decreased epithelial proliferation and increased apoptosis.[13] In a mouse model, investigators showed a predominance of gammaproteobacteria, an increase in inflammatory cytokines, and decreased epithelial growth factors associated with mucosal atrophy.[14]

- Parenteral nutrition dependence and intestinal failure-associated liver disease (IFALD)

IFALD is a state of liver dysfunction in prolonged use of PN and is diagnosed by elevated levels of conjugated bilirubin ($\geq$2 mg/dL) and liver transaminases.[15,16] IFALD is a multifactorial disease with several factors, such as inflammation, inability to sustain enteral feeds, and PN, implicated in its pathogenesis. Delay in initiating and slow advancement of enteral feeds increases the duration of PN, which can increase the risk of IFALD.[15–18]

- Central venous access duration and bloodstream infections

Central venous access is a recognized risk factor for bloodstream infections. Infection can adversely affect the outcomes in infants with NEC. Sepsis can worsen liver injury by endotoxin-induced increased production of inflammatory cytokines that cause impairment of biliary excretion, leading to cholestasis.[16] Sepsis in the context of NEC has also been shown to increase mortality.[9] Other less recognized effects of sepsis include growth restriction and increased antibiotic exposure.

CONSIDERATIONS TO ASSESS READINESS TO FEED

- Normalization of clinical signs and symptoms

Abdominal signs vary depending on the severity of NEC, including abdominal distension, redness, and tenderness, and the clinician should ensure their resolution before initiating feeds. Nasogastric decompression is started in the early stages of NEC to address gastrointestinal ileus, which occurs in response to inflammation. Elevated gastric output should subside, and the bilious or bloody nature of the gastric content should resolve before the commencement of feeds. Although the passage of stool is a sign of resolution of gastrointestinal ileus, its absence does not always reflect the ileus. Instead, it could be secondary to prolonged periods of bowel rest. The return of previously absent bowel sounds is a reliable indicator of the return of gastrointestinal motility.

- Stabilization of the general health of the infant

A safe and successful introduction of feeds depends on the infant's overall stability. Hemodynamic instability is a common feature of advanced medical NEC and surgical NEC. In unstable hemodynamic states, reallocating blood supply to other vital organs, such as the brain, compromises the splanchnic circulation due to the diving reflex. Before initiation of feeds, normalization of hemodynamic status in the absence of vasoactive medications should be achieved. As mentioned earlier, withholding feeds until the completion of the antibiotic course has not been studied prospectively. It is weak in evidence and derives further attention.

- Resolution of the radiological abnormalities

Abdominal radiographs are the other common adjunct utilized in evaluating readiness to feed following NEC. NEC is characterized by abnormal radiological signs such as dilated bowel loops, abnormal distribution of intestinal gas shadows, pneumatosis intestinalis, portal venous gas, and pneumoperitoneum. The clinician should ensure the resolution of abnormal signs on the abdominal radiograph before initiation of feeds.

FACTORS ASSOCIATED WITH FEED TOLERANCE AND ENTERAL AUTONOMY

Several factors have been recognized to impact the success of feed tolerance in infants with NEC. Some of these are related to management practices, and others to the patient characteristics as described in **Table 1**.

- Early initiation of enteral feeds after NEC

Early initiation of EN after NEC has been associated with a shorter time to achieve full feeds and a shorter central venous catheter duration. Early enteral feeding mitigates anatomic changes such as mucosal villous atrophy, seen as early as within 1 week of bowel rest. Enteral nutrition stimulates the release of hormones such as gastrin, enteroglucagon, cholecystokinin, and neurotensin, potentially enhancing intestinal adaptation by promoting motility and increasing the absorptive capacity.[19]

Bohnhorst and colleagues[20] compared outcomes of infants with NEC (Bell Stage II or higher) on an early feeding regimen with those who were fed according to the discretion of the neonatologist. In the early feeding group, feeds were reinitiated after confirming that the portal venous gas had resolved, as observed by abdominal ultrasound. Those infants who underwent early feeding reached complete enteral feeding sooner, had fewer central venous catheter days and catheter-related septicemia, and had shorter antibiotic durations. These results included infants treated medically and surgically, so it may not be entirely applicable in surgical NEC cases. However, when only those cases of surgical NEC were considered, the resumption of feeds occurred sooner in the early feeding group without an increase in complications, indicating there may still be benefits with earlier nutrition.

- Standardization of feeding regimens to reduce variability

Several recent publications describe the effect of implementing institutional feeding guidelines. Early feeding initiation after medical NEC decreases the average days to reach full enteral feeds without increasing the incidence of NEC recurrence and intestinal strictures. Through a quality improvement initiative, Patel and colleagues [21] described the effect of such feeding guidelines in their institution; the time to resume feeds after NEC decreased from 9.4 to 5.1 days, and the average number of days to reach full feeds decreased by 35%. Similarly, Arbra and colleagues[22] compared early (<7 days) and late (>7 days) feeding on patients with medical NEC and found that early reintroduction of feeding was not significantly associated with increased NEC recurrence, mortality, or stricture.

- Multidisciplinary care by intestinal rehabilitation teams

The introduction of intestinal rehabilitation teams in the care of patients with medical and surgical NEC has not only led to a dramatic improvement in survival, a decrease in the need for pediatric intestinal/liver transplantation, but also a shorter time to achieve full feeds and enteral autonomy.[23] The practice of institutional guidelines has been associated with better outcomes in feeding after NEC. Shores and colleagues [24] assessed the effectiveness of postoperative feeding guidelines in reducing the incidence and severity of IFALD among surgical infants. The investigators found that implementing institutional guidelines decreased the incidence of IFALD and the time to reach enteral autonomy. Shakeel and colleagues[25] evaluated outcomes before and after implementing institutional feeding guidelines in infants who underwent a gastrointestinal surgical procedure, including surgical NEC. The group found a reduction in the time to reach enteral autonomy from 28 days to 21 days and a reduction in the rate of central line-associated bloodstream infections from 25% to 5%.

- Special considerations in surgical NEC

The factors that affect EN after surgical NEC are shown in **Table 1**. Recognizing these factors in surgical NEC will help assess readiness for feed initiation and prognosticate feed tolerance following surgical NEC. The intestines undergo exponential growth in length and surface area throughout the gestational period, doubling in length during the last trimester. Hence, the residual bowel following an anatomic loss of intestines that occurs earlier in the gestation has a more significant potential for growth and adaptation. Preterms compared with term infants and neonates compared with older infants have better intestinal adaptation with the same residual bowel length. As one would anticipate, longer residual intestinal segments predict better recovery through a larger surface area for digestion and absorption.[26,27] Retention of the ileocecal valve is associated with a better likelihood of enteral autonomy; however, it is difficult to discern whether those benefits arise from the ileocecal valve per se or the terminal ileum.[26] The ileocecal valve might prevent the reflux of colonic contents that increase the likelihood of small intestinal bacterial overgrowth. The benefits of the ileum come from its greater ability to adapt and the site-specific characteristics such as absorption of bile salts and vitamin B12 in the terminal ileum. Similar to the ileum and ileocecal valve, retention of the colon is a predictor of improved feed tolerance. The retained colon plays an essential part in absorbing water and electrolytes; also, the short-chain fatty acids generated by the fermentation of unabsorbed carbohydrates by colonic microbiota serve as a source of energy.[28]

- Mucous fistula refeeding

Many infants with surgical NEC are left with bowel discontinuity and the creation of an ostomy with or without a mucus fistula. Although achieving full enteral feeds prior to reanastomosis in such infants is challenging, attempts toward enteral autonomy should be made with close monitoring for adequacy of growth.[29,30] The presence of mucous fistulas enables mucus fistula refeeding (MFR), a practice in which the nutrient-rich output from the proximal ostomy is reintroduced into the distal mucous fistula. MFR allows for intestinal adaptation to occur in the otherwise unused bowel. Benefits include improved growth before reanastomosis, decreased PN dependence, fewer central line days, lower rates of IFALD, and better post-surgical outcomes.[31,32] Based on the current evidence, at our center we consider MFR in infants over 1000 g body weight with small bowel ostomy and mucous fistula. Prior to MFR, a consensus is obtained from all stakeholders including surgeons and nursing, and the patency of the distal intestine is confirmed with a contrast study. Detailed instructions are provided to the nurses including the intestinal anatomy, type and depth of insertion of feeding tube, quantity and frequency of refeeding, and monitoring for complications. In most instances, the feeding tube is inserted 4 to 5 cm in to the mucous fistula, left in place for up to a week, and the entire ostomy output is refed. Infusion time is modified based on the ostomy output. At our institution, MFR is performed using a syringe pump, every 3 to 4 hours over a duration of 1 to 2 hours. The patency of the feeding tube is maintained by flushing the feeding tube and the extension tube with 1 to 2 mL of sterile water before and after refeeding.

NUTRITIONAL RECOMMENDATIONS
Parenteral nutrition

Parenteral nutrition is the primary source of support in infants following NEC during periods of intestinal rest and advancement of enteral feeds. Parenteral energy and protein needs for premature and term infants should initially target PN goals for age, and energy intake should be adjusted individually based on growth parameters. See **Table 2** with recommended macronutrient needs for term and premature infants.

Protein
Adequate protein supplementation is essential to support the growth requirements, promote cell repair following NEC, and prevent negative nitrogen balance. In a study comparing low (2.3 g/kg/d) versus high protein (3.6 g/kg/d) supplementation in very low birthweight infants with NEC, there was no difference in the incidence of cholestasis, but the high protein group demonstrated higher peak conjugated bilirubin levels (8 mg/dL vs. 3 mg/dL).[33] However, despite this marginal benefit, the effects of low protein supplementation are rift with the risk of undernutrition. Although the optimal protein needs and supplementation is debatable, it is safe to conclude that amino acids should be provided at 3 to 4 g/kg/d to promote tissue regeneration (**Table 3**).[34–36]

Lipids
IFALD significantly correlates with soybean oil-based intravenous lipid emulsions due to its predominantly proinflammatory profile. The newer generation fish oil containing lipid emulsions with their predominantly anti-inflammatory profile has been used as an alternative source of lipids in the prevention and treatment of IFALD. The most recent Cochrane systematic reviews showed only a modest benefit with a high degree of uncertainty with the use of fish oil containing multiple oil emulsions in the prevention and treatment of IFALD.[37,38] However, another meta-analysis showed that using fish oil containing multiple oil lipid-based emulsions was associated with a decrease in the

Table 2		
Energy and protein goals for parenteral nutrition		
	Preterm Infant	**Term Infant**
Energy (kcal/kg/d)	90–115[68]	85%–90% of predicted from the standard equation. See below[a]
Protein (g/kg/d)	3.5–4[34–36]	2–3[35,36]

[a] 0 to 3 mo: Estimated Energy Requirements (EER) = [89 x wt. (kg) – 100] + 175 kcal (EER = kcal/d).
Data from Refs.[34–36,68,69]

Table 3 Energy and protein goals for enteral nutrition		
	Preterm Infant	**Term Infant**
Energy (kcal/kg/d)	110–135[34,70,71]	See below[a,34,72]
Protein (g/kg/d)	3.5–4.5[34,71]	1.5 (healthy)[72] 2–3 (illness/surgery)[69]

[a] 0 to 3 mo: Estimated Energy Requirements (EER) = [89 x wt (kg) – 100] + 175 kcal (EER = kcal/d).
Data from Refs.[34,69–72]

rate of rise of bilirubin in infants with long-term PN.[39] Also, several single-center and matched-pair analysis studies have demonstrated the benefits of using pure fish oil containing lipid emulsion in treating IFALD.[17,18] Hence, in the setting of NEC, the newer generation fish oil containing lipid emulsions can be considered to provide nutrition and to reduce the risks for IFALD. However, the evidence to support this is of low certainty. The lipid-limiting strategy, where the dose of lipid emulsion is restricted to 1 to 1.5 g/kg/d, offers an inconsistent and suboptimal resolution of IFALD. Also, this strategy is associated with a high risk of essential fatty acid deficiencies.[40,41] Hence, in the current era of newer-generation lipid emulsions, the role of lipid minimization is very limited.

Glucose

Adequate glucose provision is essential to meet energy needs and optimal growth. However, higher glucose concentrations can induce hyperglycemia with resultant hyperinsulinism and steatosis and have been shown to increase the risk of IFALD. In a large retrospective review of 450 infants with long-term PN, those who developed cholestasis received higher glucose concentrations.[42] In contrast, higher glucose infusion rates (16–18 mg/kg/min) have been shown to be safe when used along with pure fish-oil-based lipid emulsion in the setting of IFALD. In these settings, despite higher glucose infusion rates, high rates of resolution of IFALD have been described.[43] The American Society for Parenteral and Enteral Nutrition recommends a glucose infusion rate of 10 to 14 mg/kg/min with a maximum range of 14 to 18 mg/kg/min[35,36]

Micronutrients

Micronutrient deficiencies are often observed, especially in the case of short bowel syndrome resulting from NEC. A retrospective study that looked at 31 children with short bowel syndrome found that zinc, copper, iron, vitamin D, and phosphorus were the most common micronutrient deficiencies while on PN and after the transition to EN.[44,45] Infants often have iron-deficiency anemia, given PN seldom contains iron. Micronutrient deficiencies may be more prevalent during the transition from PN while attempting to reach enteral autonomy.[46] Close monitoring and supplementation are strongly recommended while on PN, during the transition to EN, and once enteral autonomy is achieved.

Cyclic PN

Cyclic PN is a strategy often used to treat or prevent the development of intestinal failure-associated liver disease. Although this strategy was devised as a lifestyle-improving intervention, it is hypothesized to have several biochemical and clinical benefits. Because cyclic PN is associated with PN-free periods, it mimics the normal diurnal and feeding-fasting patterns associated with oral enteral intake. The biochemical benefits include variable hormonal secretion, and better substrate utilization, resulting in metabolic unloading of the liver, with decreased severity of intestinal failure associated liver disease.[47] The practice of cyclic PN has not been studied in infants with NEC. The downsides include increased handling of the central venous catheter, increased infection risks, and metabolic effects such as hyperglycemia and hypoglycemia.

Enteral nutrition

Initiation and Advancement
After an episode of medical or surgical NEC, it is recommended to initiate trophic feeds ($\leq$20 mL/kg/d). Based on the infant's maturity and stability, these feeds are delivered via a feeding tube or by mouth. Whether the enteral feeds should be maintained at stable trophic feeds for a short duration of 3 to 5 days before advancement in post-NEC infants has not been studied. The decision to hold steady at trophic feeds should be based on the ability of the infant to tolerate enteral feeds. Without signs of intolerance, it is safe to advance feeds daily from initiation. Enteral nutrition should be increased gradually at a rate of 10 to 20 mL/kg/d while closely monitoring for feed tolerance.[48]

Type of Enteral Feeds

i. Breast milk: Human milk is the preferred choice for initiating feeds, given its multiple beneficial bioactive compounds and growth factors that may promote intestinal adaptation and reduce intestinal damage post-NEC.[49,50] When the mother's own milk (MOM) is not available or sufficient to support the nutritional intake of the infant, pasteurized donor human milk (DHM) could be an alternative diet. The use of DHM as a substitute diet compared to the formula has been shown to decrease the risk of NEC. However, similar benefits of DHM against recurrent NEC in post-NEC setting have not been studied. Despite this lack of evidence, it is prudent to presume the safety of DHM in post-NEC states in infants who continue to be at risk for recurrent NEC. The nutritional content of DHM is lower than MOM due to several factors: the stage of lactation of donor mothers, pasteurization, and storage process.[51–53] Also, following discharge from the hospital, the availability of DHM in the community is restricted. For the above nutritional and availability reasons, once the infant is beyond the age typically associated with risk for NEC, considerations should be given to a formula when availability of MOM is restricted.

ii. Formula: The optimal formula for post-NEC feeding has not been determined. Androsky and colleagues[54] reported that early enteral feeding with an amino acid-based formula or human milk compared to a protein hydrolysate after surgery might be associated with a reduced duration of PN. Capriati and colleagues[55] reported that human milk was the most commonly used initial enteral diet in pediatric intestinal failure, usually in combination with either hydrolyzed or elemental formula. They reported that hydrolyzed formulas were no more effective than amino acid-based formulas in promoting intestinal adaptation, and these dietary variations showed no difference in the duration of PN. Medium-chain triglyceride (MCT) is readily absorbed across the enterocytes in contrast to other lipid molecules that require a complex digestion process. Hence, MCT containing formulas may be easier to digest in settings of limited absorptive capacity after resection and cholestasis.[56] However, long-chain triglycerides have resulted in better intestinal adaptation in animal models.[57] Formulas with 40% to 60% MCT and long-chain triglycerides are reported to be more advantageous and better tolerated in infants with a remaining colon.[28] Premature infants are at an increased risk for metabolic bone disease, and intestinal failure augments this risk.[58] To promote bone health, fortification of human milk is recommended for premature infants.[41] Calcium, phosphorus, and vitamin D content in elemental, partially hydrolyzed, and extensively hydrolyzed formulas is lower than that in premature formulas and may be less bioavailable, which may further increase risk of metabolic bone disease.[59–61] Close monitoring of serum alkaline phosphatase, phosphorus, and other bone indices is recommended to facilitate early detection and treatment of metabolic bone disease. Currently, the choice of the optimal formula in post-NEC feeding is led mainly by local preferences rather than scientific consensus.[55]

Mode of Feeding

Continuous feeding can maintain gastrointestinal hormones at a higher level due to saturation of the receptors, whereas bolus feeds are considered more physiologic. A systematic review looking at 9 trials (n = 919) on continuous versus bolus feeds in infants greater than 1500 g failed to show any conclusive benefit for initiation of feeds using either feeding method.[62] Wang and colleagues[63] conducted a meta-analysis looking at eight trials (707 low birthweight infants) comparing continuous versus bolus feeding and found no significant benefits but a long time to achieve full feeds in the continuously fed group. In infants with surgical NEC and short bowel syndrome, a continuous infusion is often chosen in infants with feed intolerance and shorter residual bowel length. When providing feeds via continuous infusion using human milk, the loss of nutrients, especially fat (25%–40%), should be considered as growth may be affected.[64,65]

Growth

The primary goal of nutrition in infants post-NEC is to support optimal growth. Growth should follow recommended growth charts for age and mimic that of infants without NEC.[34] Though achieving complete independence from PN and enteral autonomy is the immediate goal; it should not be attained at the expense of adequate growth. When enteral autonomy is achieved but is associated with suboptimal growth, potential causes such as pancreatic exocrine insufficiency, deceased total body sodium, and small intestinal bacterial overgrowth should be investigated and treated. In the absence of such possible reasons for growth failure, safe provision of PN should be resorted in addition to EN to avoid and correct growth failure.

FUTURE DIRECTION
Abdominal Ultrasound as a Tool for the Duration of Bowel Rest and Readiness to Feed

The utility of abdominal ultrasound in diagnosing intestinal emergencies such as NEC, volvulus, and intussusception has improved. Ultrasound (US) can help diagnose NEC where traditional radiographs are equivocal. The ultrasound has been shown to detect pneumatosis, portal venous gas, thickening of intestinal loops, altered intestinal perfusion and motility, and complex ascites undetected on X-rays.[66] However, the use of abdominal US to predict readiness to feed has not been studied in the literature. Bohnhorst and colleagues[20] studied abdominal ultrasound to determine portal venous gas resolution before feeding after NEC. The authors demonstrated that this strategy resulted in the earlier initiation of enteral feeds, resulting in benefits associated with earlier feeds. Nevertheless, the use of abdominal ultrasound as a tool to determine readiness to feed needs to be studied further before it is adopted as a mainstream strategy.

Biomarkers

Several potential biomarkers have been studied to help diagnose and evaluate the intestinal injury, such as mitochondrial DNA, serum citrulline, fecal calprotectin, fecal intestinal-fatty acid binding protein, and claudins.[67,68]

Plasma citrulline level in early diagnosis of NEC has been used as a predictor of intestinal adaptation. Enterocytes synthesize citrulline, and its level decreases with injury. Jawale and colleagues [68] evaluated through a prospective study the plasma level of citrulline among preterm infants and found that citrulline levels were lower in infants with NEC than in healthy controls. Plasma citrulline levels might be helpful to determine the enterocyte mass, particularly in surgical short bowel syndrome following NEC, to predict success with feed tolerance. Studies utilizing clinical bio-markers to indicate readiness to feed following NEC are currently lacking.

Near-Infrared Spectroscopy

Near-infrared spectroscopy (NIRS) is a noninvasive device to measure the brain and splanchnic tissue oxygen saturation. NIRS, as a screening and diagnostic tool in infants, has been studied in animal models and preterm infants in the early prediction of NEC. Heide and colleagues[69] investigated whether splanchnic tissue oxygen saturation mea-sure by NIRS could contribute to the early diagnosis of NEC through a retrospective study of premature infants with suspected NEC; their team found a high splanchnic and cerebral oxygenation may indicate NEC. On the contrary, Le Bouhellec and col-leagues[70], through a prospective observational study, evaluated the ability of NIRS to aid the diagnosis of NEC and found that the splanchnic and cerebral oxygenation were similar in patients with and without NEC. Similar to the biomarkers, studies utilizing NIRS to assess readiness to feed after NEC elicits promise have not been performed.

Probiotics

Probiotics have been extensively studied in the prevention of NEC. However, the use of probiotics in infants post-NEC has not been studied. Because NEC is characterized by altered gut permeability, the live organisms from probiotics translocating and resulting in bacteremia is a significant concern. The reports of bacteremia in patients of short bowel syndrome with central venous access receiving probiotics containing lactobacillus GG and *Saccharomyces boulardii* further strengthen these concerns.[71,72] However, some evidence emerging from animal models of short bowel syndrome sug-gests probiotics can be beneficial by increasing villus length, crypt depth, enterocyte count, and even reducing bacterial translocation.[73] A recent meta-analysis on the use of probiotics in infants with short bowel syndrome concluded that the benefits are un-proven, and the risks were significant.[74] In summary, the use of probiotics in infants following NEC is not studied. Until then, probiotics in infants following NEC should be restricted to carefully monitored research protocols.

SUMMARY

The nutritional support in infants following NEC currently reflects high variability due to a lack of strong evidence-based guidelines. Early introduction of enteral feeding following NEC promotes intestinal adaptation, and is associated with several benefits, including reduced duration of central venous access, decreased catheter-related sepsis, shorter time of hospital stay, and earlier achievement of full feeds. Standard-ized guidelines in infants post-NEC can reduce variation in nutritional practice, pro-mote antibiotic stewardship, and improve outcomes. Although enteral autonomy is the final goal in infants with NEC, it should always be accompanied by optimal growth.

Best practices

Nutrition after necrotizing enterocolitis

Best practices
- Early resumption of enteral feeds after the return of bowel function
- Standardized nutrition guidelines

- Prevent central line-associated bloodstream infections
- Highly specialized multidisciplinary care at an experienced center for infants with short bowel syndrome

What changes in current practice are likely to improve outcomes?
- Develop and adhere to standardized nutrition guidelines in infants with NEC
- Minimize the duration of antibiotics in the treatment of NEC
- Study the utility of investigative modalities such as ultrasound and near-infrared spectroscopy and biomarkers to assess readiness to feed after NEC

Major Recommendations:
- Early enteral feeding (5–7 days) should be considered after the clinical and radiological signs of NEC have resolved
- Standardization of feeding regimen and antibiotic stewardship will promote early enteral feeding
- Human milk is the preferred choice of nutrition after an episode of NEC
- In the absence of human milk, elemental or hydrolyzed formula is the preferred choice of enteral nutrition
- In neonates with bowel discontinuity secondary to complications from NEC, mucus fistula refeeding should be considered
- Once enteral nutrition is initiated, oral feeds should be encouraged as soon as the feeding cues are observed
- Use multicomponent fish oil containing ILE for the prevention of IFALD, and 100% fish oil ILE for the treatment of IFALD

FUNDING

Parvesh Garg is partially supported by the NIGMS of the NIH under Award Number U54GM115428. The content is solely the responsibility of the authors and does not necessarily represent the official views of the NIH.

ACKNOWLEDGMENT

The Mississippi Center for Clinical and Translational Research for supporting the NEC research.

REFERENCES

1. Lin PW, Stoll BJ. Necrotising enterocolitis 2006;368:13.
2. MohanKumar K, Namachivayam K, Ho TTB, et al. Cytokines and growth factors in the developing intestine and during necrotizing enterocolitis. Semin Perinatol 2017;41(1):52–60.
3. Neu J. Prevention of necrotizing enterocolitis. Clin Perinatol 2022;49(1):195–206.
4. Cristofalo EA, Schanler RJ, Blanco CL, et al. Randomized trial of Exclusive human milk versus preterm formula diets in Extremely premature infants. J Pediatr 2013; 163(6):1592–5.e1.
5. Pammi M, Cope J, Tarr PI, et al. Intestinal dysbiosis in preterm infants preceding necrotizing enterocolitis: a systematic review and meta-analysis. Microbiome 2017;5:31.
6. Kliegman RM, Fanaroff AA. Necrotizing enterocolitis. N Engl J Med 1984;310(17): 1093–103.
7. Kliegman RM, Walker WA, Yolken RH. Necrotizing enterocolitis: research Agenda for a disease of Unknown Etiology and Pathogenesis. Pediatr Res 1993;34(6): 701–8.

8. Zani A, Pierro A. Necrotizing enterocolitis: controversies and challenges. F1000 Research 2015;4:F1000. https://doi.org/10.12688/f1000research.6888.1. Faculty Rev-1373.

9. Bizzarro MJ, Ehrenkranz RA, Gallagher PG. Concurrent bloodstream infections in infants with necrotizing enterocolitis. J Pediatr 2014;164(1):61–6.

10. Ahmad I, Premkumar MH, Hair AB, et al. Variability in antibiotic duration for necrotizing enterocolitis and outcomes in a large multicenter cohort. J Perinatol 2022;1–7. https://doi.org/10.1038/s41372-022-01433-2.

11. Patole S, de Klerk N. Impact of standardised feeding regimens on incidence of neonatal necrotising enterocolitis: a systematic review and meta-analysis of observational studies. Arch Dis Child Fetal Neonatal Ed 2005;90(2):F147–51.

12. Hopkins J, Cermak SA, Merritt RJ. Oral feeding Difficulties in children with short bowel syndrome: a narrative review. Nutr Clin Pract 2018;33(1):99–106.

13. Chappell VL, Thompson MD, Jeschke MG, et al. Effects of Incremental Starvation on gut Mucosa. Dig Dis Sci 2003;48(4):5.

14. Demehri FR, Barrett M, Ralls MW, et al. Intestinal epithelial cell apoptosis and loss of barrier function in the setting of altered microbiota with enteral nutrient deprivation. Front Cell Infect Microbiol 2013;3:105.

15. Lacaille F, Gupte G, Colomb V, et al. Intestinal failure–associated liver disease: a position Paper of the ESPGHAN Working group of intestinal failure and intestinal transplantation. J Pediatr Gastroenterol Nutr 2015;60(2):272–83.

16. Fundora J, Aucott SW. Intestinal failure–associated liver disease in neonates. NeoReviews 2020;21(9):e591–9.

17. Gura KM, Premkumar MH, Calkins KL, et al. Fish oil emulsion reduces liver injury and liver transplantation in children with intestinal failure-associated liver disease: a multicenter Integrated study. J Pediatr 2021;230:46–54.e2.

18. Premkumar MH, Carter BA, Hawthorne KM, et al. High rates of resolution of cholestasis in parenteral nutrition-associated liver disease with fish oil-based lipid emulsion Monotherapy. J Pediatr 2013;162(4):793–8.e1.

19. Lucas A, Bloom SR, Aynsley-Green A. Metabolic and Endocrine consequences of depriving preterm infants of enteral nutrition. Acta Paediatr 1983;72(2):245–9.

20. Bohnhorst B, Müller S, Dördelmann M, et al. Early feeding after necrotizing enterocolitis in preterm infants. J Pediatr 2003;143(4):484–7.

21. Patel EU, Head WT, Rohrer A, et al. A quality improvement initiative to standardize time to initiation of enteral feeds after non-surgical necrotizing enterocolitis using a consensus-based guideline. J Perinatol 2022;42(4):522–7.

22. Arbra CA, Oprisan A, Wilson DA, et al. Time to reintroduction of feeding in infants with nonsurgical necrotizing enterocolitis. J Pediatr Surg 2018;53(6):1187–91.

23. Merritt RJ, Cohran V, Raphael BP, et al. Intestinal rehabilitation Programs in the management of pediatric intestinal failure and short bowel syndrome. J Pediatr Gastroenterol Nutr 2017;65(5):588–96.

24. Shores DR, Alaish SM, Aucott SW, et al. Post-operative enteral nutrition guidelines reduce the risk of intestinal failure-associated liver disease in surgical infants. J Pediatr 2018;195:140–7.e1.

25. Shakeel F, Newkirk M, Sellers A, et al. Postoperative feeding guidelines improve outcomes in surgical infants. J Parenter Enter Nutr 2020;44(6):1047–56.

26. Belza C, Fitzgerald K, de Silva N, et al. Predicting intestinal adaptation in pediatric intestinal failure: a retrospective cohort study. Ann Surg 2019;269(5):988–93.

27. Fatemizadeh R, Gollins L, Hagan J, et al. In neonatal-onset surgical short bowel syndrome survival is high, and enteral autonomy is related to residual bowel length. J Parenter Enter Nutr 2022;46(2):339–47.

28. Jeppesen PB, Mortensen PB. The influence of a preserved colon on the absorption of medium chain fat in patients with small bowel resection. Gut 1998;43(4): 478–83.

29. Smazal AL, Massieu LA, Gollins L, et al. Small Proportion of low-birth-weight infants with ostomy and intestinal failure due to short-bowel syndrome achieve enteral autonomy prior to reanastomosis. J Parenter Enter Nutr 2021;45(2):331–8.

30. Koike Y, Uchida K, Nagano Y, et al. Enteral refeeding is useful for promoting growth in neonates with enterostomy before stoma closure. J Pediatr Surg 2016;51(3):390–4.

31. Lau ECT, Fung ACH, Wong KKY, et al. Beneficial effects of mucous fistula refeeding in necrotizing enterocolitis neonates with enterostomies. J Pediatr Surg 2016; 51(12):1914–6.

32. Woods SD, McElhanon BO, Durham MM, et al. Mucous fistula refeeding promotes earlier enteral autonomy in infants with small bowel resection. J Pediatr Gastroenterol Nutr 2021;73(5):654–8.

33. Vileisis RA, Inwood RJ, Hunt CE. Prospective controlled study of parenteral nutrition-associated cholestatic jaundice: effect of protein intake. J Pediatr 1980;96(5):893–7.

34. Kleinman RE. Pediatric nutrition. Elk Grove Village, IL: American Academy of Pediatrics; 2019.

35. Crill C. Parenteral nutrition support. 2nd edition. Silver Spring, MD: American Society for Parenteral and Enteral Nutrition; 2017.

36. Squires RH. Intestinal failure. 2nd edition. Silver Spring, MD: American Society for Parenteral and Enteral Nutrition; 2017.

37. Kapoor V, Malviya MN, Soll R. Lipid emulsions for parenterally fed preterm infants. Cochrane Database Syst Rev 2019;2019(6):CD013163.

38. Kapoor V, Malviya MN, Soll R. Lipid emulsions for parenterally fed term and late preterm infants. Cochrane Database Syst Rev 2019;2019(6):CD013171.

39. Hojsak I, Colomb V, Braegger C, et al. ESPGHAN Committee on nutrition position Paper. Intravenous lipid emulsions and risk of Hepatotoxicity in infants and children: a systematic review and meta-analysis. J Pediatr Gastroenterol Nutr 2016;62(5):776–92.

40. Cober MP, Killu G, Brattain A, et al. Intravenous fat emulsions reduction for patients with parenteral nutrition–associated liver disease. J Pediatr 2012;160(3): 421–7.

41. Nehra D, Fallon EM, Carlson SJ, et al. Provision of a Soy-based intravenous lipid emulsion at 1 g/kg/d does not prevent cholestasis in neonates. J Parenter Enter Nutr 2013;37(4):498–505.

42. Costa S, Maggio L, Sindico P, et al. Preterm small for gestational age infants are not at higher risk for parenteral nutrition-associated cholestasis. J Pediatr 2010; 156(4):575–9.

43. Gura K, Premkumar MH, Calkins KL, et al. Intravenous fish oil Monotherapy as a source of Calories and fatty acids promotes age-Appropriate growth in pediatric patients with intestinal failure-associated liver disease. J Pediatr 2020;219: 98–105.e4.

44. Feng H, Zhang T, Yan W, et al. Micronutrient deficiencies in pediatric short bowel syndrome: a 10-year review from an intestinal rehabilitation center in China. Pediatr Surg Int 2020;36(12):1481–7.

45. Balay KS, Hawthorne KM, Hicks PD, et al. Low zinc status and absorption exist in infants with jejunostomies or ileostomies which persists after intestinal repair. Nutrients 2012;4(9):1273–81.

46. Yang C, fu J, Duro D, et al. High prevalence of multiple micronutrient deficiencies in children with intestinal failure: a longitudinal study. J Pediatr 2011;159(1): 39–44.e1.

47. Jensen AR, Goldin AB, Koopmeiners JS, et al. The association of cyclic parenteral nutrition and decreased incidence of cholestatic liver disease in patients with gastroschisis. J Pediatr Surg 2009;44(1):183–9.

48. Christian VJ, Polzin E, Welak S. Nutrition management of necrotizing enterocolitis. Nutr Clin Pract 2018;33(4):476–82.

49. Lönnerdal B. Bioactive proteins in human milk-potential benefits for preterm infants. Clin Perinatol 2017;44(1):179–91.

50. Miyake H, Lee C, Chusilp S, et al. Human breast milk exosomes attenuate intestinal damage. Pediatr Surg Int 2020;36(2):155–63.

51. Wesolowska A, Sinkiewicz-Darol E, Barbarska O, et al. Innovative Techniques of processing human milk to Preserve Key components. Nutrients 2019;11(5):1169.

52. Silvestre D, Ruiz P, Martínez-Costa C, et al. Effect of pasteurization on the Bactericidal capacity of human milk. J Hum Lact 2008;24(4):371–6.

53. Unger S, Stintzi A, Shah P, et al. Gut microbiota of the very-low-birth-weight infant. Pediatr Res 2015;77(1):205–13.

54. Andorsky DJ, Lund DP, Lillehei CW, et al. Nutritional and other postoperative management of neonates with short bowel syndrome correlates with clinical outcomes. J Pediatr 2001;139(1):27–33.

55. Capriati T, Nobili V, Stronati L, et al. Enteral nutrition in pediatric intestinal failure: does initial feeding impact on intestinal adaptation? Expert Rev Gastroenterol Hepatol 2017;11(8):741–8.

56. Mazzocchi A, D'Oria V, De Cosmi V, et al. The role of lipids in human milk and infant Formulae. Nutrients 2018;10(5):E567.

57. Vanderhoof JA, Grandjean CJ, Kaufman SS, et al. Effect of high Percentage medium-chain triglyceride diet on mucosal adaptation following massive bowel resection in Rats. J Parenter Enter Nutr 1984;8(6):685–9.

58. Gatti S, Quattrini S, Palpacelli A, et al. Metabolic bone disease in children with intestinal failure and long-term parenteral nutrition: a systematic review. Nutrients 2022;14(5):995.

59. Eswarakumar AS, Ma NS, Ward LM, et al. Long-term follow-up of Hypophosphatemic bone disease associated with elemental formula Use: Sustained correction of bone disease after formula change or phosphate supplementation. Clin Pediatr (Phila) 2020;59(12):1080–5.

60. Creo AL, Epp LM, Buchholtz JA, et al. Prevalence of metabolic bone disease in tube-fed children receiving elemental formula. Horm Res Paediatr 2018;90(5): 291–8.

61. Gonzalez Ballesteros LF, Ma NS, Gordon RJ, et al. Unexpected widespread hypophosphatemia and bone disease associated with elemental formula use in infants and children. Bone 2017;97:287–92.

62. Sadrudin Premji S, Chessell L, Stewart F. Continuous nasogastric milk feeding versus intermittent bolus milk feeding for preterm infants less than 1500 grams. Cochrane Database Syst Rev 2021;6:CD001819.

63. Wang Y, Zhu W, Luo BR. Continuous feeding versus intermittent bolus feeding for premature infants with low birth weight: a meta-analysis of randomized controlled trials. Eur J Clin Nutr 2020;74(5):775–83.

64. Paulsson M, Jacobsson L, Ahlsson F. Factors Influencing breast milk fat loss during Administration in the neonatal intensive care Unit. Nutrients 2021;13(6):1939.

65. Rogers SP, Hicks PD, Hamzo M, et al. Continuous feedings of fortified human milk lead to nutrient losses of fat, calcium and phosphorous. Nutrients 2010;2(3): 230–40.
66. Hwang M, Tierradentro-García LO, Dennis RA, et al. The role of ultrasound in necrotizing enterocolitis. Pediatr Radiol 2022;52(4):702–15.
67. Bindi E, Li B, Zhou H, et al. Mitochondrial DNA: a biomarker of disease severity in necrotizing enterocolitis. Eur J Pediatr Surg Off J Austrian Assoc Pediatr Surg Al Z Kinderchir 2020;30(1):85–9.
68. Jawale N, Prideaux M, Prasad M, et al, for Maimonides Neonatal Group. Plasma citrulline as a biomarker for early diagnosis of necrotizing enterocolitis in preterm infants. Am J Perinatol 2021;38(13):1435–41.
69. van der Heide M, Hulscher JBF, Bos AF, et al. Near-infrared spectroscopy as a diagnostic tool for necrotizing enterocolitis in preterm infants. Pediatr Res 2021;90(1):148–55.
70. Le Bouhellec J, Prodhomme O, Mura T, et al. Near-infrared spectroscopy: a tool for diagnosing necrotizing enterocolitis at onset of symptoms in preterm neonates with Acute gastrointestinal symptoms? Am J Perinatol 2021;38(S 01):e299–308.
71. Hennequin C, Kauffmann-Lacroix C, Jobert A, et al. Possible role of catheters in Saccharomyces boulardii fungemia. Eur J Clin Microbiol Infect Dis Off Publ Eur Soc Clin Microbiol 2000;19(1):16–20.
72. Kunz AN, Noel JM, Fairchok MP. Two cases of Lactobacillus bacteremia during probiotic treatment of short gut syndrome. J Pediatr Gastroenterol Nutr 2004; 38(4):457–8.
73. Tolga Muftuoglu MA, Civak T, Cetin S, et al. Effects of probiotics on experimental short-bowel syndrome. Am J Surg 2011;202(4):461–8.
74. Reddy VS, Patole SK, Rao S. Role of probiotics in short bowel syndrome in infants and children–a systematic review. Nutrients 2013;5(3):679–99.

Nutrition for Infants with Congenital Heart Disease

Jasmeet Kataria-Hale, MD[a], Laura Gollins, MBA, RDN, CNSC, FAND[b],
Krista Bonagurio, RDN[c], Cynthia Blanco, MD[c], Amy B. Hair, MD[b,*]

KEYWORDS

- Congenital heart disease • Nutrition • Enteral • Feeding • Parenteral nutrition
- Preoperative • Postoperative • Protocol

KEY POINTS

- Infants with congenital heart disease are at high risk of postnatal growth failure.
- Adequate perioperative nutrition can improve short- and long-term outcomes.
- The nutritional strategy should be tailored to the type of cardiac lesion and the preoperative or postoperative period using a standardized feeding protocol.
- Early enteral feeding should be initiated and coupled with parenteral nutrition to meet the fluid and nutritional needs of the infant.

INTRODUCTION

Infants with congenital heart disease (CHD) are at high risk of postnatal growth failure. Although usually born full term with a weight appropriate for gestational age, this vulnerable population often suffers from poor growth due to a multitude of factors. These include type of cardiac lesion, acute inflammatory response, increased metabolic demand, energy demands exceeding supply, intestinal malabsorption, gastroesophageal reflux, intestinal dysbiosis, and underlying chromosomal abnormalities.[1] As a result, perioperative malnutrition causes delayed wound healing, increased length of hospital stay, increased risk of infection, prolonged need for mechanical ventilation, poor neurodevelopmental outcomes, and increased mortality risk.[2–7]

Although most of the institutions have adopted guidelines for providing nutrition to the preterm infant, there is still no consensus on the optimal perioperative nutritional

Funding: C. Blanco has received funding from University Health Foundation San Antonio for neonatal clinical research.
[a] Department of Pediatrics, Division of Neonatology, Mission Hospital, 509 Biltmore Avenue, Asheville, NC 28801, USA; [b] Department of Pediatrics, Division of Neonatology, Baylor College of Medicine, Texas Children's Hospital, 6621 Fannin Street, MC: A5590, Houston, TX 77030, USA; [c] University of Texas Health Science Center, San Antonio, 7703 Floyd Curl Drive, San Antonio, TX 78229, USA
* Corresponding author.
E-mail address: abhair@bcm.edu

and feeding strategy for the infant with CHD.[8] Providers caring for these infants are faced with the unique challenges of managing fluid balance, enteral feeding and the risk of necrotizing enterocolitis (NEC), and tailoring the feeding strategy to the cardiac lesion, particularly cyanotic heart lesions or those that are ductal-dependent. In addition, the nutritional strategy for the preoperative and postoperative periods should be distinct. Despite these challenges, the provision of adequate nutrition in this high-risk population is of the utmost importance. In this article, the authors review the current literature surrounding feeding strategies and provide practical guidelines for enteral nutrition (EN) and parenteral nutrition (PN) for the infant with CHD.

PREOPERATIVE FEEDING CONSIDERATIONS

There is a lack of consensus on how to approach enteral feeding in the preoperative period. The risk of NEC from splanchnic hypoperfusion serves as a significant limitation to standardizing enteral feeding initiation across institutions.[9–12] Although uncommon in full-term infants, NEC is significantly more common in full-term infants with CHD with an incidence ranging from 1.6% to 9% depending on the lesion.[13] Despite this, studies suggest that preoperative enteral feeding does not increase the risk of NEC in infants with CHD.[14–23] When balancing the risk of withholding enteral feeding versus advancing feeds, it is reasonable to hold feeds at a volume that is well-tolerated, particularly in the preoperative period. Holding feeds at a volume of 20 to 60 mL/kg/d of unfortified milk and providing additional nutritional support via PN may be warranted preoperatively in the higher risk CHD population, particularly if awaiting surgery within the first few weeks of life. This allows for intestinal priming and caloric maximization to support adequate growth without increasing risk factors of feeding intolerance that could lead to withholding feeds altogether. A retrospective study of 546 infants demonstrates a significantly lower risk of preoperative NEC with an unfortified human milk diet. However, feeding volumes exceeding 100 mL/kg/d were associated with a significantly greater risk of preoperative NEC.[24] If an infant has a high-risk cardiac lesion such as single ventricle physiology, with close monitoring, even small volume feeds allow for crucial intestinal priming and maturation without the risk of large volume feeds that cause providers to be hesitant. A preoperative feeding guideline is provided in **Fig. 1**.

Enteral Nutrition: Feeding Initiation

Enteral feeding should be initiated as early as safely possible in all infants with CHD. There is significant evidence to suggest an improvement in short- and long-term outcomes for premature infants who receive human milk.[25–27] Donor human milk (DHM) is considered superior to formula when maternal milk is unavailable or contraindicated, especially preoperatively.[24] Although DHM is now widely available, formula is a reasonable alternative.

Trophic feeding should be initiated at 10 to 20 mL/kg/d as soon as possible and advanced by 10 to 20 mL/kg/d as tolerated.[28,29] The initiation and advancement of feeding in infants with CHD is often limited by a lack of standardized feeding protocols. As a result, initiation of feeding is delayed or quickly abandoned at the discretion of the provider. Evidence suggests that early enteral feeding promotes intestinal maturation, healthy intestinal microbiota, and future feeding tolerance.[30,31] The use of feeding protocols is favored in intensive care units as a standardized approach and leads to improvement in outcomes.[32–36] In addition to the use of a feeding protocol, the parameters for feeding intolerance should be well-defined and be used as a guide to help providers eliminate practice variation. For example, feeding intolerance can be

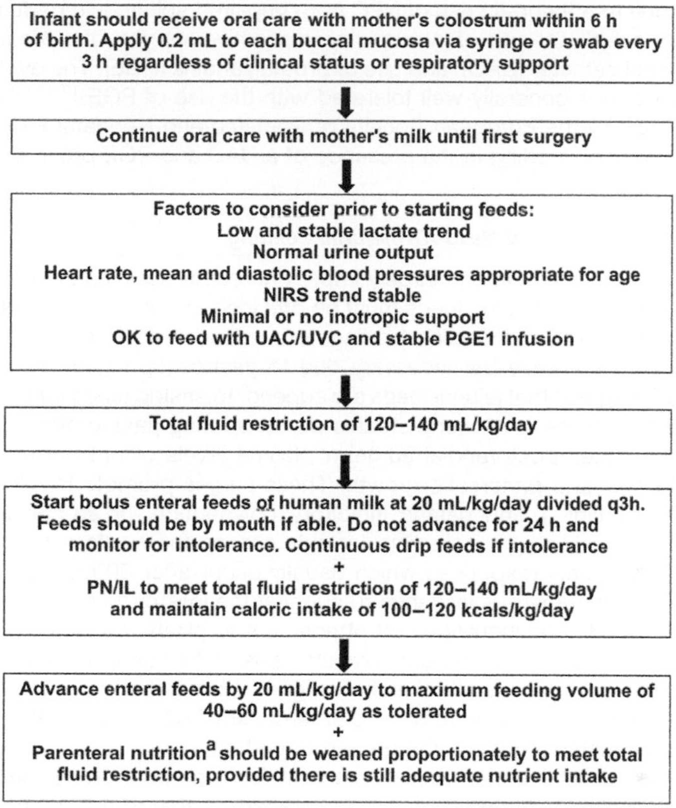

Infant should receive oral care with mother's colostrum within 6 h of birth. Apply 0.2 mL to each buccal mucosa via syringe or swab every 3 h regardless of clinical status or respiratory support

↓

Continue oral care with mother's milk until first surgery

↓

Factors to consider prior to starting feeds:
Low and stable lactate trend
Normal urine output
Heart rate, mean and diastolic blood pressures appropriate for age
NIRS trend stable
Minimal or no inotropic support
OK to feed with UAC/UVC and stable PGE1 infusion

↓

Total fluid restriction of 120–140 mL/kg/day

↓

Start bolus enteral feeds of human milk at 20 mL/kg/day divided q3h. Feeds should be by mouth if able. Do not advance for 24 h and monitor for intolerance. Continuous drip feeds if intolerance
+
PN/IL to meet total fluid restriction of 120–140 mL/kg/day and maintain caloric intake of 100–120 kcals/kg/day

↓

Advance enteral feeds by 20 mL/kg/day to maximum feeding volume of 40–60 mL/kg/day as tolerated
+
Parenteral nutrition[a] should be weaned proportionately to meet total fluid restriction, provided there is still adequate nutrient intake

Fig. 1. Preoperative feeding. IL, intralipid; NIRS, near-infrared spectroscopy; PGE1, prosta-glandins E1; PN, parenteral nutrition; UAC, umbilical arterial catheter; UVC, umbilical arterial catheter. [a]Figure 3. Parental nutrition algorithm. (*Adapted from* Kataria-Hale J, Roddy DJ, Cognata A, Hochevar P, Zender J, Sheaks P, et al. A preoperative standardized feeding protocol improves human milk use in infants with complex congenital heart disease. J Perinatol. 2021;41(3):590-7.)

defined as abdominal distension, radiographic evidence of bowel dilation or pneumatosis intestinalis and/or bloody stools with subsequent nil per os (NPO) status for greater than 24 hrs. A feeding intolerance algorithm for reevaluation and reinitiation of feeds must be implemented for consistency.

If infants are unable to be fed preoperatively, oral care with colostrum should be provided. Colostrum is rich in immune factors that are absorbed in the buccal mucosa; therefore, small amounts of colostrum should be used as immune therapy even in extremely sick infants. Although studies are still underway to determine its impact on outcomes, administering colostrum to the buccal mucosa can serve as a bridge to deliver the beneficial components of human milk in the absence of enteral feeds.[37–40] Oral care should be regularly provided to infants with CHD with care times, as shown in **Fig. 1**.[36]

Factors to Consider

There is a wide variation in feeding practices across institutions with hesitancy surrounding complex cardiac lesions, such as ductal-dependent single ventricle physiology, due to a theoretic risk of NEC from impaired splanchnic perfusion. Additional factors include the use of inotropic or vasoactive support, the presence of an umbilical arterial catheter (UAC), and use of prostaglandins (PGE). The evidence suggests that feeding is generally well tolerated with the use of PGE.[19,41,42] A position statement made by the European Society of Pediatric and Neonatal Intensive Care recommends enteral feeding in the presence of a UAC and PGE provided the infant is closely monitored.[43]

Oral, Naso-/Orogastric, and Naso-/Orojejunal Feeding

Oral feeding and stimulation can largely impact neurodevelopmental outcomes.[44,45] However, if naso- or orogastric feeds must be provided, the infusion time is important to consider. Although gravity bolus feedings are considered more physiologic, prolonged infusion times may be necessary due to gastroesophageal reflux. There is no evidence to suggest that jejunal feeds are superior to gastric feeds for feeding tolerance. In addition, there are several studies demonstrating gastric distension after a bolus feed promotes postprandial surge in plasma levels of gut hormones, which enhance intestinal and pancreatic growth. These surges promote insulin secretion, glucagon-like peptide-1 and gastric inhibitory polypeptide, or so-called incretins. Continuous feeds inhibit this enteroinsular axis altering the cyclic nature of incretin secretion and dynamic responses which usually occur after 30 minutes of a bolus feed.[46,47] In addition, there is evidence to suggest the loss of nutrients when enteral feeds are delivered continuously by fat attachment to plastic tubing and decreased protein synthesis due to altered enteroinsular axis.[48] As such, feeding intolerance and the potential for poor growth must be weighed against the known nutrient deficit with continuous feedings. In summary, oral feeds are favored when able and if not possible, bolus gastric feeds are the preferred method.

Based on the current literature, initiating enteral feeds preoperatively can be accomplished with a limited volume, especially if the infant is able to receive oral feeds as neonates usually self-regulate. Enteral feeds may be able to be liberalized preoperatively in infants with a lower risk of NEC such as those with good cardiac output, adequate systemic perfusion, and born at term with adequate fetal growth. If tolerated, infants with CHD can reach full feeds if tolerated and hemodynamically stable.

POSTOPERATIVE FEEDING CONSIDERATIONS

Much like preoperative feeding, the initiation of postoperative EN varies among centers. Infants who undergo complex cardiac surgery experience a multitude of complications that can affect feeding and ultimately growth. These include, but are not limited to, inadequate cardiac output, NEC, prolonged intubation, gastroesophageal reflux, vocal cord paralysis, open chest, and increased caloric needs secondary to a catabolic state.[15,16,18,34,41,42,49,50] As a result, clinical judgment often dictates the feeding approach, frequently leading to delayed initiation or multiple interruptions in feeding.[51,52] Infants with single-ventricle physiology, who require future surgeries, are one such group who face significant postoperative growth failure.[53] This is a particularly vulnerable group in that success of future surgeries hinges on optimal growth following stage 1 surgical palliation. In addition to initiation of feeds, the question of what to fortify with still remains. The primary concern with fortification stems from the concern for NEC with formula use in preterm infants and higher osmolality with higher caloric concentrations. Given the theoretic risk of NEC in a critically ill infant in the postoperative state, feeding should be approached with a standardized protocol.

Traditionally, fortification is added once feeds are near the goal volume.[54] This proves to be challenging in the critically ill infant as the caloric density of unfortified feeds does not meet the needs of the infant's increased metabolic demand in the postoperative state. Moreover, the total amount of fluid provided daily is often restricted due to postoperative fluid shifts and cardiac dysfunction. The delayed achievement of optimal nutrient needs sets the stage for perioperative growth failure. Early enteral feeding and early fortification with an exclusive human milk (EHM) diet has been shown to improve growth in preterm infants without CHD.[55] A recent, multi-center, randomized trial demonstrates that term infants with single-ventricle physiology who receive early fortification with an EHM diet in the postoperative stage have improved short-term growth and a decreased risk of NEC.[56] A key feature of this feeding approach is infants were exposed to a higher protein concentration and caloric density early in the feeding protocol while maintaining necessary fluid restrictions compared with the widely accepted, standard feeding approach used in preterm infants. A feeding guideline based on available literature is shown in **Fig. 2**. Although further studies are needed, it is important to consider the theoretic benefits of

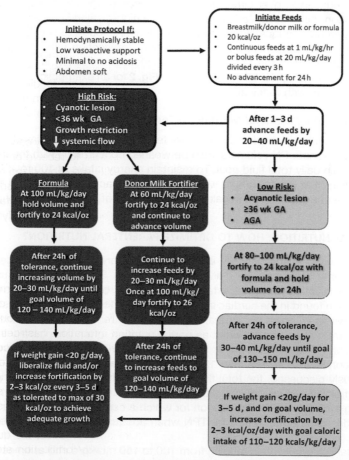

Fig. 2. Postoperative feeding protocol. (*Adapted from* Blanco CL, Hair A, Justice LB, et al. A Randomized Trial of an Exclusive Human Milk Diet in Neonates with Single Ventricle Physiology [published online ahead of print, 2022 Dec 14]. J Pediatr. 2022;S0022-3476(22)01126-X.)

postoperative outcomes related to preoperative feeding such as improved feeding tolerance, fewer complications, and therefore shorter length of hospital stay.

Daily Caloric Goals and Weight-Based Calculations

Based on a standardized protocol, EN should be advanced to a daily goal that meets fluid and caloric needs in combination with PN. Often, a central venous catheter is required to deliver the necessary macronutrients. Immediately after birth and during the initial postnatal diuresis phase, the birth weight should be used for nutrition calculations. However, daily weight gain may reflect fluid overload in the setting of CHD, at which point the weight used for nutritional calculations should be altered. It is not uncommon to establish a "dry weight" that is updated once weekly to a reasonable weight gain over that period of time. Alternatively, an expected "normal" weight gain can be used daily.

Fortification of Feeds

Total daily fluid goal is often altered based on the type of cardiac lesion. For example, infants with pulmonary over-circulation who are receiving diuretic therapy may require fluid restriction. As a result, early fortification to a higher caloric concentration should be administered to adequately meet nutrient needs. Although the evidence suggests that human milk is the best source of nutrition, fortification with formula is often needed, particularly in the face of fluid restriction. Fortification is usually initiated once 100 to 120 mL/kg/d is tolerated well. See **Fig. 2** for an example of a postoperative feeding algorithm with fortification.

Transitioning from Parenteral Nutrition to Enteral Nutrition

EN should be initiated as soon as medically feasible. Once EN is initiated, PN should begin to be weaned. PN volume should be weaned concurrently with the increase in EN to maintain daily total fluid goal. To maintain energy intake of 100 to 120 kcal/kg/d and protein of at least 3 g/kg/d with EN and PN, macronutrients in PN should be maximized and advancement in caloric concentration of EN should be considered.

PARENTERAL NUTRITION: HOW TO OPTIMIZE PARENTERAL NUTRITION?

PN is often used in the critically ill populations to prevent nutritional deficiencies when adequate EN cannot be delivered or tolerated. Supplemental PN usage and timing of PN initiation is not well established; however, based on the high percentage of malnutrition found in the cardiac infant population, initiation within the first 24 hours of life and within 24 hours postoperatively is generally recommended for the high-risk cardiac infant. PN can be provided as partial nutrition, often peripherally infused, or total nutrition (TPN) which requires a central line. Peripheral infusion is limited to a dextrose concentration less than 12.5% and osmolarity less than 900 mOsm/L.[57] As previously discussed, the total fluid goal in both the preoperative and postoperative timeframe is usually dictated by the type of congenital heart condition, often warranting a concentrated PN solution for which a central line is required. This section provides general guidelines for TPN when adequate EN cannot be delivered or sustained.

With total fluid goals often ranging from 100 to 150 mL/kg/d and at times as low as 60 to 80 mL/kg/d in the acute postoperative phase, it is important to take into consideration all other intravenous (IV) infusing fluids, medications, and blood products before writing the PN prescription.

Fig. 3 provides a guideline for initiation of PN whereby 10 large centers agreed to provide this parenteral support to infants with single-ventricle physiology.[56] The guidelines in Fig. 3 were developed based on recommendations by the American Society for Parenteral and Enteral Nutrition (ASPEN), the European Society for Pediatric Gastroenterology, Hepatology and Nutrition, and the European Society for Clinical Nutrition and Metabolism.[57–59]

Macronutrients

The nutrient goals for PN differ from those of EN due to the direct infusion of nutrients into the venous system and the decreases in diet-induced thermogenesis. PN energy needs are lower by 10% to 20% compared with enteral needs.[58] Ideal macronutrient energy distribution consists of 10% to 15% from amino acids (AA), 30% to 35% from lipids and 60% to 65% from carbohydrates.[29]

Protein: Available AA solutions specific for infants and neonates are formulated to provide similar AA profile as breastfed infants and can be found in Fig. 3. An energy supply of 30 to 40 kcals per 1 g of AA should be provided for optimal AA utilization. Research supports that AA are safe to initiate immediately after birth and continue through the preoperative and postoperative period.[59] Minimum intake of 1.5 to 3 g/kg of AA should be provided to prevent a negative nitrogen balance, and daily AA intake should not exceed 4 g/kg/d. There is currently limited evidence to suggest providing AA greater than 2.5 to 3 g/kg/d produces more favorable outcomes in the neonate or infant population.[29,58,59] There is no need to hold AA in the immediate postoperative period, unless there is severe renal dysfunction in which a short-term decrease to minimal daily intake of 1.5 g/kg/d should be considered.[59]

Dextrose: The carbohydrate energy substrate used in PN solutions is dextrose and provides 3.4 kcals/g.[57] Parenteral glucose infusion should not exceed the maximum

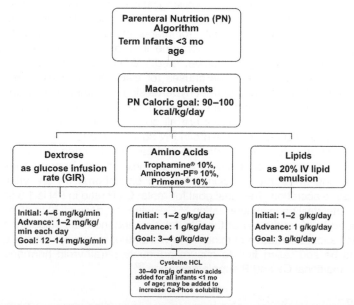

Fig. 3. Parenteral nutrition initiation and goals. (*From* Blanco CL, Hair A, Justice LB, et al. A Randomized Trial of an Exclusive Human Milk Diet in Neonates with Single Ventricle Physiology [published online ahead of print, 2022 Dec 14]. J Pediatr. 2022;S0022-3476(22) 01126-X.)

rate of glucose oxidation which is around 12 to 14 mg/kg/min for term and preterm infants.[57,60] Recommendations for initiation and advancement of glucose, represented as the glucose infusion rate (GIR), can be found in **Fig. 3**. Increase in morbidity and mortality related to hyperglycemia in the critically ill pediatric population has been well established.[60] During the acute postoperative phase, hyperglycemia (glucose > 150 mg/dL) is common due to increased catecholamine release, peripheral insulin resistance, endogenous insulin deficiency, and a persistent endogenous glucose production. A short-term GIR restriction of as low as 2 to 3 mg/kg/min or insulin administration may be required.[17,29] The dextrose content of IV medication solutions and other IV fluids should be considered when calculating GIR and adjusted in the case of persistent hyperglycemia. Once stable, GIR should be increased daily to goal as per algorithm in **Fig. 3**.

Lipids: Injectable lipid emulsions (ILE) are commercially available in 10% solution, providing 1.1 kcal/mL, 20% providing 2 kcal/mL, and 30% providing 3 kcal/mL depending on lipid components of the emulsion.[57] Per ASPEN guidelines, infant and neonatal PN should be prescribed as a two-in-one solution with ILE infusing separately due to the increased risk of calcium phosphate precipitation.[57] There is no consensus on ILE is superior based on the lipid profile unless prolonged PN is warranted and cholestasis is present. Initiation and advancement recommendations are provided in **Fig. 3**. Essential fatty acid deficiency can be avoided by providing a minimal dose of 0.5 mg/kg/d of ILE.[57] Long-chain fatty acid transport across the mitochondrial membrane is facilitated by carnitine. Carnitine supplementation of 20 to 30 mg/kg/d is recommended for preterm neonates as well as term infants requiring PN for greater than 4 weeks.[61]

Micronutrients

Maintaining electrolyte homeostasis is challenging in infants with CHD in both the preoperative and postoperative stage. Electrolyte dosing for PN follows the general guidelines for recommended daily intake for infants and can be found in **Table 1**. Fluid restriction, hemodynamic instability, hormone imbalance, inflammatory response, poor nutrition intake, prolonged hypoxia, medications, and complications such as chylothorax are among some of the causes for electrolyte disturbances. Loop diuretics are frequently prescribed to treat hypertension and heart failure in this population. Although effective, side effects such as hypokalemia, hyponatremia, hypomagnesemia, and hyperuricemia are all common. Additional supplementation via IV infusion and frequent adjustments in PN dosing are often required.

Bone mineralization is tightly controlled and can be disrupted in infants requiring long-term PN and/or loop diuretics as well as chromosomal abnormalities such as 22q11.2 deletion syndrome. Calcium (Ca) and phosphorus (P) are vital for both bone and tissue accretion. The ideal goal for molar Ca:P ratio in PN is 1.3 (mass ratio 1.7) to promote ideal bone mineralization.[62] Cysteine at a dose of 30 to 40 mg/g of AA can be added to lower the pH of the PN solution and increase solubility of Ca and P.[54,57] When supplementation of minerals is warranted, hypomagnesemia when present should be addressed first to ensure adequate parathyroid hormone function before any additional Ca and P supplementation.[62]

Monitoring

Laboratory monitoring while receiving PN will vary depending on the severity of illness and clinical status of the patient. There are no standard recommendations for monitoring micronutrients and should be tailored individually based on the duration of

Table 1
Laboratory monitoring while on parenteral nutrition

Parameter	Initial Parenteral Nutrition	Stable Parenteral Nutrition
Electrolytes, glucose, BUN, creatinine	Daily	2 times per week or as clinically indicated
Calcium, Phosphorous, Magnesium	Daily	2 times per week or as clinically indicated
PTT, PT, INR	Baseline	Weekly
Total bilirubin, direct bilirubin, Alkaline phosphatase, AST, ALT, GGT	Baseline	Weekly
Triglycerides	Daily	Weekly
Albumin, prealbumin	Baseline	Weekly
Trace minerals	N/A	1–3 monthly or as clinically indicated
Fat soluble vitamins	N/A	As clinically indicated (ie, protein losing enteropathy, chylothorax with high chest tube output)
Complete blood count with differentials	Daily	Weekly
Iron indices	As clinically indicated	At 3 mo of age

Abbreviations: AlkPhos, alkaline phosphatase; ALT, alanine aminotransferase; AST, aspartate aminotransferase; BUN, blood urea nitrogen; GGT, gamma-glutamyl transferase; INR, international normalized ratio; PTT, partial thromboplastin time; PT, prothrombin time.

Data from Ayers P, Bobo ES, Hurt RT, Mays AA, Worthington PH, eds. ASPEN Parenteral Nutrition Handbook, Third Edition. Silver Spring, MD: American Society for Parenteral and Enteral Nutrition; 2020.

PN, disease state, and clinical status. A suggested monitoring schedule can be found in **Table 1**.

GROWTH ASSESSMENT AND MONITORING

Infants with CHD comprise a high-risk population for feeding difficulties, inadequate nutrient intake, suboptimal growth, and other nutritional complications during a critical developmental period which may impact both short- and long-term outcomes.[63,64] Infants with single-ventricle physiology frequently experience a significant decrease in weight-for-age z-scores during the interstage period between neonatal surgical palliation and the second surgical stage, which affects postoperative outcomes and increases risk of morbidity due to poor nutritional status.[65–67] Close monitoring of growth and nutritional status is warranted to provide early recognition of feeding and growth difficulties to implement appropriate interventions.[64,67] Serial anthropometric measurements of weight, length, and head circumference using standard techniques and appropriate equipment should be obtained.[68,69] Term infants may be plotted on sex-specific World Health Organization (WHO) growth charts for children 0 to 2 years of age. For premature infants, anthropometric measurements should be plotted using the sex-specific Fenton (2013) growth charts until 50 weeks' postmenstrual age and then transition to the WHO growth charts using corrected gestational age. Utilization of specialized growth charts may be considered for infants with an underlying chromosomal abnormality or syndrome to evaluate anthropometric data.[67] Nutritional interventions for poor weight gain, defined as less than 20 g/d, are shown in **Fig. 2**.

PRETERM INFANTS WITH CONGENITAL HEART DISEASE: WHAT, WHEN, AND HOW MUCH TO FEED

The morbidity and mortality risk of preterm birth increases inversely with gestational age.[70,71] Infants with CHD often cannot undergo surgical repair early in the postnatal period. Although awaiting surgical repair, they are at an increased risk of experiencing medical complications related to both prematurity and CHD, thereby further delaying surgical intervention. Several studies suggest worse outcomes in preterm infants with CHD compared with those born full term[72–74] including higher risk of in-hospital mortality, NEC, sepsis, and prolonged need for invasive respiratory support.[75] In addition, preterm infants are at risk for postnatal growth failure and poor neurodevelopmental outcomes.[76–78]

The early initiation of EN with human milk in preterm infants has been shown to be beneficial for both short- and long-term outcomes.[25–27,31] However, the provision of enteral feeding in a preterm infant with CHD is challenging for a number of reasons. Given the host of potential complications related to prematurity alone, including NEC, sepsis, and intraventricular hemorrhage, many centers are reluctant to introduce enteral feeding as an additional factor. This hesitation is countered with the need for adequate preoperative nutrition and growth before surgical intervention. Feeding preterm infants by the naso-/orogastric route in the preoperative stage if the infant cannot feed by mouth. There is a theoretic risk of "intestinal angina," symptoms of which may be masked by use of a feeding tube. In this case, it may be reasonable to limit EN to trophic feeds in order to still benefit from "intestinal priming." The goal for preterm infants with CHD awaiting surgical repair is to maximize growth. If full EN cannot be achieved to provide 120 kcal/kg/d, a combination of EN and PN is recommended to achieve a minimum caloric intake of 100 to 120 kcal/kg/d.[1]

SUMMARY

Infants with CHD are at high risk of postnatal growth failure. Much like in preterm infants, there is evidence to suggest initiation of early enteral feeding with a standardized feeding protocol can improve both short- and long-term outcomes. However, the nutritional approach must be tailored to the cardiac lesion with a particular focus on the preoperative versus postoperative state. In addition, EN and PN should complement each other to meet both fluid and nutrient requirements with an emphasis on advancing enteral feeding as soon as safely possible.

Best practices

This review provides guidance on how to approach the nutritional strategy for infants with CHD.

Standardized protocols with an emphasis on early enteral feeding can improve both short- and long-term outcomes.

The nutritional strategy should be tailored to the type of cardiac lesion, gestational age, and the preoperative versus postoperative stage.

The combination of enteral and parenteral nutrition should meet the infant's daily caloric and fluid needs.

DISCLOSURE

A. Hair and C. Blanco previously received research support through a grant from Prolacta Bioscience for the Human Milk Cardiac Study.

REFERENCES

1. Justice L, Buckley JR, Floh A, et al. Nutrition considerations in the pediatric cardiac intensive care unit patient. World J Pediatr Congenit Heart Surg 2018;9(3): 333–43.
2. Wernovsky G. Current insights regarding neurological and developmental abnormalities in children and young adults with complex congenital cardiac disease. Cardiol Young 2006;16(Suppl 1):92–104.
3. Majnemer A, Limperopoulos C, Shevell MI, et al. A new look at outcomes of infants with congenital heart disease. Pediatr Neurol 2009;40(3):197–204.
4. Tabbutt S, Gaynor JW, Newburger JW. Neurodevelopmental outcomes after congenital heart surgery and strategies for improvement. Curr Opin Cardiol 2012;27(2):82–91.
5. Ravishankar C, Zak V, Williams IA, et al. Association of impaired linear growth and worse neurodevelopmental outcome in infants with single ventricle physiology: a report from the pediatric heart network infant single ventricle trial. J Pediatr 2013; 162(2):250–6.e2.
6. Mussatto KA, Hoffmann RG, Hoffman GM, et al. Risk and prevalence of developmental delay in young children with congenital heart disease. Pediatrics 2014; 133(3):e570–7.
7. Mitting R, Marino L, Macrae D, et al. Nutritional status and clinical outcome in postterm neonates undergoing surgery for congenital heart disease. Pediatr Crit Care Med 2015;16(5):448–52.
8. Howley LW, Kaufman J, Wymore E, et al. Enteral feeding in neonates with prostaglandin-dependent congenital cardiac disease: international survey on current trends and variations in practice. Cardiol Young 2012;22(2):121–7.
9. Hebra A, Brown MF, Hirschl RB, et al. Norwood WI, et al. Mesenteric ischemia in hypoplastic left heart syndrome. J Pediatr Surg 1993;28(4):606–11.
10. Harrison AM, Davis S, Reid JR, et al. Neonates with hypoplastic left heart syndrome have ultrasound evidence of abnormal superior mesenteric artery perfusion before and after modified Norwood procedure. Pediatr Crit Care Med 2005;6(4):445–7.
11. Giannone PJ, Luce WA, Nankervis CA, et al. Necrotizing enterocolitis in neonates with congenital heart disease. Life Sci 2008;82(7–8):341–7.
12. Young CM, Kingma SD, Neu J. Ischemia-reperfusion and neonatal intestinal injury. J Pediatr 2011;158(2 Suppl):e25–8.
13. McElhinney DB, Hedrick HL, Bush DM, et al. Necrotizing enterocolitis in neonates with congenital heart disease: risk factors and outcomes. Pediatrics 2000;106(5): 1080–7.
14. Kataria-Hale J, Osborne SW, Hair A, et al. Preoperative feeds in ductal-dependent cardiac disease: a systematic review and meta-analysis. Hosp Pediatr 2019;9(12):998–1006.
15. Natarajan G, Reddy Anne S, Aggarwal S. Enteral feeding of neonates with congenital heart disease. Neonatology 2010;98(4):330–6.
16. Toms R, Jackson KW, Dabal RJ, et al. Preoperative trophic feeds in neonates with hypoplastic left heart syndrome. Congenit Heart Dis 2015;10(1):36–42.

17. Slicker J, Sables-Baus S, Lambert LM, et al. Perioperative feeding approaches in single ventricle infants: a survey of 46 centers. Congenit Heart Dis 2016;11(6): 707–15.

18. Scahill CJ, Graham EM, Atz AM, et al. Preoperative feeding neonates with cardiac disease. World J Pediatr Congenit Heart Surg 2017;8(1):62–8.

19. Day TG, Dionisio D, Zannino D, et al. Enteral feeding in duct-dependent congenital heart disease. J Neonatal Perinatal Med 2019;12(1):9–12.

20. Nordenström K, Lannering K, Mellander M, et al. Low risk of necrotising enterocolitis in enterally fed neonates with critical heart disease: an observational study. Arch Dis Child Fetal Neonatal Ed 2020;105(6):609–14.

21. Kelleher ST, McMahon CJ, James A. Necrotizing enterocolitis in children with congenital heart disease: a literature review. Pediatr Cardiol 2021;42(8):1688–99.

22. O'Neal Maynord P, Johnson M, Xu M, et al. A multi-interventional nutrition program for newborns with congenital heart disease. J Pediatr 2021;228:66–73.e2.

23. Bell D, Suna J, Marathe SP, et al. Feeding neonates and infants prior to surgery for congenital heart defects: systematic review and meta-analysis. Children 2022;9(12).

24. Cognata A, Kataria-Hale J, Griffiths P, et al. Human milk use in the preoperative period is associated with a lower risk for necrotizing enterocolitis in neonates with complex congenital heart disease. J Pediatr 2019;215:11–6.e2.

25. Hair AB, Peluso AM, Hawthorne KM, et al. Beyond necrotizing enterocolitis prevention: improving outcomes with an exclusive human milk-based diet. Breastfeed Med 2016;11(2):70–4.

26. Cortez J, Makker K, Kraemer DF, et al. Maternal milk feedings reduce sepsis, necrotizing enterocolitis and improve outcomes of premature infants. J Perinatol 2018;38(1):71–4.

27. Meier PP. Human milk and clinical outcomes in preterm infants. Nestle Nutr Inst Workshop Ser 2019;90:163–74.

28. Martini S, Beghetti I, Annunziata M, et al. Enteral nutrition in term infants with congenital heart disease: knowledge gaps and future directions to improve clinical practice. Nutrients 2021;13(3):932.

29. Luca AC, Miron IC, Mîndru DE, et al. Optimal nutrition parameters for neonates and infants with congenital heart disease. Nutrients 2022;14(8):1671.

30. Lin PW, Stoll BJ. Necrotising enterocolitis. Lancet 2006;368(9543):1271–83.

31. Ballard O, Morrow AL. Human milk composition: nutrients and bioactive factors. Pediatr Clin North Am 2013;60(1):49–74.

32. Barr J, Hecht M, Flavin KE, et al. Outcomes in critically ill patients before and after the implementation of an evidence-based nutritional management protocol. Chest 2004;125(4):1446–57.

33. Petrillo-Albarano T, Pettignano R, Asfaw M, et al. Use of a feeding protocol to improve nutritional support through early, aggressive, enteral nutrition in the pediatric intensive care unit. Pediatr Crit Care Med 2006;7(4):340–4.

34. del Castillo SL, McCulley ME, Khemani RG, et al. Reducing the incidence of necrotizing enterocolitis in neonates with hypoplastic left heart syndrome with the introduction of an enteral feed protocol. Pediatr Crit Care Med 2010;11(3): 373–7.

35. Gephart SM, Hanson CK. Preventing necrotizing enterocolitis with standardized feeding protocols: not only possible, but imperative. Adv Neonatal Care 2013; 13(1):48–54.

36. Kataria-Hale J, Roddy DJ, Cognata A, et al. A preoperative standardized feeding protocol improves human milk use in infants with complex congenital heart disease. J Perinatol 2021;41(3):590–7.

37. Gephart SM, Weller M. Colostrum as oral immune therapy to promote neonatal health. Adv Neonatal Care 2014;14(1):44–51.

38. Lee J, Kim HS, Jung YH, et al. Oropharyngeal colostrum administration in extremely premature infants: an RCT. Pediatrics 2015;135(2):e357–66.

39. Sohn K, Kalanetra KM, Mills DA, et al. Buccal administration of human colostrum: impact on the oral microbiota of premature infants. J Perinatol 2016;36(2):106–11.

40. Bourgeois-Nicolaos N, Raynor A, Shankar-Aguilera S, et al. Breast milk in neonate oral care: oropharyngeal effects in extremely preterm infants. Eur J Pediatr 2022; 182(1):385–92.

41. Willis L, Thureen P, Kaufman J, et al. Enteral feeding in prostaglandin-dependent neonates: is it a safe practice? J Pediatr 2008;153(6):867–9.

42. Becker KC, Hornik CP, Cotten CM, et al. Necrotizing enterocolitis in infants with ductal-dependent congenital heart disease. Am J Perinatol 2015;32(7):633–8.

43. Tume LN, Valla FV, Joosten K, et al. Nutritional support for children during critical illness: European Society of Pediatric and Neonatal Intensive Care (ESPNIC) metabolism, endocrine and nutrition section position statement and clinical recommendations. Intensive Care Med 2020;46(3):411–25.

44. Indramohan G, Pedigo TP, Rostoker N, et al. Identification of risk factors for poor feeding in infants with congenital heart disease and a novel approach to improve oral feeding. J Pediatr Nurs 2017;35:149–54.

45. Holst LM, Serrano F, Shekerdemian L, et al. Impact of feeding mode on neurodevelopmental outcome in infants and children with congenital heart disease. Congenit Heart Dis 2019;14(6):1207–13.

46. Lucas A, Bloom SR, Aynsley-Green A. Postnatal surges in plasma gut hormones in term and preterm infants. Biol Neonate 1982;41(1–2):63–7.

47. Aynsley-Green A, Adrian TE, Bloom SR. Feeding and the development of enteroinsular hormone secretion in the preterm infant: effects of continuous gastric infusions of human milk compared with intermittent boluses. Acta Paediatr Scand 1982;71(3):379–83.

48. Rogers SP, Hicks PD, Hamzo M, et al. Continuous feedings of fortified human milk lead to nutrient losses of fat, calcium and phosphorous. Nutrients 2010;2(3): 230–40.

49. Iannucci GJ, Oster ME, Mahle WT. Necrotising enterocolitis in infants with congenital heart disease: the role of enteral feeds. Cardiol Young 2013;23(4): 553–9.

50. Iliopoulos I, Burke R, Hannan R, et al. Preoperative intubation and lack of enteral nutrition are associated with prolonged stay after arterial switch operation. Pediatr Cardiol 2016;37(6):1078–84.

51. Leong AY, Cartwright KR, Guerra GG, et al. A Canadian survey of perceived barriers to initiation and continuation of enteral feeding in PICUs. Pediatr Crit Care Med 2014;15(2):e49–55.

52. Keehn A, O'Brien C, Mazurak V, et al. Epidemiology of interruptions to nutrition support in critically ill children in the pediatric intensive care unit. JPEN J Parenter Enteral Nutr 2015;39(2):211–7.

53. Anderson JB, Iyer SB, Schidlow DN, et al. Variation in growth of infants with a single ventricle. J Pediatr 2012;161(1):16–21.e1 [quiz: e2-3].

54. Slicker J, Hehir DA, Horsley M, et al. Nutrition algorithms for infants with hypoplastic left heart syndrome; birth through the first interstage period. Congenit Heart Dis 2013;8(2):89–102.

55. Hair AB, Hawthorne KM, Chetta KE, et al. Human milk feeding supports adequate growth in infants ≤ 1250 grams birth weight. BMC Res Notes 2013;6:459.

56. Blanco C, Hair A, Justice LB, et al. A randomized trial of an exclusive human milk diet in neonates with single ventricle physiology. J Pediatr 2022. https://doi.org/10.1016/j.jpeds.2022.11.043.

57. Ayers PBE, Hurt RT, Mays AA, et al, editors. ASPEN parenteral nutrition handbook. 3rd edition. Silver Springs (MD): American Society for Parenteral and Enteral Nutrition; 2020.

58. Joosten K, Embleton N, Yan W, et al. ESPGHAN/ESPEN/ESPR/CSPEN guidelines on pediatric parenteral nutrition: energy. Clin Nutr 2018;37(6 Pt B):2309–14.

59. van Goudoever JB, Carnielli V, Darmaun D, et al. ESPGHAN/ESPEN/ESPR/CSPEN guidelines on pediatric parenteral nutrition: amino acids. Clin Nutr 2018;37(6 Pt B):2315–23.

60. Mesotten D, Joosten K, van Kempen A, et al. ESPGHAN/ESPEN/ESPR/CSPEN guidelines on pediatric parenteral nutrition: carbohydrates. Clin Nutr 2018;37(6 Pt B):2337–43.

61. Lapillonne A, Fidler Mis N, Goulet O, et al. ESPGHAN/ESPEN/ESPR/CSPEN guidelines on pediatric parenteral nutrition: lipids. Clin Nutr 2018;37(6 Pt B):2324–36.

62. Mihatsch W, Fewtrell M, Goulet O, et al. ESPGHAN/ESPEN/ESPR/CSPEN guidelines on pediatric parenteral nutrition: calcium, phosphorus and magnesium. Clin Nutr 2018;37(6 Pt B):2360–5.

63. Toole BJ, Toole LE, Kyle UG, et al. Perioperative nutritional support and malnutrition in infants and children with congenital heart disease. Congenit Heart Dis 2014;9(1):15–25.

64. Salvatori G, De Rose DU, Massolo AC, et al. Current strategies to optimize nutrition and growth in newborns and infants with congenital heart disease: a narrative review. J Clin Med 2022;11(7):1841.

65. Menon SC, McCandless RT, Mack GK, et al. Clinical outcomes and resource use for infants with hypoplastic left heart syndrome during bidirectional Glenn: summary from the Joint Council for congenital heart disease national pediatric Cardiology Quality improvement Collaborative registry. Pediatr Cardiol 2013;34(1):143–8.

66. Kelleher DK, Laussen P, Teixeira-Pinto A, et al. Growth and correlates of nutritional status among infants with hypoplastic left heart syndrome (HLHS) after stage 1 Norwood procedure. Nutrition 2006;22(3):237–44.

67. Corkins MRBJ, Bobo E, Plogsted S, et al. Pediatric nutrition support core curriculum. 2nd edition. Silver Spring (MD): American Society for Enteral and Parenteral Nutrition; 2015.

68. Poindexter BB, Cormack BE, Bloomfield FH. Approaches to growth Faltering. World Rev Nutr Diet 2021;122:312–24.

69. Kleinman REGF, editor. Pediatric nutrition. 7th edition. Elk Grove Village (IL): American Academy of Pediatrics; 2014.

70. Costeloe KL, Hennessy EM, Haider S, et al. Short term outcomes after extreme preterm birth in England: comparison of two birth cohorts in 1995 and 2006 (the EPICure studies). Bmj 2012;345:e7976.

71. Ancel PY, Goffinet F, Kuhn P, et al. Survival and morbidity of preterm children born at 22 through 34 weeks' gestation in France in 2011: results of the EPIPAGE-2 cohort study. JAMA Pediatr 2015;169(3):230–8.
72. Costello JM, Polito A, Brown DW, et al. Birth before 39 weeks' gestation is associated with worse outcomes in neonates with heart disease. Pediatrics 2010; 126(2):277–84.
73. Polito A, Piga S, Cogo PE, et al. Increased morbidity and mortality in very preterm/VLBW infants with congenital heart disease. Intensive Care Med 2013; 39(6):1104–12.
74. Laas E, Lelong N, Ancel PY, et al. Impact of preterm birth on infant mortality for newborns with congenital heart defects: the EPICARD population-based cohort study. BMC Pediatr 2017;17(1):124.
75. Dumitrascu Biris I, Mintoft A, Harris C, et al. Mortality and morbidity in preterm infants with congenital heart disease. Acta Paediatr 2022;111(1):151–6.
76. Dusick AM, Poindexter BB, Ehrenkranz RA, et al. Growth failure in the preterm infant: can we catch up? Semin Perinatol 2003;27(4):302–10.
77. Hawthorne KM, Griffin IJ, Abrams SA. Current issues in nutritional management of very low birth weight infants. Minerva Pediatr 2004;56(4):359–72.
78. Morales Y, Schanler RJ. Human milk and clinical outcomes in VLBW infants: how compelling is the evidence of benefit? Semin Perinatol 2007;31(2):83–8.

Special Populations— Surgical Infants

Stefanie Riddle, MD[a],*, Heidi Karpen, MD[b]

KEYWORDS

- Gastroschisis • Intestinal atresia • Breast milk • Dysmotility • Growth • Surgery

KEY POINTS

- Early commencement of enteral feeds has been associated with early attainment of full enteral feeds, and for those who develop short bowel syndrome/intestinal failure (SBS/IF), it increases the rate of achieving enteral autonomy.
- Human milk has many advantages specific to the postsurgical neonate: rich in immuno-globulins, nucleotides, live cells, growth factors, lactoferrin, and key oligosaccharides that may support the developing immune system and improve intestinal growth and adaptation, with fewer days on parenteral nutrition and shorter hospitalization.
- Complications such as dysmotility, hypersecretion, small intestinal bacterial overgrowth, and dysbiosis require consideration of distinct treatment options.

INTRODUCTION

Surgical disorders in neonates encompass a broad variety of diagnoses, some of which are congenital and others, such as necrotizing enterocolitis (NEC), are acquired. Congenital surgical disorders can be loosely categorized into the following groupings because these disease processes often share common surgical approaches, complications, and difficulties. Among the most common are congenital gastrointestinal disorders (CGD) such as abdominal wall defects, intestinal atresias, colorectal malformations including Hirschsprung disease and imperforate anus, intestinal malrotation and volvulus, and others that may ultimately lead to bowel resection and short bowel syndrome, complex disorders such as esophageal atresia ± tracheoesophageal fistula (EA/TEF), congenital diaphragmatic hernia, and VACTERL association, and so forth, and congenital heart disease (CHD). Despite the wide array of diagnoses and developmental underpinnings, these

[a] Department of Pediatrics, University of Cincinnati College of Medicine, Cincinnati Children's Hospital Medical Center, 3333 Burnet Avenue, Cincinnati, OH 45229, USA; [b] Emory University School of Medicine/Children's Healthcare of Atlanta, 2015 Uppergate Drive Northeast, ECC Room 324, Atlanta, GA 30322, USA
* Corresponding author. Division of Neonatology, Cincinnati Children's Hospital Medical Center, 3333 Burnet Avenue, MLC 7009, Cincinnati OH 45229.
E-mail address: Stefanie.riddle@cchmc.org

Clin Perinatol 50 (2023) 715–728
https://doi.org/10.1016/j.clp.2023.04.008
0095-5108/23/© 2023 Elsevier Inc. All rights reserved.
perinatology.theclinics.com

disorders share many common problems: increased nutritional requirements to prevent catabolism, enhance wound healing, and provide optimal growth; impaired motility and altered intestinal flora leading to feeding intolerance requiring long-term parenteral nutrition; gastroesophageal reflux and poor feeding mechanics requiring tube feedings and support; growth failure; poor barrier function and risk of infection; and other long-term sequelae. Many of these disorders may be diagnosed prenatally and are managed at centers with neonatology, pediatric surgery, nutritional support, and availability of intestinal rehabilitation programs for those with intestinal failure. This article describes current practices and difficulties in the provision of enteral and parenteral nutrition for high-risk neonates with congenital surgical conditions, and additionally highlights some of the special problems and practices related to feeding and medication management.

NUTRITIONAL REQUIREMENTS

Nutritional needs in the early neonatal period are greater than at any other time of life and present some of the greatest challenges in caring for this population. Infants with surgical conditions are at an increased risk for nutritional deficits and long-term growth failure. Many of these infants are born small for gestational age (SGA) or preterm and may have comorbid conditions such as intestinal atresias, NEC, CHD, bronchopulmonary dysplasia (BPD), sepsis, and intraventricular hemorrhage. Infants with one or more of these major morbidities are at the highest risk of growth faltering. These infants begin life with limited micronutrient and macronutrient deposition and often have a high degree of illness, which may make the provision of adequate calories and protein immediately after birth difficult. These infants may quickly descend into a nitrogen and caloric deficit due to high disease acuity and need for surgical procedures, with fluid volume limitations, and need for vasopressor support. Consequently, the surgical "at-risk" infant requires specialized nutritional support to meet their increased nutritional requirements to ensure adequate growth and meet the increased demands from critical illness.

Malnutrition is the result of inadequate energy intake or an increase in energy expenditure, causing an *energy imbalance*. Energy requirements in neonates may increase by 30% for mild-to-moderate stress and up to 50% in severe stress. Estimates of postnatal growth failure in critically ill infants range from 40% to 90% depending on the series and diagnosis. Postnatal growth failure and inadequate nutrition have been associated with poor long-term neurodevelopmental outcomes such as attention deficit disorder, aggressive behavior, and poor social and emotional development.[1,2]

There is wide practice variation in timing of surgical interventions, criteria to begin and advance enteral nutrition, and specialized practices such as mucus fistula refeeds and sham feeds. These infants depend on parenteral nutrition, often for weeks to months, which places them at increased risk of central line associated blood stream infections (CLABSIs), cholestasis and liver disease, metabolic bone disease, all of which can affect metabolism and impair growth. A recent study of infants with gastroschisis showed that growth failure for weight was present in more than 36% of infants and for length in 42% by the time of discharge. Lower weight-for-age (WAZ) at discharge was associated with prematurity, SGA/intrauterine growth restriction (IUGR) status with lower WAZ at birth, CLABSI, and longer intensive care unit (ICU) stay.[3,4]

Macronutrients and micronutrients are absorbed differentially in various locations in the small and large intestines, so individual anatomy following bowel resection can predispose to vitamin and micronutrient deficiencies. This risk of nutrient deficiency continues even if they achieve full enteral feeds and adequate somatic growth,[5–7] emphasizing the importance of multivitamin supplementation and close comprehensive follow-up.

CONTROVERSIES IN PERINATAL MANAGEMENT—GASTROSCHISIS

Abdominal wall defects are common surgical disorders in the fetus and neonate, with incidence of gastroschisis increasing in recent years.[8] Gastroschisis is characterized by a periumbilical defect of the abdominal wall, allowing herniation of abdominal contents and exposure of extruded viscera to the amniotic environment leading to intestinal damage and dysmotility. Common perinatal complications of gastroschisis including intrauterine growth restriction and bowel dilation, which has been associated in some studies with intestinal atresia, perforation, bowel necrosis, and other complicated forms of gastroschisis. Perinatal management in gastroschisis is controversial despite multiple studies to assess optimal delivery timing and route. Serial ultrasound is used for monitoring of fetal growth and well-being, as well as assessment of the integrity of the exposed bowel. Ultrasound findings of bowel wall edema, bowel dilation, and polyhydramnios may suggest bowel atresia and unfavorable outcomes.[9–12] Intrauterine growth restriction is common, with growth failure presenting as early as the midsecond trimester. Birth weight less than 10th percentile may be seen in up to 47% of neonates.[13] Contradictory evidence exists in the literature regarding the benefit of elective preterm delivery in order to prevent intrauterine fetal demise and ongoing exposure of exposed bowel to the amniotic environment.[14–16] The GOOD study (Gastroschisis Outcomes on Delivery) is a large, multicenter, randomized trial is currently ongoing with the goal of defining optimal delivery timing.[17]

Delivery room management of gastroschisis is aimed at minimizing heat and evaporative fluid loss from the eviscerated bowel. It is imperative to provide adequate intravascular volume to support intestinal perfusion and avoid hypovolemia and acidosis. Aggressive fluid resuscitation or excessive maintenance fluids should be avoided, however, because resuscitative fluid volume has been directly associated with an increased likelihood of adverse outcomes including days of postclosure mechanical ventilation, parenteral nutrition, length of stay, and bacteremia.[18] In the past, the use of empiric broad-spectrum antibiotics for extended courses was common after delivery and during reduction of the bowel. Now with greater awareness of the relationship between antibiotic use and its association with pathologic changes in the microbiome, there is a push toward more selective use of antibiotic therapy and for shorter durations.[19–21]

Reduction of the eviscerated abdominal contents and closure of the abdominal wall can occur via multiple techniques. In the optimal circumstance, primary reduction of the bowel and other organs is performed soon after the delivery. Historically, primary sutured closure was performed but a newer sutureless closure technique has become the preferred method during the last decade. Studies assessing sutureless closure have demonstrated less risk of infection, earlier time to first and full enteral feeds, less time on mechanical ventilation, and shorter duration of hospitalization.[22–24] During fetal life, without the presence of normal abdominal contents, the intra-abdominal domain often remains small and full reduction is impossible immediately after delivery. A delayed closure strategy is used in this circumstance, using a silastic silo to encase and protect the bowel allowing gradual reduction of the bowel into the abdomen. Regardless of strategy, after repair, the bowel may have ongoing inflammation or edema. The increase in intra-abdominal pressure may lead to compromise in venous return, renal perfusion, and lead to upward pressure on the diaphragm resulting in respiratory compromise. Close monitoring of fluid balance, perfusion, and respiratory status are necessary after closure.

PARENTERAL NUTRITION

Neonates have limited energy and protein stores that are rapidly depleted after birth, especially when faced with critical illness and surgical wound healing. These stores are even more limited in premature and IUGR infants. To meet nutrient requirements in surgical infants, most infants receive parenteral nutrition soon after birth and in the immediate postoperative period. Indeed, parenteral nutrition (PN) can be used as the sole source of nutrition support for neonates who cannot tolerate enteral feedings for a prolonged period.

Newborn energy intakes must meet the requirements for resting energy expenditure, energy losses, and growth. Term infants require 100 to 120 kcal/kg/d, whereas preterm infant requirements range from 110 to 160 kcal/kg/d. These requirements may be increased above these ranges in severe level of illness, with associated morbidities such as CHD, BPD, and sepsis. Infants with ostomies or SBS have increased stool losses of both protein and nonprotein calories. Providing sufficient parenteral protein beginning at birth and not prematurely discontinuing parenteral nutrition are practices that may aid in ameliorating growth faltering in infants with surgical conditions. Term infants typically require 2.5 to 3.5 g/kg/d of protein, where preterm infant requirements are much higher at 3.5 to 4.5 g/kg/d. These estimates again may fall short in infants who undergo multiple surgical procedures or who have excessive losses.

It is important not only to provide sufficient protein to prevent catabolism and promote growth but sufficient nonprotein calories to prevent them from being used for energy, as this is a very inefficient process. Typical glucose infusion rate (GIR) requirements for these infants are 12 to 15 mg/kg/min but may be as high as 17 to 18 mg/kg/min depending on energy requirements, growth, and tolerance of lipids/lipid strategies.

Lipids are a major source of energy and essential fatty acids (FAs), which are key elements especially in myelination and neurodevelopment. Long-term provision of soybean oil lipid emulsions (SO-LE) has been associated with the development of parenteral nutrition associated cholestasis (PNAC) and progression to liver disease/liver failure (PNALD) in neonates who are PN-dependent for prolonged periods of time, and several studies have shown that cholestasis can develop in infants exposed to PN for as little as 14 days.[25] SO-LE are rich in phytosterols, which have been shown to downregulate bile acid exporters[25] as well as ω-6 FAs that are proinflammatory in nature. PNAC can be reversed in many infants when they are either lipid limited to 1 g/kg/d of SO-LE[26] or switched to a fish oil lipid emulsion (FO-LE), which can only be dosed at 1 g/kg/d.[27] FO-LE is only approved for the treatment of PNAC/PNALD and typically is initiated when the direct bilirubin is greater than 2 to 4 mg/dL. Unfortunately, both of these approaches limit the amount of fat calories available to the infant and require compensation with higher GIR to maintain overall adequate intake.

SMOF-LE is a blend of soybean oil, medium chain triglycerides, olive oil, and fish oil, which is now in widespread use in neonates with surgical conditions for the prevention of PNAC/PNALD. The advantage of blended LEs is a much lower proportion of phytosterols from the SO-LE fraction (~30%) and the anti-inflammatory properties of the FO-LE. This blend approximates a ω-3/ω-6 ratio found in breast milk. There have been multiple studies assessing the safety and efficacy of SMOF-LE in premature infants as well as those with surgical conditions and early cholestasis.[28,29] Because SMOF-LE contains only 30% of the SO-LE, which is the primary source of essential FAs, it should be dosed in 2.5 to 3 g/kg/d until sufficient enteral feedings have been established to avoid essential FA deficiency. The main benefit of this approach is the ability to provide substantially more calories and decrease the risk of cholestasis in these infants.

ENTERAL NUTRITION
When to Feed

In all of these surgical populations, delays in enteral feeding leads to absence of trophic factors leading to greater complications of abnormal bacterial colonization due to antibiotic exposure and the NICU environment, ultimately leading to difficulty with adequate nutritional provision. Trophic feedings, also known as minimal enteral nutrition, gut priming, or hypocaloric feeding, are small volume feeds (typically <10–20 mL/kg/d) that are often used as a first step in feeding initiation. The benefits of trophic feeding, especially in the preterm population, are well described-enhanced enterocyte maturation, improved enzymatic function, renewal of villi and improve gut permeability and barrier function, maturation of intestinal motor function, and enteric hormone secretion.

Criteria used to determine enteral feeding readiness with return of bowel function include absence of distention, daily bowel movements, character (bilious or nonbilious) and volume of nasogastric drainage, and emesis. Ultrasound has also been used to document motility and feeding readiness in gastroschisis. In one study, utilizing ultrasound documentation of motility accelerated initiation of enteral feeds by 2 to 3 days as compared with utilizing clinical characteristics of return of bowel function.[30]

Feeding practices after gastroschisis closure or surgical interventions are highly variable.[31] Early commencement of enteral feeds has been associated with early attainment of full enteral feeds, and for those who develop SBS/IF, increases the rate of achieving enteral autonomy.[5,31–33] Minimal enteral or trophic feeds in gastroschisis have also been associated with shorter time on total parenteral nutrition (TPN), earlier achievement of full enteral feeds, and lower rates of nosocomial infection.[34] Evidence in observational studies on gastroschisis indicate that each day delays in initiation of enteral feeding by 1 day results in an increase in TPN duration by 1.55 days and length of stay (LOS) 1.39 days.

What to Feed

Although many feeding practices in the surgical population are based on experience rather than evidence, the literature strongly supports human milk as the preferred feeding choice. Human milk has many advantages specific to the postsurgical neonate: rich in immunoglobulins, nucleotides, live cells, growth factors, lactoferrin, and key oligosaccharides that may support the developing immune system and improve intestinal growth and adaptation.

The use of human milk for enteral feedings of infants following repair of gastroschisis and other CGD significantly reduced time to full feeds, days on TPN and to discharge.[35,36] Benefits have been found in days to full enteral feeds based on total breast milk dose, with fewer days on parenteral nutrition and shorter length of stay for those fed 100% breast milk, even compared with those receiving greater than 50% but not exclusive breast milk. This difference was significant, with exclusively breast milk-fed infants being discharged an average of 10 days sooner than the 50% or greater than group and 13.5 days sooner than the less than 50% group.

Significant differences have even been shown for 10% incremental increases in mother's own milk (MOM) dose.[37] When MOM is not available, use of donor breast milk as supplementation has additionally been shown to decrease length of hospital stay and central line days.[38] Growth failure is common in infants with CGD and is estimated that 28% to 36% have weight-for-length (WFL) z-score decline of greater than 0.8 from birth to discharge and that this growth failure persists for months to years after discharge[4] (Stangeby and colleagues unpublished data). Given the high risk of NEC in infants with CGD, especially gastroschisis, which approaches 10%, clinicians are often wary about fortifying enteral feedings. As most infants with CGD are late-preterm or term gestational age (GA), MOM feeds are often fortified with bridge preterm or term formulas. Some centers have advocated the use of human milk-based fortifiers (HMBF) given the risk reduction of NEC seen in the preterm population.[39,40] Until now, these HMBF have only been formulated for the preterm infant. Two recent multicenter clinical trials evaluated outcomes of infants with single ventricle physiology CHD (SVP trial) and specific CGD (gastroschisis, omphalocele, and intestinal atresias) (human milk [HM] for CGD trial) fed an exclusive human milk diet composed of MOM, PDHM, and fortified with a novel HMBF formulated specifically for the term infant compared with infants fed formula/formula fortification as part of their diet. In both studies, the overall risk of NEC was significantly reduced (3.6% vs 15.4% in SVP, 2.0% vs 7.8% in CGD), whereas WFL z-scores, direct bilirubin, and clinical sepsis were significantly improved (Clinicaltrials.gov/NCT02860702, NCT02567292).

In the absence of human milk, debate exists regarding best formula choice for surgical infants. Use of extensively hydrolyzed formulas is common and rationalized by the increased risk of protein allergy in infants following intestinal surgery.[41,42] Extensively hydrolyzed formulas may be preferable because they do not contain lactose and often have increased content of MCTs; undigested lactose has been implicated in animal models of NEC, and MCTs may be better absorbed in situations where rapid transit or bacterial overgrowth occur. Extensively hydrolyzed formulas do not satisfy many of the nutritional requirements of preterm infants, which is an important disadvantage to their use. One randomized study of hydrolyzed versus nonhydrolyzed formulas did not show improvement in tolerance or weight gain. Elemental formulas have been shown to reduce the length of parenteral nutrition dependence as compared with hydrolyzed formula, and may be an acceptable alternative when human milk is not available.[43]

How to Feed

Postoperative feeding guidelines offer a systematic approach to optimizing enteral nutrition, which may reduce variability. Use of postoperative nutrition guidelines have been shown to decrease time to full enteral feedings, decrease in days of parenteral nutrition, infection, length of hospitalization and costs, and intestinal failure-associated liver disease.[33,44,45] Development of guidelines must include input from a multidisciplinary team of neonatologists, pediatric surgeons, nurses, dieticians, and lactation consultants.[45] Despite a paucity of evidence of this association, guidelines should balance the risk of NEC in these high-risk surgical populations, and there is not a definitive best practice in terms of volume or speed of advancement. In the preterm population, standardized feeding protocols have been shown to significantly reduce the incidence of NEC and time on parenteral nutrition, shorten time to full feeds, and improve growth.[46,47] Recent evidence suggests that advancements of 20 mL/kg/d are safe and result in faster attainment of full enteral feeds, less parenteral nutrition, and shorter length of hospitalization in patients with gastroschisis and intestinal atresia.[48,49] Although postsurgical conditions represent a heterogeneous group of diagnoses, the general principles of early initiation and advancement of enteral nutrition apply to most infants undergoing intestinal surgery. At this time, feeding guidelines are not uniformly accepted in the surgical literature, although available studies did not account for adherence/compliance.[50] Intolerance to feeding advancements, including large or bilious emesis, loose or watery stools, or large volume stool or ostomy (>30 mL/kg/d) output may require slowing or stopping of feeding progression.

As there can be significant delays in offering oral feeds following abdominal surgeries or gastroschisis closure, there may also be delays in development and progression of oral feeding skills. Additionally, there may be negative oral stimuli that affect feeding readiness and success, such as oral intubation, prolonged need for nasal and oral gastric tubes, frequent suctioning, and emesis. There may also be limitations in skin-to-skin contact and avoidance of direct breast feeding, even once ready for enteral feeding initiation. Sham feeds are a strategy to promote oral feeding skills in preoperative or postoperative infants, whereby an oral feeding is offered and immediately removed before it can be digested. Limited data exists on this practice but small series and one pilot study performed on a variety of surgical diagnoses have demonstrated both safety and feasibility of sham feeds in infants with esophageal atresia and congenital gastrointestinal (GI) disorders.[51,52] Assessments for safety are ideally performed by speech or occupational therapy before the initiation of oral feeds and criteria that ensure physiologic stability should exist (time postsurgery, minimum acceptable level of respiratory support). Low-volume feeds via bottle or direct breast-feeding on an empty breast with a Replogle tube to continuous low wall suction may occur once per day, or, as skills progress, multiple attempts per day. There may be additional benefit to sham feedings with human milk, in that earlier exposure to very trophic volumes may have anti-inflammatory and other benefits associated with trophic feeds as previously described.

COMPLICATIONS AND THERAPIES
Growth Failure

In neonates, growth failure has been associated with adverse neurodevelopmental outcomes. Infants with gastroschisis are at high risk of growth failure due to preterm birth (up to 80%), frequent intrauterine growth restriction, and in utero substance exposures including tobacco and illicit substances. Unfortunately, growth failure remains common; a recent multicenter cohort study found that although one-third of infants with gastroschisis were SGA at birth, more than half were less than 10th percentile weight for age at hospital discharge.[53] On multivariable regression analysis, lower weight for age z-scores at discharge was significantly associated with prematurity, lower birth weight for age z-score, CLABSI, and longer ICU stay. Risk factors independently associated with a greater decline in weight for age z-score from birth to discharge were CLABSI, prematurity, and higher birth weight for age z-score.[4] Additionally, infants who develop short bowel syndrome and intestinal failure with prolonged parenteral nutrition reliance are at increased risk for growth failure and liver disease.[3] Traditional measurement of anthropometrics to follow growth may also insufficiently detect growth failure and does not provide information on the quality of growth. Measurement of body composition, and specifically fat mass and fat-free mass may improve their long-term outcomes with timely interventions.[54]

Gastric Acid Hypersecretion and GERD

Gastric acid hypersecretion is common in short bowel syndrome, and up to 50% of patients with gastroschisis and 90% with intestinal malrotation have gastroesophageal reflux disease and esophageal dysmotility.[55–57] The excessive acid that enters the proximal small bowel inactivates pancreatic enzymes, impairs micellar formation, and reduces carbohydrate digestion ultimately leading to malabsorption,[58] which is transient but may persist for up to 12 months postoperatively. Although there is a well-known association between H2-blocker therapy and NEC in very-low birth weight infants,[59] treatment of gastric acid hypersecretion with H2 receptor antagonists or proton pump inhibitors can improve nutrient absorption in infants following bowel resection. Treatment guidelines exist for the clinical management of gastroesophageal reflux disease (GERD) in infants and children and those with more unique physiology such as EA/TEF.[60–62]

Dysmotility

Dysmotility is also common due to structural alterations in GI anatomy, defects in enteric hormone secretion, and GI tract denervation, which can also contribute to delayed gastric emptying and gastroesophageal reflux. Normal intestinal motility requires the coordinated function of intestinal smooth muscle, the enteric nervous system, and the interstitial cells of Cajal (the "pacemaker" and transducer of neural inputs to the musculature). Alterations in the distribution of these cells have been described in gastroschisis, intestinal atresias (especially distal to the atretic segment), and Hirschsprung disease.[63–65] Therapies to address these problems can include prokinetic agents, antidiarrheal agents, and in some cases surgical interventions for the overdistended and poorly motile bowel to encourage enteral adaptation. Prokinetic agents include antidopaminergic (metoclopramide), antisertonergic (cisapride), and motilin receptor agonists (erythromycin) whose aim is to produce coordinated smooth muscle contractions to increase gastric emptying and transit in the small and large bowel.[66,67] The prokinetic effect of erythromycin is achieved at lower doses than those used for antimicrobial purposes, and some clinical studies have demonstrated improved gastric and intestinal motility; however, this has not been consistently replicated in the literature.[68,69] Adverse effects of erythromycin must also be considered, which can include hepatotoxicity, ototoxicity, and multiple drug interactions related to the cytochrome P450 enzyme system.[70] Metoclopramide is a dopamine (D2) receptor antagonist with moderate serotonin receptor activity, which has been shown to increase lower esophageal sphincter tone, improve gastric emptying and antropyloroduodenal contractions, although placebo controlled studies have failed to demonstrate efficacy.[71] Additionally, extrapyramidal reactions are a common side effect, which occur more commonly in children than adults and have led to Food and Drug Administration (FDA) labeling limiting its duration of use to 12 weeks due to the risk of tardive dyskinesia.

Infants with small bowel syndrome can also have diarrhea and malabsorption due to abnormal anatomy and rapid intestinal transit, often leading to delays and intolerance of enteral feeds. Antidiarrheal agents may include antimotility agents that slow intestinal transit, or absorbing agents that bind intestinal water and other substances to improve consistency of stools.[66] Treatment with loperamide and other opioid receptor agonists act by decreasing intestinal peristalsis, fluid secretion, and increasing absorption of fluid and electrolytes, and increasing tone in the colon and anal sphincter.[72] No comparative studies have evaluated its use in children with short bowel syndrome or intestinal failure. The liquid preparation of loperamide may contain sorbitol, which may worsen diarrhea. Agents with absorptive properties (pectin, guar gum [Benefiber, Haleon; Weybridge, Surrey, UK]) may reduce stool output and prolong transit time; however, it should not be utilized in patients suspected to have bacterial overgrowth due to the potential to worsen lactic acidosis due to carbohydrate fermentation.[73]

Small Intestinal Bacterial Overgrowth

Especially for those infants who have lost significant bowel length, higher loads of carbohydrates and dysmotility can lead to selective bacterial overgrowth of microorganisms in the small intestine. Acid suppressive therapies, especially proton pump inhibitors, are known to alter gut microbiota leading to increased risk of bacterial overgrowth.[74,75] Sequelae of overgrowth include bacterial carbohydrate fermentation leading to excess gas and water production; bile acid deconjugation resulting in poor absorption of liposoluble vitamins; bacterial macronutrient and micronutrient competition, leaving the patient with less available nutrients for absorption; villous atrophy leading to carbohydrate malabsorption; decreased short-chain fatty acid production; and intestinal and systemic inflammation. It has been shown to increase odds of bloodstream infection in children with short bowel syndrome and especially those with elevated inflammatory markers as signs of systemic stress.[76] Symptoms of small intestinal bacterial overgrowth are often nonspecific, and may include abdominal distention, increased stool frequency, weight loss, lactic acidosis, and feeding intolerance. Diagnosis may be made by hydrogen/methane breath testing, elevation of serum lactate levels, urine 4-hydroxyphenylacetic acid levels, and quantitative small bowel cultures.[77] Treatment of bacterial overgrowth centers on antibiotic therapies. Rifaximin, gentamicin, metronidazole, and others have been studied in adult and pediatric populations but limited data looking at efficacy in infants are available.[78] Treatment with antibiotics alone does not fully address the problem of intestinal dysbiosis that may exist.

Dysbiosis

Multiple factors, including dysmotility, delayed enteral nutrition, antireflux medication use, and frequent antibiotic exposure, contribute to alterations in the microbiome in infants with congenital gastrointestinal disorders making the addition of prebiotics or probiotics an appealing therapeutic option. Prebiotics are nutrients that can alter gut microbiota indirectly by favoring growth of certain bacterial species via provision of metabolites, such as the oligosaccharides contained in human milk. Probiotics are live microorganisms that, when administered in adequate amounts, confer a health benefit to the host. Probiotics are postulated to enhance mucosal barrier function and integrity, decrease inflammatory response, stabilize gut flora and limit pathogen growth, and promote enterocyte differentiation. A growing body of literature has evaluated probiotics in preterm infants, including a number of randomized clinical trials for the prevention of severe NEC, late-onset sepsis, and all-cause mortality. Currently in the United States, there are significant concerns regarding safety and efficacy due to the lack of regulatory standards for commercially available probiotic preparations and the potential for contamination with pathogenic species. Probiotic preparations may include a single bacterial strain or a combination of multiple strains and are highly variable in terms of the number of viable microorganisms. The American Academy of Pediatrics, Canadian Pediatric Society, and European Society for Paediatric Gastroenterology Hepatology and Nutrition (ESPGHAN) have all advocated for caution with regard to routine use of probiotics in preterm infants.[79–81] Small pilot studies in patients with gastroschisis and other congenital gastrointestinal disorders have demonstrated safety and feasibility, with lower relative abundance of potentially pathogenic bacterial families but no change in clinical outcomes such as feeding and length of hospitalization.

SUMMARY

Congenital gastrointestinal disorders and other surgical diagnoses require specialized nutritional support to meet their increased requirements to prevent catabolism, enhance wound healing, and provide optimal growth during times of critical illness. Growth failure may have long reaching consequences, including poor neurodevelopmental outcomes. Evidence-based practices such as early trophic feedings, use of human milk (especially MOM), and standardized feeding protocols may lead to earlier attainment of full feedings, shorter time on TPN, and shorter hospitalization. Additional complications such as GERD, dysmotility, dysbiosis require long-term multidisciplinary nutritional follow-up and care.

CLINICS CARE POINTS

- Early trophic enteral feedings are recommended to enhance many gastrointestinal functions of the post-operative neonate.
- The use of human milk should be considered the standard of care for infants undergoing surgical interventions.
- Due to a high risk for growth failure, close monitoring of both weight and linear growth are critical.
- Involvement of multi-disciplinary teams including neonatologists, dieticians, pharmacists, nursing, lactation consultants, surgeons, and gastroenterologists can enhance the care of neonates at high risk for intestinal failure.

CONFLICTS OF INTEREST

Dr H. Karpen has a research grant from Prolacta Bioscience, Inc.

REFERENCES

1. Kirolos A, Goyheneix M, Kalmus Eliasz M, et al. Neurodevelopmental, cognitive, behavioural and mental health impairments following childhood malnutrition: a systematic review. BMJ Glob Health 2022;7(7):e009330.
2. Gupta V, Trivedi A, Walker K, et al. Neurodevelopmental outcome of infants with gastroschisis at one-year follow-up. J Neonatal Surg 2015;4(2):12.
3. Strobel KM, Romero T, Kramer K, et al. Growth failure prevalence in neonates with gastroschisis : a statewide cohort study. J Pediatr 2021;233:112–8.e113.
4. Hong CR, Zurakowski D, Fullerton BS, et al. Nutrition delivery and growth outcomes in infants with gastroschisis. JPEN J Parenter Enteral Nutr 2018;42(5):913–9.
5. Gosselin KB, Duggan C. Enteral nutrition in the management of pediatric intestinal failure. J Pediatr 2014;165(6):1085–90.
6. Duro D, Kamin D, Duggan C. Overview of pediatric short bowel syndrome. J Pediatr Gastroenterol Nutr 2008;47(Suppl 1):S33–6.
7. Yang CF, Duro D, Zurakowski D, et al. High prevalence of multiple micronutrient deficiencies in children with intestinal failure: a longitudinal study. J Pediatr 2011;159(1):39–44 e31.
8. Jones AM, Isenburg J, Salemi JL, et al. Increasing prevalence of gastroschisis–14 States, 1995-2012. MMWR Morb Mortal Wkly Rep 2016;65(2):23–6.
9. Payne NR, Pfleghaar K, Assel B, et al. Predicting the outcome of newborns with gastroschisis. J Pediatr Surg 2009;44(5):918–23.
10. Ghionzoli M, James CP, David AL, et al. Gastroschisis with intestinal atresia–predictive value of antenatal diagnosis and outcome of postnatal treatment. J Pediatr Surg 2012;47(2):322–8.

11. Long AM, Court J, Morabito A, et al. Antenatal diagnosis of bowel dilatation in gastroschisis is predictive of poor postnatal outcome. J Pediatr Surg 2011; 46(6):1070–5.
12. D'Antonio F, Virgone C, Rizzo G, et al. Prenatal risk factors and outcomes in gastroschisis: a meta-analysis. Pediatrics 2015;136(1):e159–69.
13. Horton AL, Powell MS, Wolfe HM. Intrauterine growth patterns in fetal gastroschisis. Am J Perinatol 2010;27(3):211–7.
14. South AP, Stutey KM, Meinzen-Derr J. Metaanalysis of the prevalence of intrauterine fetal death in gastroschisis. Am J Obstet Gynecol 2013;209(2):114 e111–e113.
15. Sparks TN, Shaffer BL, Page J, et al. Gastroschisis: mortality risks with each additional week of expectant management. Am J Obstet Gynecol 2017;216(1):66 e61–e66 e67.
16. Youssef F, Laberge JM, Baird RJ, et al. The correlation between the time spent in utero and the severity of bowel matting in newborns with gastroschisis. J Pediatr Surg 2015;50(5):755–9.
17. Amin R, Domack A, Bartoletti J, et al. National practice patterns for prenatal monitoring in gastroschisis: gastroschisis outcomes of delivery (GOOD) provider survey. Fetal Diagn Ther 2019;45(2):125–30.
18. Jansen LA, Safavi A, Lin Y, et al. Preclosure fluid resuscitation influences outcome in gastroschisis. Am J Perinatol 2012;29(4):307–12.
19. Riddle S, Agarwal N, Haberman B, et al. Gastroschisis and low incidence of early-onset infection: a case for antimicrobial stewardship. J Perinatol 2022; 42(11):1453–7.
20. Cotten CM, Taylor S, Stoll B, et al. Prolonged duration of initial empirical antibiotic treatment is associated with increased rates of necrotizing enterocolitis and death for extremely low birth weight infants. Pediatrics 2009;123(1):58–66.
21. Alexander VN, Northrup V, Bizzarro MJ. Antibiotic exposure in the newborn intensive care unit and the risk of necrotizing enterocolitis. J Pediatr 2011;159(3): 392–7.
22. Kunz SN, Tieder JS, Whitlock K, et al. Primary fascial closure versus staged closure with silo in patients with gastroschisis: a meta-analysis. J Pediatr Surg 2013;48(4):845–57.
23. Chesley PM, Ledbetter DJ, Meehan JJ, et al. Contemporary trends in the use of primary repair for gastroschisis in surgical infants. Am J Surg 2015;209(5):901–5, discussion 905-906.
24. Fraser JD, Deans KJ, Fallat ME, et al. Sutureless vs sutured abdominal wall closure for gastroschisis: operative characteristics and early outcomes from the Midwest Pediatric Surgery Consortium. J Pediatr Surg 2020;55(11):2284–8.
25. Zaloga GP. Phytosterols, lipid administration, and liver disease during parenteral nutrition. JPEN J Parenter Enteral Nutr 2015;39(1 Suppl):39S–60S.
26. Calkins KL, Havranek T, Kelley-Quon LI, et al. Low-dose parenteral soybean oil for the prevention of parenteral nutrition-associated liver disease in neonates with gastrointestinal disorders. JPEN J Parenter Enteral Nutr 2017;41(3):404–11.
27. Bharadwaj S, Gohel T, Deen OJ, et al. Fish oil-based lipid emulsion: current updates on a promising novel therapy for the management of parenteral nutrition-associated liver disease. Gastroenterol Rep (Oxf) 2015;3(2):110–4.
28. Jackson RL, White PZ, Zalla J. SMOFlipid vs intralipid 20%: effect of mixed-oil vs soybean-oil emulsion on parenteral nutrition-associated cholestasis in the neonatal population. JPEN J Parenter Enteral Nutr 2021;45(2):339–46.

29. Repa A, Binder C, Thanhaeuser M, et al. A mixed lipid emulsion for prevention of parenteral nutrition associated cholestasis in extremely low birth weight infants: a randomized clinical trial. J Pediatr 2018;194:87–93 e81.

30. Gurien LA, Wyrick DL, Dassinger MS, et al. Use of bedside abdominal ultrasound to confirm intestinal motility in neonates with gastroschisis: a feasibility study. J Pediatr Surg 2017;52(5):715–7.

31. Aljahdali A, Mohajerani N, Skarsgard ED. Effect of timing of enteral feeding on outcome in gastroschisis. J Pediatr Surg 2013;48(5):971–6.

32. Dama M, Rao U, Gollow I, et al. Early commencement of enteral feeds in gastroschisis: a systematic review of literature. Eur J Pediatr Surg 2017;27(6):503–15.

33. Lemoine JB, Smith RR, White D. Got milk? Effects of early enteral feedings in patients with gastroschisis. Adv Neonatal Care 2015;15(3):166–75.

34. Walter-Nicolet E, Rousseau V, Kieffer F, et al. Neonatal outcome of gastroschisis is mainly influenced by nutritional management. J Pediatr Gastroenterol Nutr 2009; 48(5):612–7.

35. Gulack BC, Laughon MM, Clark RH, et al. Enteral feeding with human milk decreases time to discharge in infants following gastroschisis repair. J Pediatr 2016;170:85–9.

36. Shinnick JK, Wang E, Hulbert C, et al. Effects of a breast milk diet on enteral feeding outcomes of neonates with gastrointestinal disorders. Breastfeed Med 2016;11(6):286–92.

37. Storm AP, Bowker RM, Klonoski SC, et al. Mother's own milk dose is associated with decreased time from initiation of feedings to discharge and length of stay in infants with gastroschisis. J Perinatol 2020;40(8):1222–7.

38. Hoban R, Khatri S, Patel A, et al. Supplementation of mother's own milk with donor milk in infants with gastroschisis or intestinal atresia: a retrospective study. Nutrients 2020;12(2).

39. Cristofalo EA, Schanler RJ, Blanco CL, et al. Randomized trial of exclusive human milk versus preterm formula diets in extremely premature infants. J Pediatr 2013; 163(6):1592–1595 e1591.

40. Herrmann K, Carroll K. An exclusively human milk diet reduces necrotizing enterocolitis. Breastfeed Med 2014;9(4):184–90.

41. El Hassani A, Michaud L, Chartier A, et al. [Cow's milk protein allergy after neonatal intestinal surgery]. Arch Pediatr 2005;12(2):134–9.

42. Diamanti A, Fiocchi AG, Capriati T, et al. Cow's milk allergy and neonatal short bowel syndrome: comorbidity or true association? Eur J Clin Nutr 2015;69(1): 102–6.

43. Moschino L, Duci M, Fascetti Leon F, et al. Optimizing nutritional strategies to prevent necrotizing enterocolitis and growth failure after bowel resection. Nutrients 2021;13(2).

44. Shores DR, Alaish SM, Aucott SW, et al. Postoperative enteral nutrition guidelines reduce the risk of intestinal failure-associated liver disease in surgical infants. J Pediatr 2018;195:140–7.e141.

45. Butler TJ, Szekely LJ, Grow JL. A standardized nutrition approach for very low birth weight neonates improves outcomes, reduces cost and is not associated with increased rates of necrotizing enterocolitis, sepsis or mortality. J Perinatol 2013;33(11):851–7.

46. McCallie KR, Lee HC, Mayer O, et al. Improved outcomes with a standardized feeding protocol for very low birth weight infants. J Perinatol 2011;31(Suppl 1): S61–7.

47. Jasani B, Patole S. Standardized feeding regimen for reducing necrotizing enterocolitis in preterm infants: an updated systematic review. J Perinatol 2017; 37(7):827–33.
48. Shakeel F, Newkirk M, Sellers A, et al. Postoperative feeding guidelines improve outcomes in surgical infants. JPEN J Parenter Enteral Nutr 2020;44(6):1047–56.
49. Utria AF, Wong M, Faino A, et al. The role of feeding advancement strategy on length of stay and hospital costs in newborns with gastroschisis. J Pediatr Surg 2022;57(3):356–9.
50. Dekonenko C, Fraser JD, Deans K, et al. Does use of a feeding protocol change outcomes in gastroschisis? A report from the midwest pediatric surgery consortium. Eur J Pediatr Surg 2020;32(2):153–9.
51. Tucker A, Huang EY, Peredo J, et al. Pilot study of sham feeding in postoperative neonates. Am J Perinatol 2022;39(7):726–31.
52. Golonka NR, Hayashi AH. Early "sham" feeding of neonates promotes oral feeding after delayed primary repair of major congenital esophageal anomalies. Am J Surg 2008;195(5):659–62, discussion 662.
53. Fullerton BS, Velazco CS, Sparks EA, et al. Contemporary outcomes of infants with gastroschisis in north America: a multicenter cohort study. J Pediatr 2017; 188:192–197 e196.
54. Vlug LE, Neelis EG, Wells JCK, et al. Anthropometrics and fat mass, but not fat-free mass, are compromised in infants requiring parenteral nutrition after neonatal intestinal surgery. Am J Clin Nutr 2022;115(2):503–13.
55. Koivusalo A, Rintala R, Lindahl H. Gastroesophageal reflux in children with a congenital abdominal wall defect. J Pediatr Surg 1999;34(7):1127–9.
56. Devane SP, Coombes R, Smith VV, et al. Persistent gastrointestinal symptoms after correction of malrotation. Arch Dis Child 1992;67(2):218–21.
57. Jolley SG, Lorenz ML, Hendrickson M, et al. Esophageal pH monitoring abnormalities and gastroesophageal reflux disease in infants with intestinal malrotation. Arch Surg 1999;134(7):747–52, discussion 752-743.
58. Hyman PE, Everett SL, Harada T. Gastric acid hypersecretion in short bowel syndrome in infants: association with extent of resection and enteral feeding. J Pediatr Gastroenterol Nutr 1986;5(2):191–7.
59. Guillet R, Stoll BJ, Cotten CM, et al. Association of H2-blocker therapy and higher incidence of necrotizing enterocolitis in very low birth weight infants. Pediatrics 2006;117(2):e137–42.
60. Krishnan U, Mousa H, Dall'Oglio L, et al. ESPGHAN-NASPGHAN guidelines for the evaluation and treatment of gastrointestinal and nutritional complications in children with esophageal atresia-tracheoesophageal fistula. J Pediatr Gastroenterol Nutr 2016;63(5):550–70.
61. Rosen R, Vandenplas Y, Singendonk M, et al. Pediatric gastroesophageal reflux clinical practice guidelines: joint recommendations of the north American society for pediatric gastroenterology, hepatology, and nutrition and the European society for pediatric gastroenterology, hepatology, and nutrition. J Pediatr Gastroenterol Nutr 2018;66(3):516–54.
62. Davies I, Burman-Roy S, Murphy MS, et al. Gastro-oesophageal reflux disease in children: NICE guidance. BMJ 2015;350:g7703.
63. Auber F, Danzer E, Noche-Monnery ME, et al. Enteric nervous system impairment in gastroschisis. Eur J Pediatr Surg 2013;23(1):29–38.
64. Radhika Krishna OH, Aleem MA, Kayla G. Abnormalities of the intestinal pacemaker cells, enteric neurons, and smooth muscle in intestinal atresia. J Lab Physicians 2019;11(3):180–5.

65. Zani-Ruttenstock E, Zani A, Paul A, et al. Interstitial cells of Cajal are decreased in patients with gastroschisis associated intestinal dysmotility. J Pediatr Surg 2015; 50(5):750–4.
66. Dicken BJ, Sergi C, Rescorla FJ, et al. Medical management of motility disorders in patients with intestinal failure: a focus on necrotizing enterocolitis, gastroschisis, and intestinal atresia. J Pediatr Surg 2011;46(8):1618–30.
67. Karamanolis G, Tack J. Promotility medications–now and in the future. Dig Dis 2006;24(3–4):297–307.
68. Ng E, Shah VS. Erythromycin for the prevention and treatment of feeding intolerance in preterm infants. Cochrane Database Syst Rev 2008;3:CD001815.
69. Curry JI, Lander AD, Stringer MD. A multicenter, randomized, double-blind, placebo-controlled trial of the prokinetic agent erythromycin in the postoperative recovery of infants with gastroschisis. J Pediatr Surg 2004;39(4):565–9.
70. Chicella MF, Batres LA, Heesters MS, et al. Prokinetic drug therapy in children: a review of current options. Ann Pharmacother 2005;39(4):706–11.
71. Tolia V, Calhoun J, Kuhns L, et al. Randomized, prospective double-blind trial of metoclopramide and placebo for gastroesophageal reflux in infants. J Pediatr 1989;115(1):141–5.
72. Baker DE. Loperamide: a pharmacological review. Rev Gastroenterol Disord 2007;7(Suppl 3):S11–8.
73. Puwanant M, Mo-Suwan L, Patrapinyokul S. Recurrent D-lactic acidosis in a child with short bowel syndrome. Asia Pac J Clin Nutr 2005;14(2):195–8.
74. Sieczkowska A, Landowski P, Zagozdzon P, et al. Small bowel bacterial overgrowth associated with persistence of abdominal symptoms in children treated with a proton pump inhibitor. J Pediatr 2015;166(5):1310–1312 e1311.
75. Sieczkowska A, Landowski P, Zagozdzon P, et al. The association of proton pump inhibitor therapy and small bowel bacterial overgrowth in children. Eur J Gastroenterol Hepatol 2017;29(10):1190–1.
76. Cole CR, Frem JC, Schmotzer B, et al. The rate of bloodstream infection is high in infants with short bowel syndrome: relationship with small bowel bacterial overgrowth, enteral feeding, and inflammatory and immune responses. J Pediatr 2010;156(6):941–947 e941.
77. Avelar Rodriguez D, Ryan PM, Toro Monjaraz EM, et al. Small intestinal bacterial overgrowth in children: a state-of-the-art review. Front Pediatr 2019;7:363.
78. Shah SC, Day LW, Somsouk M, et al. Meta-analysis: antibiotic therapy for small intestinal bacterial overgrowth. Aliment Pharmacol Ther 2013;38(8):925–34.
79. Poindexter B, Committee On F, Newborn. Use of probiotics in preterm infants. Pediatrics 2021;147(6). e2021051485.
80. van den Akker CHP, van Goudoever JB, Shamir R, et al. Probiotics and preterm infants: a position paper by the European society for paediatric gastroenterology hepatology and nutrition committee on nutrition and the European society for paediatric gastroenterology hepatology and nutrition working group for probiotics and prebiotics. J Pediatr Gastroenterol Nutr 2020;70(5):664–80.
81. Marchand V. Using probiotics in the paediatric population. Paediatr Child Health 2012;17(10):575–6.

Controversies and Conundrums in Newborn Feeding

Jennifer McAllister, MD, IBCLC*, Scott Wexelblatt, MD,
Laura Ward, MD, IBCLC

KEYWORDS

- Breastfeeding • Newborn weight loss • Supplementation • Ankyloglossia
- Late preterm

KEY POINTS

- Breastfeeding is the biologic norm for newborn nutrition, and clinicians should promote evidence-based practices that support breastfeeding in the hospital.
- Guidance and discussions regarding controversial breastfeeding topics should be informed by evidence, whereas acknowledging there is a lack of high-quality studies for some breastfeeding topics.
- There are few medical indications for formula supplementation, and if necessary, supplementation should be offered judiciously.

INTRODUCTION

Breastfeeding and the provision of human milk are the standard and biological norm for infant feeding, health, and nutrition. Maternal and infant short- and long-term benefits are well documented. Breastfeeding confers a decreased risk of sudden unexpected infant death (SUID), infant mortality, respiratory and gastrointestinal infections, asthma, eczema, obesity, and autoimmune diseases including type I diabetes, ulcerative colitis, Crohn's disease, and leukemia (**Fig. 1**).[1] Improved neurodevelopmental outcomes and performance on intelligence tests have also been demonstrated in children who are breastfed.[2] People who breastfeed are at lower risk for diabetes, hypertension, and malignancies including breast, ovarian, endometrial, and thyroid cancers (see **Fig. 1**).[1] Despite these well-known benefits, many parents face individual, institutional, and societal challenges leading to the failure of achieving their breastfeeding goals, and racial, socioeconomical, and educational disparities exist.[3]

Department of Pediatrics, University of Cincinnati College of Medicine, Cincinnati Children's Hospital Medical Center Perinatal Institute, 3333 Burnet Avenue, ML 7009, Cincinnati, OH 45229, USA
* Corresponding author.
E-mail address: jennifer.mcallister@cchmc.org

Clin Perinatol 50 (2023) 729–742
https://doi.org/10.1016/j.clp.2023.04.003
0095-5108/23/© 2023 Elsevier Inc. All rights reserved.

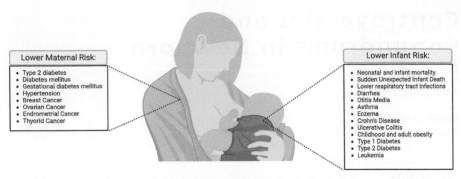

Lower Maternal Risk:
- Type 2 diabetes
- Diabetes mellitus
- Gestational diabetes mellitus
- Hypertension
- Breast Cancer
- Ovarian Cancer
- Endrometrial Cancer
- Thyorid Cancer

Lower Infant Risk:
- Neonatal and infant mortality
- Sudden Unexpected Infant Death
- Lower respiratory tract Infections
- Diarrhea
- Otitis Media
- Asthma
- Eczema
- Crohn's Disease
- Ulcerative Colitis
- Childhood and adult obesity
- Type 1 Diabetes
- Type 2 Diabetes
- Leukemia

Fig. 1. Maternal and infant outcomes associated with breastfeeding.

The American Academy of Pediatrics (AAP), World Health Organization (WHO), and American College of Obstetricians (ACOG) are consistent in their recommendation of exclusive breastfeeding for the first 6 months of life.[1] Data suggest that if 90% infants were compliant with this recommendation, the United States would save billions of dollars per year and prevent over 900 annual deaths.[4] In 2019, 83.2% of all babies born in the United States were ever breastfed, but 19.2% of breastfed newborns received formula supplementation within the first 2 days of life, which may contribute to the sharp declines in exclusive breastfeeding that are seen at 3 and 6 months.[5] The care that the mother and infant receive in the first postpartum days influences future breastfeeding success,[6] and targeted interventions during the birth hospitalization can help reduce the prevalence of formula supplementation. However, providers and families often face medical concerns and breastfeeding difficulties that challenge breastfeeding success within the first few days after birth.

The objective of this article is to review evidence for common controversies in newborn feeding and medical challenges that may impact newborn feeding practices and recommendations. Literature published within the last decade is included. Because these topics can be controversial and encounter a wide variety of practice variation, we attempt to provide a concise presentation of the research available and highlight areas in which there are no studies or evidence to provide recommendations or support.

BABY-FRIENDLY HOSPITAL INITIATIVE

In 1991, the WHO and the United Nations International Children's Emergency Fund (UNICEF) launched the Baby-Friendly Hospital Initiative (BFHI) to empower health care facilities to better support breastfeeding.[7] Based on the Ten Steps to Successful Breastfeeding, BFHI has been implemented worldwide and is associated with improvement in short- and long-term breastfeeding outcomes including breastfeeding initiation, exclusivity, and duration.[8,9] In the United States, BFHI has also had similar positive impacts on breastfeeding,[10–12] and it is considered the gold standard of evidence-based practices for maternity facilities.[9] Adoption of Baby-Friendly hospital practices has also been associated with reduction of racial disparities and inequities in breastfeeding duration and exclusivity[13] addressing historical and societal factors. The ten steps were most recently updated in 2018, and BFHI has been acknowledged and endorsed by organizations including the AAP, ACOG, and the Academy of Breastfeeding Medicine.[1,3,9] Despite the overwhelming evidence of the positive impact of BFHI on breastfeeding outcomes, there have been barriers to the implementation of the practice across US hospitals. The influence of reduced or free formula from industry, costs associated with Baby-Friendly designation and increased resources for breastfeeding support, and a lack of advocacy from key stakeholders has led to slow adoption.[14]

BREASTFEEDING CONTROVERSIES

Although breastfeeding is the biological norm for infant feeding, it may be challenging, and parents often struggle to reach their breastfeeding goals. The postpartum period can be a time of isolation, and in the age of social media, many parents use and value pro-breastfeeding communities and other online sources of information for breastfeeding support.[15] Although social media can be a method to promote breastfeeding awareness and attitudes, misinformation regarding breastfeeding practices can be widespread, and there may be a disconnect between evidence-based practices and information the public receives on social media websites. Consequently, vulnerable parents may seek solutions to breastfeeding problems that may not be appropriate for their infant.[16] It is important to understand the difficulties parents face and to provide empathetic listening while also providing evidence-based support.

Ankyloglossia

Ankyloglossia, or tongue-tie, is the condition where the lingual frenulum, which is the fold of tissue that attaches the ventral surface of the tongue to the floor of the mouth, is unusually anterior, thick, tight, or short resulting in restricted tongue mobility.[17] The prevalence of ankyloglossia has been reported to be between 3% and 11%[17,18] and is thought to have a genetic component.[18] Although publications and research about ankyloglossia have surged over the last several years,[19] the condition is not new, and association between tongue-tie and breastfeeding problems have been recognized for over 500 years.[20,21] Limitation of tongue movement by a restricted sublingual frenulum may contribute to an ineffective latch, suckling problems, decrease in breast milk transfer, and maternal nipple pain and trauma.[18,22,23]

Identification of ankyloglossia should include a review of breastfeeding efficacy by a trained professional as well as assessment of the tongue mobility through a standardized and objective tool.[24] Several validated tools have been developed to assess tongue mobility and vary in degree of complexity.[23] Interventions for ankyloglossia range from expectant management to surgical procedures. There is limited evidence on breastfeeding outcomes regarding conservative approaches, but maternal breastfeeding self-efficacy, nipple pain, and milk transfer can improve over time with surgical intervention.[25] Frenotomy is the division or release of the lingual frenulum and is the procedure of choice for ankyloglossia, as it is quick, easy to perform, and has a very low complication rate.[18] It is typically performed with straight, sharp scissors, which is the gold standard approach, but the use of scalpels, electrocautery, and laser is becoming more frequent.[18,23] Because tongue-tie is a functional diagnosis, the presence of a lingual frenulum alone should not guide decision for surgical intervention.

A Cochrane review in 2017 evaluated the safety and efficacy of frenotomy in improving ability to feed orally among infants younger than 3 months of age with tongue-tie and feeding problems.[18] Five randomized control trials were included in the review, and findings demonstrated that frenotomy is safe and was associated with reduced maternal nipple pain but failed to show consistent improvement in infant breastfeeding outcomes.[18] However, in all of the included studies, frenotomy was offered and often performed in all controls which limited the quality of the results. Only one study evaluated severity of ankyloglossia and reported improvement in breastfeeding after frenotomy in those identified as having severe tongue-tie. A recent review by Hatami and colleagues from Australia sought to determine association between ankyloglossia severity using standardized assessment tools and post-frenotomy breastfeeding outcomes. They reported that frenotomy improved breast-feeding and speech outcomes but were unable to conclude if severity assessment scores correlated with outcomes due to the quality of evidence available.[26] Further high-quality, randomized controlled trials (RCTs) with appropriate study design and follow-up are needed to inform decision-making for surgical intervention in breast-feeding infants with ankyloglossia.

Pacifiers and Artificial Nipples

When first published in 1990, an original recommendation of the Ten Steps to Successful Breastfeeding advised avoidance of pacifiers and artificial nipples for breast-feeding infants due to the concern that if exposed to an artificial nipple, an infant may experience nipple confusion, or a preference of one method of feeding over another. Pacifiers have historically been used to calm infants, and they provide a mechanism for nonnutritive sucking which is a normal, biological need for infants.[7,27] The use of pacifiers has also been shown have a protective effect on SUID leading to the AAP recommending pacifier use during sleep.[28] The conflicting advice from these two prominent and influential organizations has led to confusion among parents and providers. Several studies have evaluated the impact of pacifier use on breastfeeding outcomes. A Cochrane review in 2016 demonstrated that pacifier use in healthy term infants did not significantly affect the prevalence or duration of exclusive and partial breastfeed-ing up to 4 months of age regardless of timing of pacifier introduction.[27] Concern has also been raised regarding nipple confusion and the impact on breastfeeding for in-fants supplemented with a bottle, but evidence evaluating this issue is lacking. Some studies have shown that nutritive suck patterns differ in babies that are supple-mented with a bottle,[29] but the evidence for an impact of bottle feeding on breastfeed-ing duration and frequency is mixed.[30] In 2018, after review of the available literature, the WHO and UNICEF revised the 10 Steps and recommended counseling about the use and risks of feeding bottles, teats, and pacifiers rather than complete avoidance. In the updated BFHI document, they state that pacifier use does not seem to impact breastfeeding, and benefits and concerns for different supplemental feeding methods including bottles are outlined.[7]

Substance Use

Rates of substance use among pregnant people has risen in the past decades, and decisions surrounding feeding of newborns born to people with substance use disor-ders can be challenging. According to the National Survey on Drug Use and Health in 2019, 18.4% of pregnant women aged 15 to 44 reported the use of illicit substances, tobacco products, or alcohol within the past month, which is likely an underestimate of the true prevalence of substance use in this population.[31–33] Both the mother and in-fant stand to benefit significantly from breastfeeding, but these benefits must be thoughtfully weighed against the risks associated with potential infant exposure to a substance through lactation. During pregnancy, drug concentrations in the fetal serum are at steady state and equilibrate with maternal serum concentrations, but in the postpartum and breastfeeding period, exposure of a substance through breast milk is typically less than 10% of the exposure in utero.[34] Pharmacokinetic data in lactating women are sparse, and oral bioavailability is variable for many substances. The amount of a substance ingested through breast milk can be estimated using relative infant dose (RID), which is generally presented as a percentage of the mother's dose.[35] In general, an RID of 5% to 10% is an accepted reference range associated with a low risk of an adverse drug reaction in an infant.[34] Reported RID for many substances can be found through a variety of resources including LactMed, a database supported by the National Library of Medicine (https://www.ncbi.nlm.nih.gov/books/NBK501922/). In general, recommendations for breastfeeding in mothers with substance use should consider the RID of the substance, the mother's engagement in substance use treatment, and the known safety and potential long-term effects of exposure to the substance through breast milk.

Opioids

For infants with chronic exposure to opioids *in utero*, breastfeeding has been shown to reduce severity of opioid withdrawal symptoms, need for pharmacologic treatment for severe withdrawal, increased maternal confidence and bonding, and decreased maternal stress.[36–38] Breastfeeding should be recommended and encouraged for women engaged in medication-assisted treatment regardless of dose of medication for treatment of opioid use disorder.

Nicotine

Nicotine and other compounds from tobacco smoke transfer to the newborn through breast milk, but nicotine cessation products such as patches and gum may be a safer alternative while breastfeeding. Mothers should be counseled to stop or decrease smoking or vaping while breastfeeding, and if they continue, they should breastfeed before smoking or vaping to minimize the amount of transmission to the infant.[1]

Cannabis

Similarly, delta-9-tetrahydrocannabinol, the psychoactive compound in cannabis, is transferred through the breast milk at variable amounts depending on the strength of cannabis and chronicity of use.[39] Data are lacking on the effects of tetrahydrocannabinol (THC) exposure to infants through breast milk, and women should be discouraged from using cannabis while breastfeeding.[1,40]

Alcohol

Alcohol concentrations in breast milk parallel blood alcohol levels, and the highest levels of alcohol are found in breast milk 30 to 60 minutes after consumption.[1] Intake should be limited to two standard drinks per day, and mothers should wait 2 hours after drinking to breastfeed her infant.[40]

MEDICAL CONUNDRUMS

The evidence-based recommendation of exclusive breastfeeding for the first 6 months of life is due to the associated decrease in the risk of several outcomes, including lower respiratory tract infections, severe diarrhea, otitis media, and obesity.[1] There is speculation that these issues may be mediated by gut dysbiosis, and there is evidence that exclusive breastfeeding is associated with a more diverse, healthier microbiome at 6 months.[41] In addition, an association between decreased breastfeeding duration with early formula supplementation has been shown.[12] Early supplementation may result in decreased breastfeeding demand and subsequent increased milk stasis, potentially interfering with the establishment of successful breastfeeding. Although there are medical indications for supplementation of breastfed infants,[42] it can be challenging to find the correct balance between avoiding unnecessary supplementation while ensuring it is provided when needed. These are difficult, important decisions that need to be made during a short hospital stay, often before the establishment of a full milk supply. Furthermore, there are maternal and infant risk factors that increase the risk of poor breastfeeding outcomes (**Table 1**), and it is essential for the clinician to consider the breastfeeding dyad as a unit when making feeding recommendations.

Newborn Weight Loss

Weight loss in the neonatal period is "universally recognized, but poorly understood."[43] Unfortunately, there is little consensus on what constitutes a "safe" amount of weight loss. Excessive weight loss is often defined as $\geq$10% of birth weight and warrants further evaluation due to the associated risk of complications including hypernatremia, dehydration, and hypoglycemia.[44,45] In 2015, Flaherman and colleagues developed weight loss nomograms from a large cohort of healthy infants greater than 36 weeks gestation during the birth hospitalization. These nomograms (available online at www.newbornweight.org) account for delivery mode, feeding type, and hour of life and may help identify newborns with a concerning weight loss trajectory. Of note, excessive neonatal weight loss was not atypical in this cohort, with about 5% who were born vaginally and 12% who were born by cesarean section (C/S) losing greater than 10% of their birthweight by 48 hours of life, and 25% of those born by C/S losing greater than 10% of birthweight by 72 hours of life. Although this degree of weight loss was not infrequent, it is important to recognize that compared with international cohorts, excessive weight loss was more prevalent in US babies, and weight gain in the first week was substantially lower,[46] suggesting that while this degree of weight loss may be "typical" in the United States, it may not be "normal." It is also important to note that these nomograms do not predict outcomes after discharge, and they have low sensitivity in predicting excessive weight loss after hospital discharge.[47] Thus, it is important to identify risk factors for delayed lactogenesis and low milk supply in breastfeeding mothers that can predispose the infant to excessive weight loss and for whom continued lactation support should be prioritized (see **Table 1**).

If supplementation with formula is necessary in the breastfed infant, there is evidence that small volumes may not significantly impact longer term breastfeeding duration. In 2013, Flaherman and colleagues reported results from a small RCT in which breastfed infants were randomized to receive small volumes (10 mL) of formula

Table 1
Risk factors/predictors for excessive neonatal weight loss, delayed lactogenesis, and insufficient milk supply

Maternal Factors	Infant Factors
Extremes of maternal age (<20, >35)	Prematurity or early-term gestation
Primiparity	Poor infant feeding behaviors
Metabolic issues (obesity, polycystic ovarian syndrome, thyroid disease, diabetes, hypertension, preeclampsia)	Need for breastfeeding aids (nipple shield, supplemental nursing system)
Postpartum hemorrhage	Large for gestational age, small for gestational age
Infertility, assisted reproductive technology	Supplementation
Cesarean delivery, prolonged delivery	Infant latch difficulty/nipple pain or trauma
Breast anatomy issues (insufficient glandular tissue, previous breast surgery)	Infant medical issues (eg, hypoglycemia, neurologic problems, respiratory difficulty)
Early postpartum hormonal contraception (<6 wk)	Oral anatomic abnormalities

following breastfeeding until the onset of copious milk production, or to continued exclusive breastfeeding once a predefined weight loss threshold was met.[48] Infants in the early limited formula group were more likely to be exclusively breastfed at 3 months compared with controls, and there were no differences reported between groups at 6 months.[49] However, if infants were still receiving formula at 1 week of age, they were significantly less likely to be still breastfed at 6 and 12 months.[49] Therefore, it is recommended to avoid supplementation unless it is medically indicated, but if it is necessary, small volumes should be given with a plan to discontinue as soon as appropriate. In addition, lactation support should be provided until exclusive breastfeeding can be established. Breastfeeding mothers whose infants require supplementation should initiate milk expression to protect their supply until supplementation is discontinued.[50]

Late Preterm

Late preterm infants born between 34 0/7 and 36 6/7 weeks gestation comprise the majority of the infants born prematurely and are considered an at-risk population.[51] Although a significant body of evidence surrounds the nutritional needs of very low birthweight infants, little is published on late preterm infants. Many room-in with their mothers in the newborn nursery, and consequently may be managed as if they were full-term infants which may put them at risk for both short-term and long-term morbidities.[51,52]

Although breast milk is considered the optimal nutrition, late preterm infants may have increased caloric needs, and they often require supplementation to achieve adequate growth. In addition, late preterm infants commonly experience feeding difficulties due to their immature or ineffective latch.[53] They may be less robust at the breast compared with their term counterparts, and it may be difficult to achieve appropriate nutritional goals through direct breastfeeding alone. Suboptimal feeding skills coupled with an increased incidence of delayed lactogenesis and conditions associated with low milk supply in their mothers (see **Table 1**)[54] put late preterm infants at increased risk for readmission due to inadequate intake, dehydration, hyperbilirubinemia, and poor weight gain.[52,55] Therefore, late preterm infants may require individualized feeding plans to ensure adequate caloric intake and intensive lactation support to assist their mothers in reaching their breastfeeding goals.

Nipple shields may facilitate direct breastfeeding in late preterm infants; however, data are lacking about the utility in the term population.[56,57] In addition, breast compression during latching may improve milk transfer for late preterm infants.[56] If a late preterm infant is not directly breastfeeding effectively or if supplementation is required, milk expression is recommended to promote and protect milk supply.[56] For this population, certain pump strategies may result in a higher milk volume. A biphasic pump pattern and "hands-on pumping," or massage during mechanical expression, may result in more effective milk drainage and subsequent milk volumes.[58,59] Test weights before and after direct breastfeeding can estimate the volume of milk transferred at the breast and may help inform clinicians in establishing a feeding plan for after discharge.[53] Families should be counseled to continue pump sessions until the infant transitions to exclusive at-the-breast feedings and lactation support tools are no longer needed. In addition, milk expression should be gradually decreased over time to ensure an appropriate supply based on the infant's needs.[53,56] If supplementation is required, expressed mother's milk is preferred, then alternatively, pasteurized donor milk if available, or formula.[1,50] Sometimes breast milk alone may not meet the late preterm infant's metabolic needs. In these cases, increased calories may be achieved with fortification of breast milk or by supplementing with preterm formula after breastfeeding.[51] The evidence for the use of increased caloric density following discharge in preterm infants is conflicting, and most studies did not include late preterm infants born after 35 weeks.[55,60] There is some evidence that cup feeding is associated with longer breastfeeding duration in preterm infants compared with bottle feeding.[60] In summary, discharge feeding plans should be individualized, accounting for maternal milk supply and feeding goals, as well as infant feeding skills and nutritional needs.

Jaundice

Almost all infants have hyperbilirubinemia, or jaundice, during the newborn period due to increased production of bilirubin from heme degradation, decreased conjugation of bilirubin secondary to liver immaturity, and increased reabsorption of bilirubin in the intestine.[61,62] Bilirubin is an antioxidant and may have an evolutionary neuroprotective property.[62] There are no large, randomized trials evaluating breastfeeding or feeding practices, and the impact on treatment for this very common newborn problem.

It is important to understand the etiology of hyperbilirubinemia when making recommendations regarding feeding in an infant with jaundice. Hyperbilirubinemia that seems in the first 24 hours of life is pathologic and most commonly is due to hemolytic disease of the newborn. Although there is a strong association between exclusive breastfeeding and hyperbilirubinemia,[61] there is no evidence to support supplementation to decrease the need for exchange transfusion or to decrease the length of treatment of jaundice.[50] The onset of hyperbilirubinemia on the second day of life through the first week of life has been labeled "breastfeeding" jaundice but may be better termed "suboptimal intake jaundice."[61] This type of hyperbilirubinemia results from decreased stool frequency and an increased enterohepatic circulation of bilirubin.[61] Situations of low milk supply or inefficient breastfeeding may contribute to jaundice (see **Table 1**), but poor intake of any milk, including formula, may also result in hyperbilirubinemia by this mechanism. In one study, newborns who received formula feedings had decreased readmissions for phototherapy compared with those who were exclusively breastfed.[63] However, another small single-center study showed that breastfeeding more than eight times a day was associated with a decrease in the need for readmission for hyperbilirubinemia.[64] In addition, interrupting phototherapy to allow for breastfeeding has not been shown to hinder the effectiveness of phototherapy.[65] Improving feeding volumes with lactation support, hand expression or pumping, and supplementation when necessary, are important interventions to prevent and treat jaundice due to inadequate intake.[61] Finally, hyperbilirubinemia seen in infants at 2 to 3 weeks of age has been termed "breastmilk" jaundice, and the etiology is unknown but thought to be multifactorial.[61] Cessation of breastfeeding is not necessary to prevent high levels of hyperbilirubinemia secondary to breast milk jaundice, and supplementation with formula should not be recommended if infants are adequately breastfeeding with appropriate intake and weight gain.[61,66]

HYPOGLYCEMIA

Hypoglycemia is a common issue for many newborns and is most often seen in infants born large for gestational age, small for gestational age, infants of diabetic mothers, and late preterm infants.[67] Prevention and treatment of hypoglycemia start with feeding and often supplementation, and infants with persistent hypoglycemia may require admission to the neonatal intensive care unit (NICU) for intravenous glucose infusion which may negatively impact breastfeeding. Dextrose gel is an inexpensive oral supplement given to newborns as an intervention to improve hypoglycemia and prevent admission to the NICU with the goal of maintaining exclusive breastfeeding.

There have been multiple RCTs evaluating dextrose gel and impact on breastfeeding outcomes with mixed results, but few have been performed in the United States. The first randomized, double-blind, placebo-controlled trial, the Sugar Babies study, was performed in New Zealand and was effective in preventing the primary outcome of hypoglycemia but failed to show improvement in exclusive breastfeeding.[68] However, the study population had a very high baseline exclusive breastfeeding rate (approximately 90%) which is much higher than most US centers, and results may not be generalizable to other populations with lower breastfeeding rates.[68] More recently, the Hypoglycaemia Prevention with Oral Dextrose study was a randomized double-blinded trial performed in Australia and New Zealand which included 2149 babies. This study demonstrated improvement in hypoglycemia with a number needed to treat of 21 to prevent one occurrence of hypoglycemia, but there was not a reduction in NICU admissions due to hypoglycemia.[69] Alternatively, in India in 2020, a large open-label RCT evaluating dextrose gel showed a decrease in NICU admissions for hypoglycemia.[70] A Cochrane review published in 2022 aimed to assess the effectiveness of oral dextrose gel in correcting hypoglycemia in newborn infants during the birth hospitalization and reducing long-term neurodevelopmental impairment. The investigators concluded that dextrose gel improves the incidence of hypoglycemia and may result in a slight reduction in the risk of major neurologic disability at age 2 years or older without any adverse events from the intervention.[71] In addition, dextrose gel treatment likely reduces the incidence of separation from the mother for treatment of hypoglycemia and increases the likelihood of exclusive breastfeeding after discharge.[71]

SUMMARY

Breastfeeding is the biologic norm for infant feeding with overwhelming benefits for both the mother and infant. There are medical, social, and societal challenges that impact the attainment of breastfeeding goals and influence decisions and recommendations for optimal newborn feeding. Medical issues including jaundice, hypoglycemia, newborn weight loss, and infants who are born late preterm are common problems encountered during the birth hospitalization, and it is crucial newborn providers be knowledgeable about evidence-based practices including recommendations from international and national organizations. Breastfeeding controversies can be perpetuated through misinformation from social media and family influences as well as a lack of high-quality, generalizable studies. Clinicians must balance parental wishes with available evidence and expert opinion when providing recommendations regarding infant feeding.

FUTURE DIRECTIONS

Further research is needed on controversial newborn feeding topics where there is a lack of high-quality evidence to guide intervention and practice. In addition, medical providers must acknowledge parental concerns about newborn feeding and have open communication to develop trust to help inform the best, evidence-based care. Finally, local, regional, and national efforts to educate, support, and promote exclusive breastfeeding are required to improve long-term health outcomes.

Best practices

What is the current practice for newborn feeding?

Breastfeeding is the biologic norm for newborn feeding, but there are many common newborn issues that can make breastfeeding more difficult, and many people do not achieve their breastfeeding goals.

What changes in current practice are likely to improve outcomes?

Guidelines from professional organizations outline ways to support breastfeeding in the hospital and help determine mother–infant dyads at risk for breastfeeding difficulties. Clinical tools that evaluate newborn weight loss, jaundice, and interventions such as dextrose gel for newborn hypoglycemia should be used to help guide decisions regarding newborn feeding.

Major Recommendations

Evidence-based practices should be followed to support breastfeeding and newborn feeding, and where there is a paucity of evidence, clinical guidelines, and standardized care should be used.

CLINICS CARE POINTS

- Implementation of the World Health Organization's Ten Steps to Successful Breastfeeding and the Baby-Friendly Hospital Initiative has a positive impact on breastfeeding outcomes in the United States.
- Breastfeeding is recommended for mothers engaged in medication-assisted treatment for opioid use disorder to improve maternal and infant outcomes.
- Infants with hyperbilirubinemia do not require formula supplementation if they are adequately breastfeeding with appropriate intake and weight gain, and discontinuation of breastfeeding is not necessary to prevent or decrease breastmilk jaundice.

DISCLOSURE

The authors have nothing to disclose.

REFERENCES

1. Meek JY, Noble L, Section on B. Policy statement: breastfeeding and the use of human milk. Pediatrics 2022;150(1).
2. Horta BL, Loret de Mola C, Victora CG. Breastfeeding and intelligence: a systematic review and meta-analysis. Acta Paediatr 2015;104(467):14–9.
3. Barriers to breastfeeding: supporting initiation and continuation of breastfeeding: ACOG committee opinion, number 821. Obstet Gynecol 2021;137(2):e54–62.
4. Bartick M, Reinhold A. The burden of suboptimal breastfeeding in the United States: a pediatric cost analysis. Pediatrics 2010;125(5):e1048–56.
5. Breastfeeding Among U.S. Children Born 2012-2019, CDC National Immunization Survey. Available at : https://www.cdc.gov/breastfeeding/data/nis_data/results.html. Accessed September 6, 2022. Accessed.
6. Babakazo P, Donnen P, Akilimali P, et al. Predictors of discontinuing exclusive breastfeeding before six months among mothers in Kinshasa: a prospective study. Int Breastfeed J 2015;10:19.
7. Protecting, promoting and supporting breastfeeding: the Baby-friendly Hospital Initiative for small, sick and preterm newborns. Geneva: World Health Organization and the United Nations Children's Fund (UNICEF); 2020. Licence: CC BY-NC-SA 3.0 IGO.
8. Perez-Escamilla R, Martinez JL, Segura-Perez S. Impact of the Baby-friendly Hospital Initiative on breastfeeding and child health outcomes: a systematic review. Matern Child Nutr 2016;12(3):402–17.

9. Hernandez-Aguilar MT, Bartick M, Schreck P, et al. ABM clinical protocol #7: model maternity policy supportive of breastfeeding. Breastfeed Med 2018; 13(9):559–74.

10. Munn AC, Newman SD, Mueller M, et al. The impact in the United States of the baby-friendly hospital initiative on early infant health and breastfeeding outcomes. Breastfeed Med 2016;11:222–30.

11. Feltner C, Weber RP, Stuebe A, et al. In: Breastfeeding Programs and Policies, Breastfeeding Uptake, and Maternal Health Outcomes in Developed Countries [Internet]. Rockville, MD: Agency for Healthcare Research and Quality (US); 2018.

12. Perrine CG, Scanlon KS, Li R, et al. Baby-Friendly hospital practices and meeting exclusive breastfeeding intention. Pediatrics 2012;130(1):54–60.

13. Merewood A, Bugg K, Burnham L, et al. Addressing racial inequities in breastfeeding in the southern United States. Pediatrics 2019;143(2).

14. Semenic S, Childerhose JE, Lauziere J, et al. Barriers, facilitators, and recommendations related to implementing the Baby-Friendly Initiative (BFI): an integrative review. J Hum Lactation 2012;28(3):317–34.

15. Amalia N, Orchard D, Francis KL, et al. Systematic review and meta-analysis on the use of probiotic supplementation in pregnant mother, breastfeeding mother and infant for the prevention of atopic dermatitis in children. Australas J Dermatol 2020;61(2):e158–73.

16. Grond SE, Kallies G, McCormick ME. Parental and provider perspectives on social media about ankyloglossia. Int J Pediatr Otorhinolaryngol 2021;146:110741.

17. Kelly Z, Yang CJ. Ankyloglossia. Pediatr Rev 2022;43(8):473–5.

18. O'Shea JE, Foster JP, O'Donnell CP, et al. Frenotomy for tongue-tie in newborn infants. Cochrane Database Syst Rev 2017;3:CD011065.

19. Bin-Nun A, Kasirer YM, Mimouni FB. A dramatic increase in tongue tie-related articles: a 67 Years systematic review. Breastfeed Med 2017;12(7):410–4.

20. Obladen M. Much ado about nothing: two millenia of controversy on tongue-tie. Neonatology 2010;97(2):83–9.

21. Ruben RJ. Development of otorhinological care of the child. Acta Otolaryngol 2004;124(4):536–9.

22. Todd DA, Hogan MJ. Tongue-tie in the newborn: early diagnosis and division prevents poor breastfeeding outcomes. Breastfeed Rev 2015;23(1):11–6.

23. LeFort Y, Evans A, Livingstone V, et al. Academy of breastfeeding medicine position statement on ankyloglossia in breastfeeding dyads. Breastfeed Med 2021; 16(4):278–81.

24. Ingram J, Copeland M, Johnson D, et al. The development and evaluation of a picture tongue assessment tool for tongue-tie in breastfed babies (TABBY). Int Breastfeed J 2019;14:31.

25. Douglas P. Making sense of studies that claim benefits of frenotomy in the absence of classic tongue-tie. J Hum Lactation 2017;33(3):519–23.

26. Hatami A, Dreyer CW, Meade MJ, et al. Effectiveness of tongue-tie assessment tools in diagnosing and fulfilling lingual frenectomy criteria: a systematic review. Aust Dent J 2022;67(3):212–9.

27. Jaafar SH, Ho JJ, Jahanfar S, et al. Effect of restricted pacifier use in breastfeeding term infants for increasing duration of breastfeeding. Cochrane Database Syst Rev 2016;8:CD007202.

28. Moon RY, Carlin RF. Hand I, task force on sudden infant death S, the committee on F, newborn. Sleep-related infant deaths: updated 2022 recommendations for reducing infant deaths in the sleep environment. Pediatrics 2022;150(1).

29. Batista CLC, Rodrigues VP, Ribeiro VS, et al. Nutritive and non-nutritive sucking patterns associated with pacifier use and bottle-feeding in full-term infants. Early Hum Dev 2019;132:18–23.

30. Zimmerman E, Thompson K. Clarifying nipple confusion. J Perinatol 2015;35(11): 895–9.

31. 2019 National Survey on Drug Use and Health: National findings. Available at: https://www.samhsa.gov/data/report/2019-nsduh-detailed-tables. Accessed October 2022.

32. Smith BL, Hall ES, McAllister JM, et al. Rates of substance and polysubstance use through universal maternal testing at the time of delivery. J Perinatol 2022; 42(8):1026–31.

33. Hall ES, McAllister JM, Kelly EA, et al. Regional comparison of self-reported late pregnancy cigarette smoking to mass spectrometry analysis. J Perinatol 2021; 41(10):2417–23.

34. Verstegen RHJ, Anderson PO, Ito S. Infant drug exposure via breast milk. Br J Clin Pharmacol 2022;88(10):4311–27.

35. Rowe H, Baker T, Hale TW. Maternal medication, drug use, and breastfeeding. Child Adolesc Psychiatr Clin N Am 2015;24(1):1–20.

36. Abdel-Latif ME, Pinner J, Clews S, et al. Effects of breast milk on the severity and outcome of neonatal abstinence syndrome among infants of drug-dependent mothers. Pediatrics 2006;117(6):e1163–9.

37. Welle-Strand GK, Skurtveit S, Jansson LM, et al. Breastfeeding reduces the need for withdrawal treatment in opioid-exposed infants. Acta Paediatr 2013;102(11): 1060–6.

38. Chu L, McGrath JM, Qiao J, et al. A meta-analysis of breastfeeding effects for infants with neonatal abstinence syndrome. Nurs Res 2022;71(1):54–65.

39. Bertrand KA, Hanan NJ, Honerkamp-Smith G, et al. Marijuana use by breastfeeding mothers and cannabinoid concentrations in breast milk. Pediatrics 2018; 142(3).

40. Reece-Stremtan S, Marinelli KA. ABM clinical protocol #21: guidelines for breastfeeding and substance use or substance use disorder, revised 2015. Breastfeed Med 2015;10(3):135–41.

41. Ho NT, Li F, Lee-Sarwar KA, et al. Meta-analysis of effects of exclusive breastfeeding on infant gut microbiota across populations. Nat Commun 2018;9(1): 4169.

42. Kellams A, Harrel C, Omage S, et al. ABM clinical protocol #3: supplementary feedings in the healthy term breastfed neonate, revised 2017. Breastfeed Med 2017;12:188–98.

43. Davanzo R, Cannioto Z, Ronfani L, et al. Breastfeeding and neonatal weight loss in healthy term infants. J Hum Lactation 2013;29(1):45–53.

44. Lavagno C, Camozzi P, Renzi S, et al. Breastfeeding-associated hypernatremia: a systematic review of the literature. J Hum Lactation 2016;32(1):67–74.

45. Miyoshi Y, Suenaga H, Aoki M, et al. Determinants of excessive weight loss in breastfed full-term newborns at a baby-friendly hospital: a retrospective cohort study. Int Breastfeed J 2020;15(1):19.

46. Nommsen-Rivers LA, Dewey KG. Growth of breastfed infants. Breastfeed Med 2009;4(Suppl 1):S45–9.

47. Smith AP, Ward LP, Heinig MJ, et al. First-day use of the newborn weight loss tool to predict excess weight loss in breastfeeding newborns. Breastfeed Med 2021; 16(3):230–7.

48. Flaherman VJ, Aby J, Burgos AE, et al. Effect of early limited formula on duration and exclusivity of breastfeeding in at-risk infants: an RCT. Pediatrics 2013;131(6): 1059–65.

49. Flaherman VJ, Cabana MD, McCulloch CE, et al. Effect of early limited formula on breastfeeding duration in the first year of life: a randomized clinical trial. JAMA Pediatr 2019;173(8):729–35.

50. Feldman-Winter L, Kellams A, Peter-Wohl S, et al. Evidence-based updates on the first week of exclusive breastfeeding among infants >/=35 weeks. Pediatrics 2020;145(4).

51. Asadi S, Bloomfield FH, Harding JE. Nutrition in late preterm infants. Semin Perinatol 2019;43(7):151160.

52. Moyer LB, Goyal NK, Meinzen-Derr J, et al. Factors associated with readmission in late-preterm infants: a matched case-control study. Hosp Pediatr 2014;4(5): 298–304.

53. Meier P, Patel AL, Wright K, et al. Management of breastfeeding during and after the maternity hospitalization for late preterm infants. Clin Perinatol 2013;40(4):689–705.

54. Shapiro-Mendoza CK, Tomashek KM, Kotelchuck M, et al. Effect of late-preterm birth and maternal medical conditions on newborn morbidity risk. Pediatrics 2008;121(2):e223–32.

55. Young PC, Korgenski K, Buchi KF. Early readmission of newborns in a large health care system. Pediatrics 2013;131(5):e1538–44.

56. Boies EG, Vaucher YE. ABM clinical protocol #10: breastfeeding the late preterm (34-36 6/7 Weeks of gestation) and early term infants (37-38 6/7 Weeks of gestation), second revision 2016. Breastfeed Med 2016;11:494–500.

57. Chow S, Chow R, Popovic M, et al. The use of nipple shields: a review. Front Public Health 2015;3:236.

58. Meier PP, Engstrom JL, Janes JE, et al. Breast pump suction patterns that mimic the human infant during breastfeeding: greater milk output in less time spent pumping for breast pump-dependent mothers with premature infants. J Perinatol 2012;32(2):103–10.

59. Morton J, Hall JY, Wong RJ, et al. Combining hand techniques with electric pumping increases milk production in mothers of preterm infants. J Perinatol 2009;29(11):757–64.

60. Flint A, New K, Davies MW. Cup feeding versus other forms of supplemental enteral feeding for newborn infants unable to fully breastfeed. Cochrane Database Syst Rev 2016;(8):CD005092.

61. Flaherman VJ, Maisels MJ, Academy of Breastfeeding M. ABM clinical protocol #22: guidelines for management of jaundice in the breastfeeding infant 35 Weeks or more of gestation-revised 2017. Breastfeed Med 2017;12(5):250–7.

62. Hansen R, Gibson S, De Paiva Alves E, et al. Adaptive response of neonatal sepsis-derived Group B Streptococcus to bilirubin. Sci Rep 2018;8(1):6470.

63. Wickremasinghe AC, Kuzniewicz MW, McCulloch CE, et al. Efficacy of subthreshold newborn phototherapy during the birth hospitalization in preventing readmission for phototherapy. JAMA Pediatr 2018;172(4):378–85.

64. Chen YJ, Yeh TF, Chen CM. Effect of breast-feeding frequency on hyperbilirubinemia in breast-fed term neonate. Pediatr Int 2015;57(6):1121–5.

65. Sachdeva M, Murki S, Oleti TP, et al. Intermittent versus continuous phototherapy for the treatment of neonatal non-hemolytic moderate hyperbilirubinemia in infants more than 34 weeks of gestational age: a randomized controlled trial. Eur J Pediatr 2015;174(2):177–81.

66. Kemper AR, Newman TB, Slaughter JL, et al. Clinical practice guideline revision: management of hyperbilirubinemia in the newborn infant 35 or more weeks of gestation. Pediatrics 2022;150(3).

67. Committee on F, Newborn, Adamkin DH. Postnatal glucose homeostasis in late-preterm and term infants. Pediatrics 2011;127(3):575–9.

68. Harris DL, Weston PJ, Signal M, et al. Dextrose gel for neonatal hypoglycaemia (the Sugar Babies Study): a randomised, double-blind, placebo-controlled trial. Lancet 2013;382(9910):2077–83.

69. Harding JE, Hegarty JE, Crowther CA, et al. Evaluation of oral dextrose gel for prevention of neonatal hypoglycemia (hPOD): a multicenter, double-blind randomized controlled trial. PLoS Med 2021;18(1):e1003411.

70. Gupta K, Amboiram P, Balakrishnan U, et al. Dextrose gel for neonates at risk with asymptomatic hypoglycemia: a randomized clinical trial. Pediatrics 2022;149(6).

71. Edwards T, Liu G, Battin M, et al. Oral dextrose gel for the treatment of hypoglycaemia in newborn infants. Cochrane Database Syst Rev 2022;3:CD011027.

The Role of the Neonatal Registered Dietitian Nutritionist: Past, Present, and Future

Stephanie Merlino Barr, MS, RDN, LD[a],*,
Rosa K. Hand, PhD, RDN, LD, FAND[b], Tanis R. Fenton, PhD, RDN[c],
Sharon Groh-Wargo, PhD, RDN[a,b]

KEYWORDS

- Registered dietitian nutritionist • Staffing ratio • Staffing • Infant • Nutrition • Growth
- Neonatal

KEY POINTS

- Neonatal registered dietitian nutritionists (RDNs) play a critical role in improving outcomes of preterm and critically ill infants.
- There is a need for data connecting neonatal RDN staffing ratios to patient outcomes to define ideal staffing ratios.
- Responding neonatal RDNs want a 29% increase in current neonatal intensive care unit RDN staffing levels to better achieve their current and desired responsibilities.

INTRODUCTION

"How did we actually live without these key workers in the nurseries?" This is a quote referring to neonatal registered dietitian nutritionists (RDN) by Dr Reginald Tsang, a distinguished and trailblazing neonatologist, reflecting on half a century of practice in the historical introduction to the latest edition of *Nutritional Care of Preterm Infants.*[1] In this article, the authors review the emergence of the role of the neonatal RDN, present the results of a recent national survey of neonatal RDN staffing and responsibilities, and discuss both the implications of the survey and suggest a call to action going forward.

[a] Department of Pediatrics, MetroHealth Medical Center, 2500 MetroHealth Drive, Cleveland, OH, 44102, USA; [b] Department of Nutrition, Case Western Reserve University, 10900 Euclid Avenue, Cleveland, OH 44106, USA; [c] Cumming School of Medicine, University of Calgary, 3280 Hospital Drive Northwest, Calgary, Alberta T2N 4Z6, Canada
* Corresponding author.
E-mail address: smerlino@metrohealth.org

Clin Perinatol 50 (2023) 743–762
https://doi.org/10.1016/j.clp.2023.04.010
0095-5108/23/© 2023 Elsevier Inc. All rights reserved.

BACKGROUND

In the United States, RDNs, also called registered dietitians (or less formally, dietitians), complete coursework in food, nutrition, and social/communication sciences, a supervised practice experience of at least 1000 hours and must pass a national standardized examination.[2–4] Once credentialed by the Commission on Dietetic Registration (CDR), RDNs must complete at least 75 hours of continuing education every 5 years.[4,5] Some states have additional licensure or certification of RDNs.[4] Beginning in 2024, newly credentialed RDNs will also be required to hold a master's degree.[6] The scope of the practice for an RDN includes nutrition-related assessment, diagnosis, intervention, monitoring, and evaluation in a variety of practice settings, from community nutrition to intensive care.[4] Since 2014, the Centers for Medicare and Medicaid Services have allowed RDNs to hold order-writing privileges for therapeutic diets (including enteral and parenteral nutrition), if the hospital or long-term care facility grants these privileges and if state law allows.[4,7,8] For the remainder of this article, the authors use the term RDN when data are specific to the United States and dietitian when referring to data from other countries. CDR also credentials the nutrition and dietetics technician, registered (NDTR), who work in supportive roles with RDNs. NDTRs either hold a 2 year degree that includes 450 hours of supervised practice or a bachelor's degree and have passed a national examination.[2,4,5,9]

RDNs are increasingly recognized as vital members of the health care team, with extensive and varied roles and responsibilities.[10] The importance of dietitians as team members is particularly true in the neonatal intensive care unit (NICU) setting. A survey conducted in the United States almost 20 years ago found that approximately 40% of American NICUs had neonatal RDNs.[11] A 2005 study reported that 76% of responding NICUs involved RDNs in care with the largest RDN presence in NICUs with high patient acuity.[12] In 2009, Hans and colleagues reported that nearly 80% of respondents to their survey had neonatal RDNs in level II and level III nurseries.[13] Recent staffing surveys in Canada, Australia, and New Zealand have estimated that approximately 90% to 100% of level III NICUs have access to the services of a neonatal dietitian.[14,15] These findings suggest that dietitian involvement has become a standard practice in the NICU.[16]

Although there is good evidence for the increasing presence of RDNs in NICUs, there are less data about their specific roles, responsibilities, and workload, which are often quantified by staffing ratios (NICU beds per full-time equivalents [FTEs]). Staffing ratios can affect the capacity at which RDNs are able to provide patients and families with high-quality nutrition care, which is of particular importance in the NICU given the high acuity of the patients.[15,17] Factors that are likely to influence RDN staffing ratios include the type of services provided, number of beds, percent occupancy, patient acuity, length of stay, level of staff experience, accreditation specifications, and hospital initiatives.[10]

NICUs that use dietitians are more likely to consistently monitor neonatal growth and use optimum nutrition practices.[15] Dietitian-led implementation of evidence-based nutrition support practices in NICUs has been shown to improve nutrient intake, growth, and clinical outcomes, reduce length of stay and related costs, and reduce intravenous nutrition costs and prescription errors.[12,15] NICUs that do not use an RDN are more likely to provide inappropriate feedings such as unfortified breast milk or full-term formula to very low birth weight infants.[12] Neonatal RDNs are necessary for optimizing specialized nutrition support for infants with metabolic abnormalities, identifying and treating those with acquired vitamin and mineral deficiencies, and preventing malnutrition.[15] Neonatal RDNs are exclusively focused on the development and implementation of evidence-based, individualized nutrition care, so their presence improves provision of the highest quality nutrition care to this high-risk population.

Despite their presence and these important roles, there has been no identified ideal neonatal RDN staffing ratio for the NICU. One publication from 1989 suggested 30 beds per 1 FTE RDN.[18] The 2021 US News and World Report for pediatric hospital rankings awards one point for a staffing ratio of 20 or more NICU beds per FTE RDN and two points for fewer than 20 NICU beds per FTE RDN.[19] These rankings are only applicable to the select group of children's hospitals that are eligible for inclusion; only 198 hospitals participated in the 2020 to 2021 survey.[19] Importantly, these ratios are not evidence-based and were removed from the 2022-23 methodology for the US News and World Report for Best Children's Hospitals; there is now a point awarded for NICU-dedicated registered dietitians with no staffing ratio defined.[20] Reported ratios have varied widely, ranging from 21 to 60 NICU beds per FTE RDN.[12] According to data tracked by one of the authors (SGW) for nearly 20 years for the Ohio Neonatal Nutritionists (a nonprofit organization of NICU RDNs practicing in the state) staffing ratios in Level III–IV NICUs recently averaged 34 patient beds per FTE RDN, although level III and level IV units differed at 36:1 and 28:1, respectively. These ratios have remained unchanged over the last 2 decades, although personal observations suggest that roles and responsibilities have increased.

Questions regarding ideal staffing for RDNs in all clinical settings are not new.[21,22] There is currently no methodology to effectively predict clinical RDN staffing needs and currently no validated staffing ratio model that is universally accepted.[21] Two large studies that used self-reported time diaries suggest that in the inpatient setting, as much as 50% of RDN time is spent on activities that are not directly related to patient care.[22,23] Neither of these studies examined both time and patient outcomes.[22,23]

This dearth of staffing data is not a deficiency unique to neonatal nutrition or the dietetics profession. In the nursing profession, individual publications have shown that fewer patients per nurse have been associated with lower patient rates of failure to rescue, mortality, decubitus ulcers, pneumonia, and sepsis as well as lower rates of dissatisfaction and burnout among nurses.[24,25] However, a Cochrane review found little evidence to support staffing ratios for improving patient or staff outcomes.[26] Therefore, patient-to-nurse ratios, including those mandated at the state or country level, are often based on consensus rather than evidence.[26] Thus, the lack of high-quality evidence related to staffing ratios for neonatal RDNs is not unique.

In summary, there is evidence that the contributions of RDNs to NICU patient care are important, but there is a paucity of data about contemporary neonatal RDN roles and responsibilities and the associated staffing ratios. To address this need, the authors conducted a cross-sectional survey that was constructed to assess the current staffing and the roles and responsibilities of neonatal dietitians and dietetic technicians in the United States and Canada. This manuscript reports the United States data only.

METHODS
Describing Neonatal Nutrition Responsibilities and Staffing Characteristics: A National Survey of Neonatal Registered Dietitian Nutritionist Practice

The survey was designed by the authors and administered using Qualtrics Software.[27] Before full distribution, it was beta-tested with a group of experienced Ohio neonatal RDNs. Survey participants were neonatal RDNs, NDTRs, and NICU medical leadership across the United States. US survey participants were recruited via email lists to target RDN and NDTR recruitment and included PediRD, the Pediatric Nutrition

Dietetic Practice Group, the NICU Dietitians Facebook group, the Virginia Neonatal Nutrition Association, the Ohio Neonatal Nutritionists, Northeast Ohio Neonatal Nutritionists, the Minnesota Neonatal Nutrition Conference, the Dr Diane Anderson Neonatal Nutrition Conference, and Astarte. For additional US recruitment, the authors emailed NICU medical directors whose email addresses were publicly available via neonatologysolutions.com. The recruitment email contained a forwardable survey link and was distributed starting in October 2021. The survey was open for 4 weeks total. As an incentive for survey completion, RDNs and NDTRs were able to provide their email separately and confidentially to be entered into a drawing for one of five copies of the book "Academy of Nutrition and Dietetics Pocket Guide to Neonatal Nutrition, 3rd edition."

The authors obtained an exempt determination from the Case Western Reserve University institutional review board (IRB, #20211081). Survey participants viewed a consent information page, and consent was implied by continuing in the survey.

The survey collected hospital-level data from RDNs, NDTRs, and physicians, and individual-level data from RDNs and NDTRs. Hospital-level data included hospital size, type (delivery or children's), NICU level, availability of a human milk and/or formula room, and RDN and NDTR staffing. Individual-level data included compensation and benefits (optional), job responsibilities, and ideal time allocation of job responsibilities. Skip logic was used so that participants only saw relevant questions; thus, the number of administered questions was variable.

To match multiple responses from a single hospital and account for data clustering, the authors required participants to name their hospital and hospital zip/postal code. In data cleaning, a non-neonatal RDN investigator determined if represented institutions were academic or nonacademic hospitals depending on if they had pediatric residencies or neonatal fellowships, then de-identified the responses and created a unique hospital-level code for use in analysis and before sharing with the neonatal RDN investigators. A response rate was not calculated at the individual level, as responding RDNs may have been exposed to the recruitment email in multiple listservs. Instead, an institution-level response rate was performed following data-cleaning, using participant-provided institution data, and a public listing of US-based NICUs.

Statistical analyses were performed using R 4.1.0 (R Core Team, 2021). In the descriptive statistics performed, means and standard deviations (SDs) were used to describe normally distributed data, whereas median and interquartile ranges were used to describe non-normal data. In comparing differences between levels of NICUs, the Kruskal–Wallis test was performed for nonparametric data, and t test or analysis of variance (ANOVA) was performed for parametric data. Proportions, chi square, and Fisher's exact tests were used for categorical data. A significance level of 0.05 was used for all analyses.

RESULTS
Responding Hospital Results

Hospital-level characteristics are described in **Table 1**. A total of 162 hospitals were represented in the survey; 51 institutions had level IV NICUs, 103 had level III, and 8 had level II. With an estimated 1384 NICUs in the United States, the NICU response rate was estimated to be 12%; response rates by NICU level were as follows: 3% of Level II, 16% of Level III, and 45% of level IV NICUs were represented in our survey. **Fig. 1** depicts the density of responding NICUs based on the estimated number of NICUs in each state. A median of 13% (IQR 9%–21%) NICUs responded in each represented state. There were no responses from the states of: Alaska, Alabama,

	Overall	Level 4	Level 3	Level 2	$p^{a,b,c}$
Table 1 Institution-level demographics					
N	162	51	103	8	
Hospital type hosting NICU (%)[d]					<.05
Children's hospital: Main campus	55 (34)	37 (73)	18 (18)	0 (0)	
Children's hospital: Satellite campus	7 (4)	1 (2)	6 (6)	0 (0)	
Delivery hospital	100 (62)	13 (26)	79 (77)	8 (100)	
Academic institution (%)[d]					
Pediatric residency	86 (53)	45 (88)	41 (40)	0 (0)	<.05
Neonatal fellowship	62 (38)	36 (71)	26 (25)	0 (0)	<.05
Number of licensed NICU beds[a]	46 [30, 65]	65 [52, 84]	38 [28, 49]	10 [10, 13]	<.05
Average daily NICU census[a]	34 [20, 55]	60 [48, 70]	29 [18, 37]	7 [5, 9]	<0.05
Annual NICU admissions[a]	699 [519, 1000]	875 [699, 1278]	550 [431, 709]	NA	<.05

[a] Nonnormal distribution, described with median (interquartile range); *P* value assessed using the Kruskal–Wallis test.
[b] Normal distribution, described with mean (standard deviation); *P* value assessed using a one-way *t* test or ANOVA.
[c] Categorical variables *P* value assessed using a chi square test or Fisher's exact test.
[d] All reported percentage responses are valid percentage responses and thus do not include missing values in the denominator. Missingness varies by question.

Louisiana, Mississippi, New Mexico, Vermont, or Wyoming; Wyoming did not a level III or IV NICU at the time of the survey.

Formula rooms were available for 80% of the responding hospitals, and those providing the highest level of care were most likely to have a formula room (level 4:

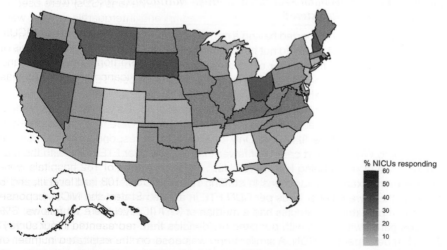

Fig. 1. Density of responding NICUs based on estimated NICUs in each state. Median of 13.3% (9.5%–20%) NICUs responded in represented states

Table 2
Summary of milk and formula room practices at responding institutions

	Overall	Level 4	Level 3	Level 2	$P^{a,b,c}$
n	162	51	103	8	
Formula room present (% yes)[d]	111 (80)	41 (93)	68 (76)	2 (40)	<0.05
Formula room serves which populations (% yes)[d]					<0.05
All of pediatrics	64 (46)	37 (84)	27 (30)	0 (0)	
NICU only	47 (34)	4 (9)	41 (46)	2 (40)	
No formula room	28 (20)	3 (7)	22 (24)	3 (60)	
Formula room serving multiple hospitals (% yes)[d]	5 (5)	2 (5)	3 (5)	0 (0)	0.95
Milk room access (% yes)[d]	73 (53)	33 (73)	38 (43)	2 (40)	<0.05
Milk room in hospital (% yes)[d]	63 (46)	30 (67)	32 (36)	1 (20)	<0.05
Plan to build milk room in hospital (% yes)[d]	12 (16)	4 (29)	8 (14)	0 (0)	0.29
Milk room serving NICU only (% yes)[d]	40 (54)	14 (42)	25 (63)	1 (100)	0.15
Milk room serving multiple hospitals (% yes)[d]	2 (3)	1 (3)	1 (3)	0 (0)	0.98

[a] Nonnormal distribution, described with median (interquartile range); P value assessed using the Kruskal–Wallis test.
[b] Normal distribution, described with mean (standard deviation); P value assessed using a one-way t-test or ANOVA.
[c] Categorical variables P value assessed using a chi square test or Fisher's exact test.
[d] All reported percentage responses are valid percentage responses, and thus do not include missing values in the denominator. Missingness varies by question.

93%; level 3: 76%; and level 2: 40%) (**Table 2**). Although 28 (20%) responding NICUs reported not having a formula room, of these NICUs, four reported having a milk room onsite, one reported having access to a milk room not onsite, and three reported having plans to create a milk room. The remaining 20 NICUs that reported not having a formula room (14%) did not report having access to a milk room or having plans to build one.

Staffing Ratios for Neonatal Registered Dietitian Nutritionists and Nutrition and Dietetics Technician, Registered

Every responding NICU reported having a neonatal RDN in their unit and no responses were received from units that did not have a neonatal RDN. The RDN staffing ratio was calculated by dividing the number of licensed beds by the total reported RDN FTEs. For all respondents, the median staffing ratio was 33.6 beds per FTE RDN (interquartile range [IQR] 24.0, 45.0) (**Table 3**). Level IV NICUs had the lowest median staffing ratio at 26.2 (20.3, 41.5) beds per FTE RDN, followed by level III NICUs with a median staffing ratio of 35.5 (27.9, 46.2) beds per FTE RDN, meaning there were fewer beds per RDN FTE in level IV than in level III NICUs. Only 11% ($n = 14$) of responding NICUs met the US News and World Report criteria of fewer than 20 beds per FTE RDN, with the majority of those ($n = 10$) being level IV NICUs.

The authors examined variations in staffing ratios in academic and nonacademic hospitals; there were fewer beds per RDN FTE in academic centers. NICUs in hospitals without pediatric residencies had a median of 37.7 (IQR 26.5, 47.3) beds per FTE RDN compared with those with pediatric residencies that had a median of 30.0 (IQR 22.1, 41.4) beds per FTE RDN. A similar trend was observed in hospitals with (median 30.0, IQR 21.5, 41.3 beds per FTE RDN) and without (median 35.0, IQR 26.6, 47.3 beds per FTE RDN) neonatal fellowships.

Table 3

Reported and desired neonatal registered dietitian nutritionist and nutrition and dietetics technician, registered staffing

	Overall	Level 4	Level 3	Level 2	$P^{a,b,c}$
N	162	51	103	8	
RDN FTE for NICU[a]	1.0 [1.0, 2.0]	2.50 [2.0, 3.1]	1.0 [0.9, 1.5]	0.2 [0.2, 0.5]	<0.05
RDN staffing ratio (NICU beds per FTE RDN)[a]	33.6 [24.0, 45.0]	26.2 [20.3, 41.5]	35.5 [27.9, 46.2]	30.0 [20.0, 40.0]	<0.05
NDTR in NICU (% yes)[d]	10 (7.5)	5 (11.6)	5 (5.9)	0 (0.0)	0.47
NDTR FTE[b]	1.7 (1.9)	1.9 (2.6)	1.4 (1.3)	0.0 (0.0)	0.72
NDTR staffing ratio (NICU beds per FTE NDTR)[b]	81.5 (69.0)	124.3 (75.3)	47.3 (44.5)	NA	0.10
Desired NICU beds per FTE RDN	24.0 [19.2, 30.5]	22.1 [17.7, 26.0]	25.0 [20.0, 32.7]	NA	
Desired additional RDN FTE to achieve desired staffing ratio	0.5 [0, 0.7]	0.5 [0, 1]	0.5 [0, 0.51]	NA	

[a] Nonnormal distribution, described with median (interquartile range); P value assessed using the Kruskal–Wallis test.
[b] Normal distribution, described with mean (standard deviation); P value assessed using a one-way t test or ANOVA.
[c] Categorical variables P value assessed using a chi square test or Fisher's exact test.
[d] All reported percentage responses are valid percentage responses and thus do not include missing values in the denominator. Missingness varies by question.

A total of 10 NICUs reported having NDTRs, five being level III NICUs (6% of responding level III NICUs) and five being level IV NICUs (12% of responding level IV NICUs) (see **Table 3**). The NDTR staffing ratio, calculated as number of licensed beds divided by NDTR FTEs, was only calculated for institutions that reported both NDTR and licensed bed data ($n = 9$). The mean NDTR staffing ratio was 47.3 (SD 44.5) beds per FTE NDTR for Level III NICUs and 124.3 (SD 75.3) beds per FTE NDTR for level IV NICUs. All NDTR staffing ratio data were reported from NICUs that used RDNs.

Individual Neonatal Registered Dietitian Nutritionist Results

Individual demographics of respondents are described in **Table 4**, and individual position information is described in **Table 5**. A total of 186 individual RDNs took this survey with 72% ($n = 134$) completing the survey. Only one NDTR responded to our survey, and thus their response is not reported here. Most RDN respondents were female (98%), white (93%), and non-Hispanic (94%). Our respondents had a weighted average age of 41.5 years. A total of 60% of responding neonatal RDNs had a master's degree or higher and 58% (89/153) had a specialty certification. The most common certification among respondents was the Certified Nutrition Support Clinician (31%, 47/153). Responding RDNs worked on average 37 h/wk with an average of 31 h/wk assigned to NICU-related responsibilities. A total of 64% (97/151) of responding RDNs worked all their scheduled time in NICU-related responsibilities. A total of 85% of responding RDNs identified as being full-time employees with 14% being part time and 1% being pro re nata (PRN), as necessary.

Responsibilities results
The authors asked questions regarding daily responsibilities by grouping tasks into five categories: clinical, outpatient, administrative, research, and education. Responding neonatal RDNs typically spend 75% of their time in clinical work (**Fig. 2**).

Clinical responsibilities
There was complete agreement from responding neonatal RDNs that creating an initial nutrition plan and completing a follow-up nutrition plan are important for NICU outcomes. Most (97%, $n = 138/142$) responding neonatal RDNs reported that they participated in daily patient rounds; all those who stated they rounded reported that they felt rounding was very (91%, $n = 126/138$) or moderately (9%, $n = 12/138$) important to NICU outcomes. In addition to daily rounding, neonatal RDNs reported that they also participated in discharge rounds (45%, $n = 64$), surgical/gut rehabilitation rounds (11%, $n = 16$), chronic lung rounds (10%, $n = 14$), and bone health rounds (7%, $n = 10$).

Neonatal RDN time spent on screening for urgency of nutrition care or follow-up varied among respondents with 11% ($n = 15/143$) spending a substantial amount of time, 22% ($n = 32/143$) a moderate amount of time, 48% ($n = 69/143$) a small amount of time, and 19% ($n = 27/143$) rarely or never spending time in this task. Those who reported spending a substantial or moderate amount of time performing nutrition screening, 75% ($n = 35/47$) stated it was very important to NICU outcomes, 23% ($n = 11/47$) moderately important, and 2% ($n = 1/47$) minimally important.

Individual inpatient counseling, group education, and discharge education responsibilities varied between responding neonatal RDNs. Of all neonatal RDNs that reported performing inpatient nutrition counseling, 65% ($n = 70/108$) stated it was very important to NICU outcomes, 32% reported it was moderately important, and 3% stated it was minimally important to outcomes. The majority (94%, $n = 29/31$) that did not

Table 4
Individual-registered dietitian nutritionist demographics

	Overall	Level 4	Level 3	Level 2	$p^{a,b,c}$
N	186	67	112	7	
Female[f] (%)[d]	150 (98)	56 (98)	89 (98)	5 (100)	0.93
Race (% white[g])[d]	137 (93)	55 (98)	77 (89)	5 (100)	0.08
Identify as Hispanic, Latino, or Spanish (% yes)[d]	6 (4)	2 (4)	4 (5)	0 (0)	0.86
Age, in years[b,e]	42	39	41	42	0.39
Years as credentialed RDN[a]	13 [6, 22]	14 [5, 23]	13 [6, 20]	10 [10, 14]	0.99
Years in current NICU position[a]	6 [3, 12]	6 [2, 12]	7 [3, 12]	6 [1, 7]	0.65
Years in neonatal nutrition[a]	9 [4, 14]	9 [3, 15]	9 [4, 14]	9 [6, 9]	0.80
% RDN career in current NICU position[b]	56 (26)	55 (25)	56 (26)	44 (35)	0.56
% RDN career in neonatal nutrition[b]	67 (25)	69 (27)	66 (23)	57 (37)	0.52
Education: Master's degree or higher (% yes)[d]	92 (60)	32 (56)	58 (64)	2 (40)	0.42
Total specialty certifications (%)[d]					0.62
0	64 (42)	26 (46)	34 (37)	4 (80)	
1	66 (43)	22 (39)	43 (47)	1 (20)	
2	20 (13)	8 (14)	12 (13)	0 (0)	
3	3 (2)	1 (2)	2 (2)	0 (0)	
Any specialty certifications (% yes)[d]	89 (58)	31 (54)	57 (63)	1 (20)	0.13
Member of the Academy of Nutrition and Dietetics (% yes)[d]	58 (38)	21 (37)	33 (36)	4 (80)	0.14

[a] Nonnormal distribution, described with median (interquartile range); P value assessed using the Kruskal–Wallis test.
[b] Normal distribution, described with mean (standard deviation); P value assessed using a one-way t test or ANOVA.
[c] Categorical variables P value assessed using a chi square test or Fisher's exact test.
[d] All reported percentage responses are valid percentage responses and thus do not include missing values in the denominator. Missingness varies by question.
[e] Age was collected as a categorical variable by decade due to IRB specifications. A weighted average was calculated from valid responses.
[f] Gender was originally asked if individuals identified as female, male, other, or if they preferred not to respond. All responses were either female or male, and thus, this information was presented as a binary variable.
[g] Race was originally asked if individuals identified as white, Black or African American, American Indian or Alaska Native, Asian, Native Hawaiian or Pacific Islander, or other. Owing to very small numbers of responses in multiple racial groups, the variable was transformed to a binary one to maintain respondent anonymity.

Table 5
Registered dietitian nutritionist position characteristics

	Overall	Level 4	Level 3	Level 2	$P^{a,b,c}$
N	186	67	112	7	
Scheduled h/wk[a]	40 [36, 40]	40 [40, 40]	40 [36, 40]	40 [32, 40]	0.15
Scheduled NICU h/wk[a]	36 [24, 40]	40 [35, 40]	32 [20, 40]	13 [6, 25]	<0.05
% Time dedicated to NICU[a]	100 [75, 100]	100 [100, 100]	100 [75, 100]	34 [18, 63]	<0.05
Job classification (%)[d]					0.87
Full time	133 (85)	51 (88)	78 (83)	4 (80)	
Part time	22 (14)	6 (10)	15 (16)	1 (20)	
PRN	2 (1)	1 (2)	1 (1)	0 (0)	
Position under Nutrition and Food Services (% yes)[d]	136 (88)	50 (86)	81 (88)	5 (100)	0.66
Manager title (%)[d]					0.55
Nutrition manager or other RDN	145 (93)	54 (93)	86 (93)	5 (100)	
NICU nurse manager	4 (3)	1 (2)	3 (3)	0 (0)	
Physician	4 (3)	3 (5)	1 (1)	0 (0)	
Other	3 (2)	0 (0)	3 (3)	0 (0)	

[a] Nonnormal distribution, described with median (interquartile range); *P* value assessed using the Kruskal–Wallis test.
[b] Normal distribution, described with mean (standard deviation); *P* value assessed using a one-way *t* test or ANOVA.
[c] Categorical variables *P* value assessed using a chi square test or Fisher's exact test.
[d] All reported percentage responses are valid percentage responses and thus do not include missing values in the denominator. Missingness varies by question.

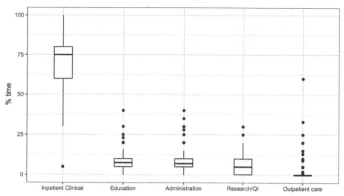

Fig. 2. Proportion of timer per month spent in various categories of NICU responsibilities.

perform individual inpatient counseling said that someone else performed this responsibility. Group educations classes were not an activity typically performed by neonatal RDNs with only 13% of responding neonatal RDNs ($n = 18/140$) performing this task. Most of the responding neonatal RDNs stated that someone else was responsible for group education classes (66%, $n = 81/122$), although 13% ($n = 16/122$) stated that this responsibility was not completed in their unit by them or anyone else. Discharge education classes were performed by 80% of responding neonatal RDNs ($n = 112/140$) with most respondents saying this was very important (79%, $n = 89/112$) or moderately important (20%, $n = 22/112$).

Charting requirements were reported as number of days from admission for initial note and number of days for follow-up. The median number of days reported required for a note to be written following a new admission was 3 days and 7 days for a follow-up, with no difference between level III and level IV units. Approximately 48% of responding neonatal RDNs stated that they found charting to be very important for NICU outcomes ($n = 57/141$), 43% moderately important ($n = 50/141$), and 10% minimally important ($n = 14/141$).

Our survey had limited responses ($n = 8$) from neonatal RDNs in level II NICUs. Approximately one-fifth (21%, $n = 30/139$) of responding neonatal RDNs indicated that they directly provide coverage for a level II NICU, another third (32%, $n = 42/130$) indicated another dietitian is responsible for level II NICU coverage. Most of the neonatal RDNs consulting in level II NICUs indicated that this care is very important for patient outcomes (56%, $n = 22/39$), whereas 31% ($n = 15/49$) stated it was moderately important and 4% ($n = 2/49$) minimally important.

Outpatient responsibilities results
Only 19% of responding neonatal RDNs ($n = 26/143$) reported having regular outpatient clinic responsibilities directly related to NICU follow-up. The median proportion of time spent in outpatient clinic on an average month was 0% in responding neonatal RDNs (see **Fig. 2**).

Administrative responsibilities results
Administrative responsibilities made up for a minority of overall time spent by responding neonatal RDNs with a reported median of 7% of time spent in these activities in an average month (see **Fig. 2**). Proportions of time spent in specific administration responsibilities are displayed in **Fig. 3**.

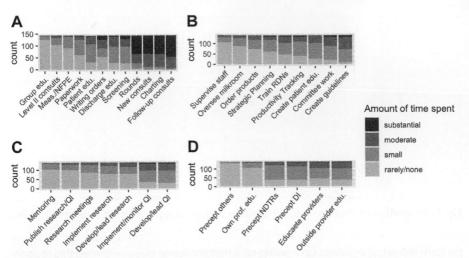

Fig. 3. Proportion of neonatal RDN time currently spent on weekly tasks. (*A*) Clinical responsibilities; (*B*) Administrative responsibilities; (*C*) Research responsibilities; (*D*) Education responsibilities.

Research responsibilities results

Responding neonatal RDNs reported a median of 5% of time spent on research activities in an average month (see **Fig. 2**). Most responding neonatal RDNs reported that they rarely or never spent any time on the following research activities: mentoring others in research (74%, $n = 104/141$), publishing research (70%, $n = 99/141$), research meetings (60%, $n = 85/141$), implementing research (56%, $n = 79/141$), and developing/leading research (56%, $n = 79/141$). Most of the responding neonatal RDNs stated that they spent a small amount of time regularly on developing/leading quality improvement (QI) projects (48%, $n = 67/141$) and implementing QI projects (45%, $n = 63/141$). Proportions of time spent in specific research activities are depicted in **Fig. 3**. Neonatal RDNs that worked at academic hospitals (defined as hospitals that have a pediatric residency or neonatal fellowship) reported spending more time on research-related activities compared with those who worked at nonacademic institutions (data not shown).

Education responsibilities results. After clinical responsibilities, education-related responsibilities required the second largest proportion of time spent for neonatal RDNs with a median of 7.5% of work time spent on education in a typical month (see **Fig. 2**). Educating health care providers both within and outside of responding neonatal RDNs institutions and precepting dietetic interns were the most frequently reported educational activities of responding neonatal RDNs (see **Fig. 3**).

Compared with neonatal RDNs working at nonacademic hospitals, those working in academic hospitals more frequently reported spending a moderate to substantial amount of time educating health care providers at their own institutions (33% vs 17%), educating providers at other institutions (38% vs 13%), precepting dietetic interns (24% vs 11%), and precepting dietetic technician interns (15% vs 11%).

Neonatal RDNs at academic institutions more frequently reported spending a moderate to substantial amount of time on their own professional education compared with those at nonacademic institution (7% vs 0%). However, most of the all responding neonatal RDNs reported rarely or never spending their work time on their own professional education (76%, $n = 106/140$).

DISCUSSION

The authors found that neonatal RDNs are responsible for performing a wide variety of activities that based on previous research are likely contributing to positive patient outcomes. There is wide variation in neonatal RDN staffing. The authors have identified areas where the depth and breadth of the neonatal RDN role could be expanded. Based on our responses, there is currently insufficient staffing of neonatal RDNs to accomplish all responsibilities deemed important by respondents.

Why Registered Dietitian Nutritionists

Neonatal RDNs are vital members of the NICU team that contribute to better patient outcomes and improvements in the NICU workflow. In a survey of practice, Cormack and colleagues reported that the neonatal dietitian is able to standardize neonatal nutrition care by designing and encouraging consistent nutrition protocols and practice while also monitoring growth and other outcomes.[15] This standardized care is associated with a reduction in length of stay, a reduction in days on intravenous nutrition, and a reduction in occurrence of necrotizing enterocolitis all of which reduce hospital costs.[15] Dietitians are able to perform nutrition-specific tasks such as prescribing enteral and intravenous nutrition, which can release medical staff time. These activities, taken together are likely to be cost neutral or possibly result in cost savings.[15] Having adequate neonatal RDN personnel is critically important, however, to date the ideal neonatal RDN staffing has not been identified.

Actual Neonatal Registered Dietitian Nutritionist Staffing Ratios

All responding NICUs reported using a neonatal RDN. Although this could be in part due to recruitment methodologies of this survey, it is also likely reflective of the increasing presence of RDNs in NICUs. Although the 2021 US News and World Report rankings for pediatric hospitals awards two points for fewer than 20 beds per FTE RDN, only 11% of responding NICUs met this ratio, with the majority meeting this guideline ($n = 10/14$) being level IV NICUs.

There was a clear trend that level IV NICUs had lower bed:FTE RDN ratios, a finding consistent with unpublished data by one of the authors (SGW) on behalf of the Ohio Neonatal Nutritionists over the past several decades. A difference in RDN staffing ratios between levels of NICUs may be reflective of both the patient acuity as well as the differing job responsibilities in clinical, academic, managerial, and research realms. It is interesting to note that the time of individual neonatal RDNs devoted to the NICU differs by NICU level as well, with level IV neonatal RDNs typically spending all 100% of their professional time in the NICU, compared with level II neonatal RDNs spending a median of 33% of their time in NICU-related work.

Although level IV neonatal RDNs reported a lower desired RDN staffing ratio (ie, fewer beds per FTE RDN) compared with level III neonatal RDNs, respondents in level III NICUs desired a higher percent increase of RDN staffing. Lower staffing ratios seem to be more common in higher acuity settings, but there seems to be a perceived larger gap in adequate staffing in level III NICUs. Additional FTEs would presumably allow the RDN to spend increased time on responsibilities identified in **Fig. 4**. Identifying neonatal RDN staffing ratios that correlate with improved NICU patient outcomes is a current gap in the literature.

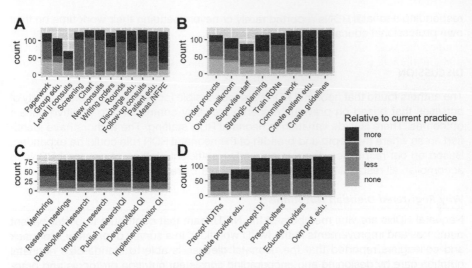

Fig. 4. Proportion of neonatal RDN time spent of tasks in ideally staffed NICU. (*A*) Clinical responsibilities; (*B*) Administrative responsibilities; (*C*) Research responsibilities; (*D*) Education responsibilities.

Clinical responsibilities

Our survey identified clinical responsibilities that neonatal RDNs frequently performed and believed to be important to patient outcomes. Unsurprisingly, there was complete agreement that creating an initial nutrition plan and completing a follow-up nutrition plan are both frequently performed tasks important for patient outcomes. There was similar agreement on the neonatal RDN involvement in multidisciplinary rounds. The presence of RDNs on rounds allows for nutrition-related education for trainees, facilitates interdisciplinary discussion on complex cases, and promotes improved nutrition administration and nutrition-related outcomes.[28]

Screening and charting

The Joint Commission states that patients must be screened for nutritional risk (standard AOP.1.4) and that those who are identified at risk should receive nutrition therapy (standard COP.5.1).[29] The authors found discordance in the responses for who performed screening, how much time individual neonatal RDNs used to perform screening, and the level of importance assigned to this task. Screening patients for nutrition risk may be an area that can be automated, performed by an alternative provider (eg, NDTR), or may be unnecessary if all patients are routinely assessed. Removing the responsibility for screening from the neonatal RDN might allow these professionals more time to perform tasks at a higher level of practice.

The Joint Commission states that the documentation of assessment and intervention must be standardized within a hospital, but there are no specific charting mandates for RDNs. Although there is no mandate for charting standards commonly reported by our participants, there may be practical explanations for this finding. First, having a 3-day requirement for an initial note allows for staffing flexibilities over weekends. In addition, the first 48 hours of an NICU admission are often composed of fluid and electrolyte management that is either protocolized or is driven by physician management.

Most of the responding neonatal RDNs stated that they found charting to be either moderately or very important for NICU outcomes. Similarly, most of the responding RDNs reported that they would spend similar amounts of time charting in an ideally staffed NICU (see **Fig. 4**). Although the authors did not capture actual hours spent on individual tasks, other studies have shown that the most time-demanding activity for medical/surgical nurses was documentation. In a time and motion study of medical/surgical nurses, it was observed that documentation took 33% of the nurses' time, whereas only 19.3% of time was spent in patient care.[30] Our survey found that there were many areas in the clinical and nonclinical realms in which responding neonatal RDNs were interested in spending more time (see **Fig. 4**). This increased involvement would likely require a substantial readjustment of daily workload or additional staffing hours to be feasible.

Level II neonatal intensive care units

Our limited responses from level II neonatal RDNs may be a result of our recruitment methods but may be reflective that many level II NICUs do not use full-time or specifically dedicated neonatal RDNs. As level II NICUs typically care for infants older than 32 weeks' post-menstrual age and above 1500 g, there may be a perceived lesser need for routine specialized nutrition care. Late preterm infants have prematurity-related challenges that may impair feeding abilities and growth which result in nutritional deficits; therefore, they are likely to benefit from specialized nutrition support during the NICU stay and at discharge.[31]

Feed preparation

The 2021 US World News Ranking states that NICUs must offer "a dedicated area within the facility for milk and formula preparation."[19] Evidence suggests that neonatal care is improved when NICUs have specialized milk rooms.[32,33] Neonatal RDNs are uniquely qualified to create and manage these types of facilities, and it may be a good opportunity for career advancement and/or role expansion. As described in **Table 2**, there were differences in feed preparation facilities between NICU levels with level 4 NICUs more frequently having greater access to centralized milk preparation rooms compared with level 3 and 2 NICUs. Fewer beds per FTE RDN would be necessary for the appropriate management of these milk rooms, which require daily staffing, quality control, product management, and recipe creation, among other tasks.

Areas where registered dietitian nutritionists want to do more clinically

Neonatal RDNs uniformly wanted to increase their clinical activities in individual nutrition counseling, individual discharge education, and group education, which may reflect a desire for more direct patient care to have meaningful influence on an individual patient's medical course and health outcomes. Given the numerous responsibilities and limited staffing of neonatal RDNs, some efficiencies might be gained by providing some education in a group setting. Alternatively, neonatal RDNs could oversee the development of a group education curriculum that could be implemented by an NDTR or other health professional. Group sessions may allow for NICU parents to feel less isolated and perhaps increase visitation but may not be appropriate for all families and may be limited when social distancing is required.[34]

Research responsibilities

Our findings indicate that research is not a major component of current neonatal RDN responsibilities, although it is a consistent area of interest for increased involvement. Research-related activities made up for only a small component of time allotted activities, which was true regardless of being at an academic or nonacademic facility. Neonatal RDN involvement in research may be dependent on other health care professionals' expectations, protected time, and funding for research. Research is a topic on the examination for the RDN credential; however, the focus is on understanding research to implement evidence-based practice rather than a requirement to conduct one's own research.[35,36] Various publications have reviewed the barriers to research among RDNs, which include lack of training as well as structural barriers such as limited to no time dedicated for research in the workplace.[37,38] Two studies that have examined the path of allied health clinicians generally and RDNs specifically who are successful in combining research with clinical practice identified mentoring found a supportive workplace environment (including protected time for research) and personal characteristics as important contributors to success.[38,39] Supporting neonatal RDNs with protected time, training, and resources would likely allow for increased participation in research.

Education responsibilities

Neonatal RDNs working in academic hospitals with pediatric residencies and/or neonatal fellowships more frequently reported spending time educating providers at their own and other institutions as well as precepting dietetic interns and dietetic technician interns compared with neonatal RDNs who worked at nonacademic hospitals. Providing interprofessional neonatal nutrition education is an important task that neonatal RDNs should be performing to improve the quality of nutrition-related care that patients receive.[40] Leaders in the profession recommend that neonatal RDNs should be involved in both the bedside education and nutrition curriculum development of medical trainees at all levels.[40,41]

Although dietitians at academic institutions reported dedicating time to their own professional education, most of all responding neonatal RDNs reported rarely spending their work time on their own professional education. Continuing education is not only required for RDNs to keep their credential but also essential to promote evidence-based practices and to keep pace with the evolving nature of neonatal care. The survey finding of RDNs rarely spending work time on their own professional education was surprising and concerning and may reflect a lack of support from the workplace.

Nutrition and dietetics technician, registered

Our manuscript is the first to describe NDTR staffing ratios in the NICU environment, although only a minority of responding NICUs reported using NDTRs. The scope of practice for NDTRs is to work with an RDN to provide patient/client care or working independently when providing more general nutrition advice or in food service. NDTRs can assess patients and provide and monitor interventions but do not make nutrition diagnoses.[4] In the NICU, NDTRs have duties such as gathering and plotting anthropometric measurements and nutrition intakes, providing discharge education, and working in milk laboratories. Utilization of NDTRs may benefit NICU functioning and allow for neonatal RDNs to feasibly evolve their professional responsibilities.

Desired staffing ratios results

Responding neonatal RDNs reported their opinion of the ideal nutrition staffing for their NICU (see **Table 3**). Overall, respondents wanted a 29% increase in current RDN staffing levels. The desired increase in staffing varied by NICU level; neonatal RDNs who worked in level IV units reported a desired 19% increase in staffing and level III neonatal RDNs a 43% increase. There were insufficient responses to report desired staffing in level II NICUs.

Desired time spent in specific responsibilities in an ideal staffing scenario relative to current time spent is depicted in **Fig. 4**. Relative to current responsibilities, neonatal RDNs reported they wanted to spend more time on direct individual patient care (eg, performing nutrition focused physical exam, individual patient education), creating guidelines and patient education materials, educating providers, and on their own professional education. Neonatal RDNs also reported that they wanted to spend more time in nearly all research-related responsibilities.

Limitations

Limitations of our research include our inability to calculate an individual response rate. Our overall institutional response rate was similar to that seen in most electronic surveys of RDNs[37,42] and among health professionals in general.[43]

The authors used the following evidence-based strategies to increase response rate among health professionals; recruitment messages were sent from organizations with which the respondents had affiliations, reminder messages were sent, and incentives for participation were offered.[43,44] When these strategies have been used, response rate has not been demonstrated to be a good indicator of nonresponse bias[44]; therefore, the authors believe that they are able to draw conclusions despite a low response rate. Importantly, our estimated representation of 45% of all level IV US NICUs far exceeds typical response rates for electronic surveys. Given our high response rate from level IV NICUs, our results are likely most representative of level IV neonatal RDN roles and staffing, particularly in comparison to level II NICUs and NICUs without a dedicated RDN. The authors only had responses from units with neonatal RDNs, which may not accurately reflect RDN staffing in all US NICUs.

Our survey was administered in October 2021, when COVID was waning in the United States between the delta and omicron surges. The authors are unable to determine how COVID-related staff resignations or other changes may have influenced our data and have little pre-COVID data with which to compare.

SUMMARY

Neonatal RDNs are vital members of the NICU team and have the potential to expand on their roles in research, education, and clinical realms. Structural supports for neonatal RDNs are needed for this role expansion, including additional staffing of neonatal RDNs and NDTRs, protected time for nonclinical activities, and support of continuing professional education. Future questions that the authors are exploring with these data include compensation rates of neonatal RDNs, comparing US neonatal RDN staffing and responsibilities with Canadian practices and comparing neonatal RDNs with other areas of dietetics. The authors found that responding neonatal RDNs have an overall median staffing ratio of 33.6 beds per FTE but desire a 29% increase in RDN staffing. Determining ideal neonatal RDN staffing ratios should be further explored with a priority of connecting staffing ratios to patient outcomes and modeling predictors of staffing needs.

CLINICS CARE POINTS

- Neonatal registered dietitian nutritionsits have education and experience that make them uniquely qualified to lead the medical team in providing nutrition-focused care in the Neonatal Intensive Care Unit.

- Registered dietitian nutritionists contribute nutrition knowledge and translate nutrition evidence into clinical care of high-risk newborns.

- More evidence is needed on registered dietitian nutritionist staffing requirements that promote improved outcomes and to inform staffing decisions.

DISCLOSURE

There are no financial conflicts of interest to disclose.

REFERENCES

1. Tsang RC. A historical perspective. In: Koletzko B, Cheah FC, Domellof M, et al, editors. World Rev Nutr Diet 2021;122:1–4.
2. Accreditation Council for Education in Nutrition and Dietetics. About Accredited Programs. Accessed 27 April, 2022. https://www.eatrightpro.org/acend/accredited-programs/about-accredited-programs.
3. Commission on Dietetic Registration. RD Examination—Eligibility Requirements. Accessed 27 April, 2022. https://www.cdrnet.org/rd-eligibility.
4. Andersen D, Baird S, Bates T, et al. Academy of nutrition and dietetics: revised 2017 scope of practice for the registered dietitian nutritionist. J Acad Nutr Diet 2018;118(1):141–65.
5. Commission on Dietetic Registration. Of Interest to Newly Registered Dietitians and Dietetic Technicians. Accessed 27 April, 2022. https://www.cdrnet.org/form-of-interst-to-newly-registered-dietitians-and-dietetic-technicians.
6. Commission on Dietetic Registration. 2024 Graduate Degree Requirement—Registration Eligibility. Accessed 27 April, 2022. https://www.cdrnet.org/graduatedegree.
7. Academy of Nutrition and Dietetics. Therapeutic Diet Orders: State Status and Regulation. Published December 2021. https://www.eatrightpro.org/advocacy/licensure/therapeutic-diet-orders-state-status-and-regulation. Accessed 27 April, 2022.
8. Peterson S, Dobak S, Phillips W, et al. Enteral and parenteral order writing survey—a collaborative evaluation between the academy of nutrition and dietetics' dietitians in nutrition support dietetics practice group and the American society for parenteral and enteral nutrition (ASPEN) dietetics practice section. Nutr Clin Pract 2020;35(3):377–85.
9. Commission on Dietetic Registration. DTR Examination—Eligibility Requirements. https://www.cdrnet.org/certifications/registration-eligibility-requirements-for-dietetic-technicians. Accessed 27 April, 2022.
10. Hess L. Evolution of clinical dietetic staffing: past, present, and future. Top Clin Nutr 2007;22(1):20–7.
11. Thompson M, Price P, Stahle DA. Nutrition services in neonatal intensive care: a national survey. J Am Diet Assoc 1994;94(4):440–1.
12. Olsen IE, Richardson DK, Schmid CH, et al. Dietitian involvement in the neonatal intensive care unit: more is better. J Am Diet Assoc 2005;105(8):1224–30.
13. Hans DM, Pylipow M, Long JD, et al. Nutritional practices in the neonatal intensive care unit: analysis of a 2006 neonatal nutrition survey. Pediatrics 2009;123(1):51–7.
14. Fenton T, Geggie J, Warners J, et al. Nutrition services in Canadian neonatal intensive care: the role of the dietitian. J Can Diet Assoc 2000;61:172.
15. Cormack B, Oliver C, Farrent S, et al. Neonatal dietitian resourcing and roles in New Zealand and Australia: a survey of current practice. Nutr Diet J Dietit Assoc Aust 2020;77(3):392–9.
16. Sneve J, Kattelmann K, Ren C, et al. Implementation of a multidisciplinary team that includes a registered dietitian in a neonatal intensive care unit improved nutrition outcomes. Nutr Clin Pract 2008;23(6):630–4.
17. Nevin-Folino N, Ogata BN, Charney PJ, et al. Academy of Nutrition and Dietetics: revised 2015 standards of practice and standards of professional performance

for registered dietitian nutritionists (competent, proficient, and expert) in pediatric nutrition. J Acad Nutr Diet 2015;115(3):451–60.

18. Mayfield SR, Albrecht J, Roberts L, et al. The role of the nutritional support team in neonatal intensive care. Semin Perinatol 1989;13(2):88–96.

19. Olmsted M, Powell R, Murphy J, et al. Methodology U.S. News & World Report 2021-22 Best Hospitals: Specialty Rankings. U.S. News & World Report's Best Hospitals; 2021. Available at: https://health.usnews.com/media/best-hospitals/BH_Methodology_2021-22.

20. Olmsted M, Powell R, Murphy J, et al. Methodology U.S. News & World Report 2022-23 Best Hospitals: Specialty Rankings. U.S. News & World Report's Best Hospitals; 2022. Available at: https://health.usnews.com/media/best-hospitals/BCH_Methodology_2022-23.pdf.

21. Marcason W. What is ADA's staffing ratio for clinical dietitians? J Am Diet Assoc 2006;106(11):1916.

22. Hand RK, Jordan B, DeHoog S, et al. Inpatient staffing needs for registered dietitian nutritionists in 21st century acute care facilities. J Acad Nutr Diet 2015;115(6):985–1000.

23. Phillips W. Clinical nutrition staffing benchmarks for acute care hospitals. J Acad Nutr Diet 2015;115(7):1054–6.

24. Aiken LH, Clarke SP, Sloane DM, et al. Hospital nurse staffing and patient mortality, nurse burnout, and job dissatisfaction. JAMA 2002;288(16):1987–93.

25. Duffield C, Diers D, O'Brien-Pallas L, et al. Nursing staffing, nursing workload, the work environment and patient outcomes. Appl Nurs Res ANR 2011;24(4):244–55.

26. Butler M, Schultz T, Halligan P, et al. Hospital nurse-staffing models and patient- and staff-related outcomes. Cochrane Database Syst Rev 2019;4. https://doi.org/10.1002/14651858.CD007019.pub3.

27. Qualtrics. Published online 2005. Available at: https://www.qualtrics.com.

28. Casey LM, Strauss J, Dhaliwal KK, et al. NeoCHIRP: a model for intestinal rehabilitation in the neonatal intensive care unit. Nutr Clin Pract 2021;36(6):1320–7.

29. Joint Commission International. Joint Commission International Accreditation Standards for Hospitals.; 2021. https://www.jointcommissioninternational.org/-/media/jci/jci-documents/accreditation/hospital-and-amc/jci-errata-standards-only_7th-ed-hospital.pdf. Accessed 24 September, 2022.

30. Hendrich A, Chow MP, Skierczynski BA, et al. 36-hospital time and motion study: how do medical-surgical nurses spend their time? Perm J 2008;12(3):25–34.

31. Lapillonne A, O'Connor DL, Wang D, et al. Nutritional recommendations for the late-preterm infant and the preterm infant after hospital discharge. J Pediatr 2013;162(3, Supplement):S90–100.

32. Steele C, Bixby C. Centralized breastmilk handling and bar code scanning improve safety and reduce breastmilk administration errors. Breastfeed Med 2014;9(9):426–9.

33. Steele C, Short R. Centralized infant formula preparation room in the neonatal intensive care unit reduces incidence of microbial contamination. J Am Diet Assoc 2008;108(10):1700–3.

34. Hall SL, Ryan DJ, Beatty J, et al. Recommendations for peer-to-peer support for NICU parents. J Perinatol 2015;35(1):S9–13.

35. Accreditation Council for Education in Nutrition and Dietetics. 2022 Standards for Dietetic Internships. Published September 1, 2021. Available at: https://www.eatrightpro.org/-/media/eatrightpro-files/acend/accreditation-standards/2022standardsdi-82021–1.pdf?la=en&hash=A20E5B7F7C5FDB8C83F20766CB524D1AD44A52C4. Accessed 2 May, 2022.

36. Accreditation Council for Education in Nutrition and Dietetics. 2022 ACEND Accreditation Standards for Nutrition and Dietetics Graduate Degree Programs (GP) (Future Education Model). Published November 1, 2021. https://www.eatright-pro.org/-/media/eatrightpro-files/acend/fem-2022/fem-graduate-reformat.pdf?la=en&hash=B6EC9DE14313A95B819F1899EE970563F92AD251. Accessed 2 May, 2022.

37. Dougherty CM, Burrowes JD, Hand RK. Why registered dietitian nutritionists are not doing research-perceptions, barriers, and participation in research from the academy's dietetics practice-based research network needs assessment survey. J Acad Nutr Diet 2015;115(6):1001–7.

38. Boyd M, Gall SB, Rothpletz-Puglia P, et al. Characteristics and drivers of the registered dietitian nutritionist's sustained involvement in clinical research activities: a mixed methods study. J Acad Nutr Diet 2019;119(12):2099–108.

39. Harvey D, Plummer D, Nielsen I, et al. Becoming a clinician researcher in allied health. Aust Health Rev 2016;40(5):562–9.

40. Hark LA, Deen D. Position of the academy of nutrition and dietetics: interprofessional education in nutrition as an essential component of medical education. J Acad Nutr Diet 2017;117(7):1104–13.

41. Van Horn L, Lenders CM, Pratt CA, et al. Advancing nutrition education, training, and research for medical students, residents, fellows, attending physicians, and other clinicians: building competencies and interdisciplinary coordination. Adv Nutr 2019;10(6):1181–200.

42. Augustine MB, Swift KM, Harris SR, et al. Integrative medicine: education, perceived knowledge, attitudes, and practice among academy of nutrition and dietetics members. J Acad Nutr Diet 2016;116(2):319–29.

43. VanGeest J, Johnson TP. Surveying nurses: identifying strategies to improve participation. Eval Health Prof 2011;34(4):487–511.

44. Groves RM, Peytcheva E. The impact of nonresponse rates on nonresponse bias: a meta-analysis. Public Opin Q 2008;72(2):167–89.

Moving?

Make sure your subscription moves with you!

To notify us of your new address, find your **Clinics Account Number** (located on your mailing label above your name), and contact customer service at:

Email: **journalscustomerservice-usa@elsevier.com**

800-654-2452 (subscribers in the U.S. & Canada)
314-447-8871 (subscribers outside of the U.S. & Canada)

Fax number: **314-447-8029**

Elsevier Health Sciences Division
Subscription Customer Service
3251 Riverport Lane
Maryland Heights, MO 63043

*To ensure uninterrupted delivery of your subscription, please notify us at least 4 weeks in advance of move.

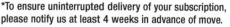

Printed and bound by CPI Group (UK) Ltd, Croydon, CR0 4YY

03/10/2024

01040468-0006